MANAGEMENT GUIDELINES
FOR WOMEN'S HEALTH
NURSE PRACTITIONERS

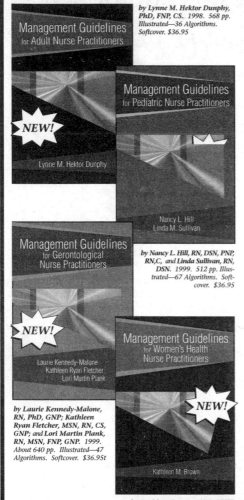
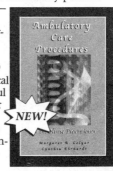

MANAGEMENT GUIDELINES FOR WOMEN'S HEALTH NURSE PRACTITIONERS

Kathleen Brown, RN, PhD, NP

 F. A. DAVIS COMPANY • Philadelphia

F.A. Davis Company
1915 Arch Street
Philadelphia, PA 19103

Printed in Canada

Last digit indicates print number: 10 9 8 7 6 5 4 3 2 1

Acquisitions Editor: Joanne P. DaCunha, RN, MSN
Production Editor: Michael Schnee
Cover Designer: Louis J. Forgione

Library of Congress Cataloging-in-Publication Data

Brown, Kathleen, 1950–
    Management guidelines for women's health nurse practitioners/Kathleen Brown.
        p.   cm.
    Includes bibliographical references and index.
    ISBN 0-8036-0292-8 (alk. paper)
    1. Nurse practitioners.   2. Clinical competence.
    I. Title.
    [DNLM: 1. Genital Diseases, Female.   2. Nurse Practitioners.   3. Obstetrics.   4. Women's Health.   WP 140
    B878m 1999]
    RT82.8.B75   1999
    610.73′678—dc21
    DNLM/DLC
    for Library of Congress   99-26449
                                                                          CIP

DEDICATION

To the readers, who provide the best care possible for women, in an increasingly complex health-care environment.

To all the women with whom I have interacted in my professional life. You taught me everything that I know, and I am now passing that on to others.

PREFACE

Management Guidelines for Women's Health Nurse Practitioners was written as a quick reference source for nurse practitioners (NPs) in clinical practice, to help guide patient-NP interaction. The book is useful for any NP dealing with women's health issues in clinical situations.

Unit I, "The Healthy Woman," gives information on health promotion for women throughout the life span, including recommendations—from government and private organizations—for health screenings for women. The nutrition section discusses appropriate nutrition for adolescent women, adult women, and infants.

Unit II, "Assessment," covers history taking and the physical examination of women. Emphasis is placed on a history that is appropriate for clinical encounters with women, as well as procedures for breast and pelvic examinations.

Unit III, "Treating Illness," covers, using a systems approach, common presentations that bring women to a clinical practice, including diseases and abnormalities of the breast, infections of the breast and reproductive tract, benign diseases of the reproductive tract, and carcinomas. Discussion also addresses amenorrhea, infertility, pelvic relaxation, abnormal vaginal bleeding, and many other areas. A section devoted to contraception includes discussion of contraceptive methods plus ideas for counseling women about each method. An entire chapter on menopause includes signs and symptoms, risk assessment, health promotion (including hormone replacement therapy), and alternatives to medical therapy. The chapter called "Symptom-Based Problems" discusses common clinical presentations of women such as abdominal pain, pelvic pain, dysmenorrhea, dyspareunia, headache, and cyclic mastalgia.

Each system in Unit III discusses diseases or dysfunctions commonly seen in women. For example, the section on the musculoskeletal system discusses fibromyalgia, osteoporosis, rheumatoid arthritis, and lupus erythematosis.

The last two chapters of the book cover pregnancy and the postpartum period. The chapter on pregnancy includes physiologic adaptations, anticipatory guidance provided through antenatal care, management of common complaints of pregnancy, and complications of pregnancy. The postpartum chapter discusses assessment of the postpartum patient and common postpartum complications.

Unit III is written in an easy-to-follow monograph format. Each topic is discussed in the following sequence:

- Definition
- Etiology
- Occurrence
- Age
- Ethnicity
- Contributing factors
- Signs and symptoms
- Diagnostic tests
- Differential diagnosis
- Treatment
- Follow-up
- Sequelae
- Prevention/prophylaxis
- Referral
- Education

Every section of Unit III includes flowcharts (algorithms) designed to assist the reader with clinical decision making. Many of the sections include tables and charts that provide valuable information at a glance.

This book contains many appendixes with useful information; these are designed for use by the NP. The appendixes include women's health organizations' telephone numbers and websites, immunization schedules, history and physical forms, consent forms, teaching and counseling guidelines, laboratory values, and more. The book closes with patient handouts designed to be copied by the NP and given to appropriate patients. The patient handouts include information on sexually transmitted diseases, self-examinations, explanations of test results, nutritional guidelines, stress-management techniques, exercise diagrams, contraception (including emergency contraception), protecting fertility, infertility, menopause, hormone replacement therapy, PMS, osteoporosis, prevention of heart disease, urinary incontinence, pregnancy and work, and more. These handouts may be copied, modified as the reader wishes, and distributed to women, who will find them useful.

This book was written by a women's health NP with 20 years of clinical experience. The author is sharing with the reader her experience in providing individualized care for women. Twenty years of active listening and "practicing," in the true sense of the word, is passed on to the reader. The book provides the practicing NP with helpful guidelines for everyday clinical situations. It assists the NP in forming plans for care, provides guidelines for referral to other health-care professionals, gives suggestions for counseling and teaching, and provides useful NP appendixes and patient handouts.

Kathleen Brown

ACKNOWLEDGMENTS

A special acknowledgment to Bruce Kaufmann, MD, without whom my clinical life would not have been possible.

Thank you to Diane Blodgett for her patience and her encouragement in assisting with the writing of this book.

K.B.

CONTENTS

UNIT **I**

THE

HEALTHY

WOMAN

CHAPTER 1

PHYSIOLOGIC AND
PSYCHOLOGIC
CHANGES

Introduction

In women's health, nurse practitioners (NPs) work with women of all ages. An understanding and appreciation of the milestones in women's development provides one key to establishing a therapeutic and holistic professional relationship. An approach to interviewing and examining an adolescent female differs from an approach to women experiencing menopause. Since each clinical situation is unique, the NP must consider many factors, such as education, reason for entry into the health-care setting, past experiences with health-care providers, and previous life experience. Developmental level and physiologic change are also considerations. Table 1–1 includes a synopsis of age-specific health goals followed by a discussion of major physiologic and psychologic events experienced by the majority of women.

Physiologic Changes

MENSTRUATION

At the beginning of the normal female menstrual cycle, the follicular phase, the hypothalamus, in response to low levels of estrogen, which thickens the uterine lining, produces follicle-stimulating hormone (FSH) releasing hormone, which stimulates the anterior lobe of the pituitary gland to release FSH. FSH causes several egg-

TABLE 1-1   AGE-SPECIFIC HEALTH GOALS FOR WOMEN

Adolescence
- Maintain physical, mental, emotional, and social growth at optimum levels.
- Develop positive health behavior patterns in physical fitness, nutrition, exercise, work, recreation, sex, and relationships.

Young Adulthood
- Move from dependent adolescence to independent adulthood.
- Achieve employment.
- Develop healthy social relationships.

Middle Adulthood
- Develop good health habits; detect disease early and treat disease.
- Reevaluate values, family situations, and career choices.
- Evaluate goal achievement.

Older Adulthood
- Adjust to menopause.
- Detect and treat any chronic illness.
- Continue achievement of life goals.

Elderly Years
- Prepare for retirement.
- Prepare for biologic, psychologic, and social changes.

Advanced Years
- Maintain independence.
- Continue to be physically and mentally active.

containing follicles in one of the two ovaries to develop and also stimulates estrogen manufacture by the follicles. As the estrogen level in the bloodstream rises, the anterior pituitary gland is signaled to decrease its production of FSH and to release luteinizing hormone (LH). During the ovulatory phase, the estrogen level rises, FSH level declines and then peaks along with the level of LH. LH suppresses the growth of all but one of the follicles, which then matures and releases an ovum. During the luteal phase, the empty follicle releases estrogen and progesterone. Progesterone helps prepare the uterine lining for implantation should the ovum be fertilized. Increasing levels of progesterone inhibit LH release. If fertilization does not occur, the corpus luteum decays and the manufacture of estrogen and progesterone decreases. The withdrawal of these two hormones causes the blood supply to the upper layer of endometrial cells to shed, along with blood from the broken vessels. During the first 1 or 2 days of menstruation, the hypothalamus again responds to the relative absence of estrogen and the cycle begins again (Fig. 1-1).

Body changes for young women that begin to occur between age 9 and 16 years include an increase in body hair, weight gain, growth spurts, growth of the uterus and vagina, and changes in body proportions. Breast buds begin to develop around age 11 years, influenced by the secretion of estrogen by the ovaries and prolactin by the pituitary.

Menarche, first menstruation, typically occurs after the development of pubic hair and breast development and after a growth spurt in height. Ova are contained within the ovaries at birth, with the average young woman having 75,000. Ovaries begin a heightened manufacture of estrogen at about age 11 and begin to take a

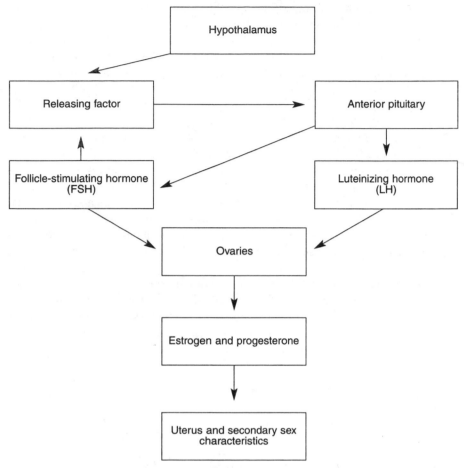

FIGURE 1–1 Physiologic changes leading to menses.

cyclic form for approximately 18 months prior to menarche. Researchers suggest that menstruation requires a critical weight (between 94 and 103 lb) and a critical fat-to-lean body composition ratio (22%–24%).

The average age of first menstruation has been steadily declining in the United States and is now 12.3 years with a range from 9 to 17 years. One-third of young women now reach menarche at or before age 11. Improved diet, hygiene, and health are likely responsible for the lowering of the first age of menstruation.

CLIMACTERIC

Climacteric, a gradual aging process in both sexes, includes changes affecting the entire body. Only women experience menopause, which refers specifically to the

cessation of ovulation and menstruation. The gradual reduction of levels of progesterone and estrogen is a result of decreased production of these hormones by
the ovaries. The average age for menopause is 51 years (Fig. 1–2). The primary
physiologic changes begin when the follicles stop maturing. The anterior pituitary
continues to release hormones, but the ovaries lose their responsiveness and so a
reduction of estrogen level results. Some estrogen continues to be produced by the
follicles and the adrenal glands, but it is not sufficient to trigger a menstrual cycle.
Menopause indicates the end of menstruation.

Unless the reason for menopause is surgical, estrogen and progesterone levels reduce gradually. Of three types of estrogen, the level of only one of these, estradiol, decreases dramatically at menopause. Estrone and estriol levels decline somewhat, but not as significantly as the level of estradiol. Note: The postmenopausal
body makes different kinds of estrogen; the ovaries synthesize less and the adrenal
glands synthesize more. Estrogen is also produced in fat cells and by cholesterol.
FSH and LH levels increase in menopause, and a consequence of this increase, although the mechanism is not understood, may be "hot flashes" (Fausto-Sterling,
1985).

Approximately 75% of all menopausal women experience hot flashes, a sudden increase in blood flow to the skin, which seems to be triggered by pituitary releases of LH. Hypothalamic neurons controlling the release of LH are located near
the temperature-regulating center, suggesting that an LH surge and hot flashes

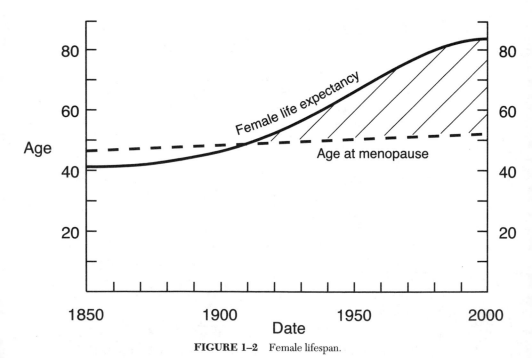

FIGURE 1–2   Female lifespan.

may be a result of hypothalamic functioning. Hot flashes eventually disappear as the body adjusts to the changing levels of LH and estrogen. Hot flashes are the primary reason for women seeking therapy for menopause. Hot flashes, prevalent in the first 2–3 years after menopause, usually last 2–5 minutes (see Chapter 9).

In the absence of circulating estrogen, the vaginal mucosa may become thin and dry. Bone loss, which begins before menopause, may accelerate after menopause. Cardiac disease is the chief cause of death in men and women. Before menopause, coronary heart disease (CHD) rates are lower in women than in men, but after menopause the mortality rate in women approaches that of men (see Chapter 9).

The popular idea that menopause is difficult and troublesome has not been borne out by research. In Massachusetts, 2500 randomly sampled women between the ages of 45 and 55 were followed by the Massachusetts Women's Health Study. This important prospective study reveals that women's health status and use of health services were predicted by premenopausal health factors and not by menopause. Menopause was not a predictor of either psychologic or physical well-being. According to the study, most women "report feeling neutral or relieved when they stop menstruating and increasingly positive as their menopause proceeds" (Adler, 1991).

Developmental Tasks

ADOLESCENCE

Adolescence is a time of transition from childhood to adulthood. Adolescents are closely tied to their parents yet spend more and more time with their peers. In a search for their identity, adolescents are decidedly self-centered. Accompanying the self-centeredness is a sense of invulnerability. Many adolescents believe that unwelcome events "cannot happen" to them. Adolescents make important decisions about sexual behavior in a framework of self-centeredness and invulnerability (see Appendix).

PREGNANCY

Most women in our society continue to want babies and continue to have them, although women now want fewer babies than their mothers and grandmothers did. They also have children at a later age and space them at more convenient intervals. Although all pregnant women undergo the same general physiologic changes, the subjective experience of pregnancy varies widely. How a woman experiences her pregnancy depends on her past experience and her present environment. How a pregnant woman reacts to the changes in her body depends on the meaning of the pregnancy to her and on her environment, including cultural, social, economic, and physical conditions.

YOUNG ADULTHOOD

In young adulthood, the main concerns are marriage and career. Young adults se-
lect partners for life simultaneously with choosing and developing career paths.

MIDDLE ADULTHOOD

Middle adulthood brings a time of concern for health. Injuries are the leading cause
of death for females until age 34, most often motor vehicle–related injuries, falls,
and violence. Domestic assault is a major unrecognized source of preventable injury
in women. Women in middle adulthood complain, in order of frequency, about:
stress, arthritis, excessive weight, migraine or chronic headaches, and tiredness.

From the 20s until retirement, the main concerns of most adults include how
much they will produce, how they will make a valuable contribution, and how they
will achieve success. Adults who are satisfied with their jobs are generally satisfied
with their lives, and those who like their lives generally like their jobs. Middle adulthood can be a time of combining employment and motherhood, separation and di-
vorce, and "midlife crisis."

OLDER ADULTHOOD

There has been a lack of serious attention to the understanding of the midlife and
maturing stages in the lives of women. A number of feminist writers criticize the
usual approach to the discussion of a woman's middle and later years, with its
overemphasis on biologic changes and a use of language that pathologizes normal
aging processes in women. In medical texts, women are equated with reproductive
capabilities and as these capabilities wane, terms such as "atrophy," "wasting," and
"estrogen-deficient" are used.

Contemporary older women disconfirm and defy stereotypes of them as worn
out and unattractive. For most women, life continues to be vital after age 50, 60,
and 70, and sometimes even beyond that. The dividing lines between young adulthood, middle age, and old age have become increasingly unclear because people
live longer and behave differently from their parents and grandparents.

A number of social and personal issues influence aging in women. Widows
constitute almost 5% of the U.S. population. The mean age for widowhood is 66;
of the 5.9 million women over 65 living alone, 80% are widows. An estimated
100,000 people in the United States over the age of 55 get divorced. Poverty can
be a serious problem for widows and divorced women over 65.

Older women constitute the fastest-growing portion of the U.S. population. Of
every 10 or 11 persons in the United States, 1 is over 65 years of age, compared to
only 4% in 1900; 84% of women and 70% of men are alive at age 65. Women over
50 constitute 38% of all adult women in the United States, and within the next 20
to 25 years it is estimated that almost 20% of the U.S. population will be made up
of women over 50. At age 64, women currently outnumber men by 100 to 83. By

the age of 85, women outnumber men by 100 to 39. Among women over 50 years of age in this country, 89% are European-American, 9% are African-American, and 2% are Latina or Asian-American. Of all elderly men and women, 95% live in the community—by themselves, with spouses, with family, or with friends. Thus only 5% are in nursing homes.

BIBLIOGRAPHY

Boston Women's Health Collective: The New Our Bodies Ourselves. Touchstone, New York, 1992.

Fowls, D (ed): A Profile of Older Americans. American Association of Retired Persons, Washington, D.C., 1993.

Gilligan, C: In a Different Voice: Psychological Theory and Women's Development. Harvard University Press, Cambridge, MA, 1982.

Griffith-Kenney, J: Contemporary Women's Health. Addison-Wesley, Menlo Park, CA, 1986.

Mann, J: The Difference: Growing Up Female in America. Warner Books, New York, 1994.

Sherman, B and Korenman, S: Hormonal characteristics of the human menstrual cycle throughout reproductive life. J Clin Invest 55(4):699–706, 1975.

Speroff, L, Glass, R, and Nathan, K: Clinical Gynecologic Endocrinology and Infertility. Williams and Wilkins, Baltimore, 1981.

Voda, A: Menopause: A normal view. Clinical Obstet Gynecol 35(4):923–933, 1992.

CHAPTER **2**

PROMOTING HEALTH

Introduction

By definition nurse practitioners (NPs) in women's health spend a majority of their clinical day dealing with the promotion of health. One of the many differentiations between nursing practice and medical practice is the emphasis nursing places on health promotion. NPs holding advanced degrees in nursing work toward the development of strong policies and procedures in any clinical setting that will influence women to maintain or promote health. The following discussion of the role of the NP in promoting health in women is followed by definitions of levels of prevention and screening recommendations.

Role of the NP

NPs provide excellent health care based on the skills of history taking, clinical examination, diagnosis, and nursing interventions. The women's health NP is a registered nurse prepared through a formal course of study to deliver primary health care to women throughout the life cycle. The dynamic role of the women's health NP changes with societal needs. The NP provides comprehensive, coordinated, and continuous care to women in collaboration with other members of the health-care team. NPs are responsible and accountable for the outcomes of their practice.

Today women are the majority of consumers and providers of health care. As women become increasingly more knowledgeable, independent, and assertive, they view health-care providers as consultants, teachers, and resources for current information about health concerns. Women expect to be active participants in their health care from identifying signs and symptoms to deciding on a treatment plan. They believe, and rightly so, that they know more about their bodies and life-styles than anyone else and therefore can best decide which treatment option is most suitable for them. The NP's role as a client advocate is to adequately inform the woman

10

about all relevant health issues and to support her decisions. The NP determines the type and amount of information the woman wants and the degree of participation and responsibility the woman is willing to assume in health-care decisions. As an advocate, the NP must be familiar with current diagnostic and treatment techniques. The advocate must keep current on research in the field and must be able to explain clearly to the woman treatments, potential consequences, side effects, risks, and benefits. Alternative treatments that may fit the woman's life-style should also be considered. Supporting the woman's right to choose and the choices she makes is an important NP function (see Appendix).

Levels of Prevention

Health promotion involves activities directed toward sustaining or increasing a level of well-being. Primary prevention involves activities directed toward decreasing the probability of becoming ill. Secondary prevention focuses on direct screening to promote early diagnosis and treatment of disease. Tertiary prevention minimizes disability (Table 2–1).

Screening tests refer to the application of tests to large populations of asymptomatic people with the hope of identifying disease or potential disease. The disease being screened for should be associated with significant morbidity or mortality in the population being served. There must be effective treatment for the disease, and the screening test must be accurate, simple, acceptable, and safe for the screened population.

Accuracy of the test is measured by sensitivity, which is the proportion of positive tests among those known to have the disease. Specificity reflects the portion of negative tests among those who have the disease. The positive predictive value refers to the likelihood that people with positive results actually have the disease in question. This latter category is how the practitioner interprets test results: What is the probability that this positive result is a true one?

When screening is applied to large numbers of people, follow-up for positive results is an important consideration. If many women do not have the disease, but are exposed to a diagnostic workup, the disease must be sufficiently present in the population to avoid an unacceptable rate of false-positive screenings. There must be a commitment of resources to a follow-up screening program. There must be ability to notify patients of positive test results and the ability to further evaluate and test those with positive results.

TABLE 2–1 LEVELS OF PREVENTION

Primary	Secondary	Tertiary
Decreasing probability of illness	Screening to promote diagnosis and treatment	Minimizing disability

Age

The age of a woman is an important consideration in providing health care. Age is related to risk factors, morbidity, and mortality. Young women are at greatest risk for death from accidents and violence. For middle-aged women, accidents and violence continue to be important causes of death, but heart disease, cancer, and suicide also become important causes of female mortality. As women age, heart disease, cancer, stroke, diabetes, pulmonary disease, and liver disease are causes of death. In elderly women the causes of death are cancer, cardiovascular disease, pneumonia, diabetes, and respiratory disease.

Screening Recommendations

BREAST CANCER

The three screening tests for breast cancer include the following: self breast examination (SBE), clinical examination by a practitioner, and mammogram. Studies on the effectiveness of SBE in detecting tumors range from 25% to 50%. The effectiveness of clinical breast examination used alone is approximately 45%, with its accuracy depending on the practitioner and the difficulty of the examination. Most studies correlate clinical breast examination with mammography and have found a reduction in breast cancer mortality in women over the age of 50. The benefit of mammogram for women under the age of 50 is smaller than for women over the age of 50. For women under the age of 50, decisions about when to begin mammography screening must be made after consideration of the risk-benefit question. (Refer to Chapter 7 for the section on breast cancer for risks.)

COLON AND RECTAL CANCER

Screening tests include a rectal examination, fecal occult blood testing, and sigmoidoscopy. Rectal examination allows for detection of carcinoma in a very limited area. Fecal occult blood testing determines the presence of blood in stools, presumably from an early cancer. Positive tests can be produced by recent consumption of rare red meat and by some medications, such as aspirin and iron, as well as by hemorrhoids. Follow-up for positive tests is colonoscopy or a combination of sigmoidoscopy and barium enema. A recent study shows that currently used methods of fecal occult blood testing detect fewer than 50% of colon cancers. The American Cancer Society recommends annual rectal examination of all adults beginning at age 40, fecal occult blood testing annually beginning at age 50, and sigmoidoscopy every 3 to 5 years beginning at age 50. Special attention should be paid to people at high risk for colon cancer, that is, those with one or more of the following risk factors: significant family history; personal history of breast, endometrial, or ovarian cancer; polyps; or ulcerative colitis.

CERVICAL CANCER

The screening test for cervical cancer is the Papanicolaou (Pap) smear. The risk factor for cervical cancer is sexual activity, in particular, with multiple partners. A consensus was developed by a number of professional organizations, including the American Cancer Society, the National Cancer Institute, the American College of Obstetricians and Gynecologists, and the American Medical Association, recommending annual Pap smears for all women who are sexually active or have reached the age of 18. When three Pap smears have been "normal," Pap testing may be done less frequently, with the usual recommendation being every 3 years. Women over the age of 65 do not seem to benefit as much from screening if previous smears have been consistently normal.

OVARIAN CANCER

Ovarian cancer has a high mortality rate. Unfortunately, no effective screening modality has been identified. Pelvic examination is inadequate for detecting the disease in an early phase. The level of cancer antigen 125 (CA 125) is elevated in women with ovarian cancer, but it is not clear whether levels are sufficiently elevated early enough in the disease process to make surgery more effective for eradication of the disease. Ultrasound has been considered, but the low incidence of the disease prohibits its use for screening.

ENDOMETRIAL CANCER

The American Cancer Society recommends endometrial sampling for high-risk women at menopause. Risk categories include infertility, obesity, history of ovarian failure, abnormal uterine bleeding, unopposed estrogen therapy, and tamoxifen treatment.

SKIN CANCER

The major concern in skin cancer is malignant melanoma. The screening modality is complete physical examination of the skin. High-risk groups are people with a history of skin cancer, those who work outdoors, and those exposed to chemical skin carcinogens.

HEART DISEASE

Cardiovascular disease is the leading cause of death for both men and women in the United States. The American Heart Association recommends a baseline electrocardiogram (ECG) at age 20 with repeat ECGs at ages 40 and 60. However, resting ECGs have a low sensitivity and specificity for underlying cardiovascular disease in healthy asymptomatic people; little information exists about ECG findings in women. Exercise ECG is advocated by some for routine screening in women over 40 or for those at risk for heart disease.

HYPERTENSION

Reduction of hypertension decreases the incidence of several leading causes of death such as coronary heart disease (CHD), stroke, and congestive heart failure (CHF). The American Heart Association calls for routine blood pressure measurement at least every 2 years for people with a diastolic below 85. Those with higher readings require more frequent evaluations. Risk factors for hypertension are African-American ancestry, significant family history, previous hypertension, and obesity. At-risk women should be evaluated at least annually.

CHOLESTEROL

Low serum cholesterol level in men reduces the incidence of CHD. Similar benefits are presumed to apply to women. Serum cholesterol level should be measured in all adults over the age of 20 at least once every 5 years. Low levels of high-density lipoprotein (HDL) are associated with increased risk for CHD, and high HDL level appears to be protective against CHD. Therefore, measurement of the HDL level should be ordered with total cholesterol screening.

DIABETES

Diabetes is relatively common and often asymptomatic. Routine screening for nonpregnant women can lead to early detection. Urine testing for glucose is a poor screening tool. Periodic fasting serum glucose measurement in high-risk individuals, that is, women who are obese, have a significant family history of diabetes, or have gestational diabetes, should be performed as recommended by the American Diabetes Association.

TUBERCULOSIS

Routine tuberculin skin testing is recommended for all persons. The tuberculin skin test can be useful in apparently healthy individuals, especially children and young adults. Healthy individuals with a high risk of exposure to tuberculosis, such as those in the health-related professions, should be screened annually.

Table 2–2 shows recommendations for screening low-risk women.

ADULT IMMUNIZATION

Vaccination has proved to be the most effective and cost-efficient means to prevent infectious diseases. In most circumstances, the benefits of appropriate indicated vaccination overwhelmingly outweigh the risks.

Adolescents and Young Adults—Ages 15–24 Years

- If immunization was not complete or not done in childhood, give a three-dose series of diphtheria and tetanus. Give the first two doses at least 4

TABLE 2-2 SCREENING TESTS FOR LOW-RISK WOMEN

Age 18–40	Age 40–50	Age 50–65	65 and Older
SBE monthly	SBE monthly	SBE monthly	SBE monthly
BE by practitioner annually --------------------applies to all age groups -------------------------->			
Annual Pap	Annual Pap	Annual Pap	Pap as indicated
Physical examination q 3 yr	Physical examination q 3 yr	Physical examination q 3 yr	Annual physical
BP q 2 yr	BP q 2 yr	BP q 2 yr	BP as indicated
Serum cholesterol q 5 yr ----------------------applies to all age groups -------------------------->			
Periodic fasting glucose ----------------------applies to all age groups -------------------------->			

weeks apart and the third dose 6–12 months after the second dose. For those who have completed the three-dose series, give a booster every 10 years.
- All persons born after 1956 should have received measles vaccine. Because of an outbreak of measles on college campuses in 1989, a two-dose live measles, mumps, and rubella (MMR) vaccine has been recommended. Young adults attending college should have documentation of having received two doses of live MMR vaccine after their first birthday. Persons are considered immune to rubella only if they have a record of immunization or laboratory evidence of immunity.
- Influenza vaccine should be recommended for women who provide community service.
- Hepatitis B vaccine is recommended for all young adults. Immunization consists of two intramuscular (IM) doses 4 weeks apart and a third dose 5 months after the second dose. Protection lasts 7 years.

Adults—Ages 25–64 Years

- Give a booster of tetanus and diphtheria every 10 years.
- One dose of measles vaccine is recommended for all adults born in 1957 or later. Laboratory confirmation of rubella immunization is required.
- Consider hepatitis B immunization for all health-care workers, institutionalized patients, and patients at risk for sexually transmitted diseases. Screen all pregnant women for hepatitis B.
- Influenza vaccine is recommended for women who provide community service or women who are at risk for transmitting the virus to others.

TABLE 2-3   ADULT IMMUNIZATIONS

Age 15–24	Age 25–64	Age 65 and Older
Incomplete Immunizations:		
3-dose series of diphtheria and tetanus booster q 10 yr	Tetanus/diphtheria q 10 yr	Influenza vaccine
Influenza vaccine	Influenza vaccine	Pneumococcal vaccine q 6 yr
Hepatitis B—3-dose series	Hepatitis B vaccine	Tetanus/diphtheria q 10 yr
	Proof of rubella immunity	
Complete Immunizations:		
Proof of 2-dose live MMR vaccine and rubella immunity	Measles vaccine—1 dose	
Diphtheria/tetanus booster q 10 yr		
Influenza vaccine		

From: The National Coalition for Adult Immunizations, 4733 Bethesda Ave., Suite 750, Bethesda, MD.

Adults 65 or Older

- This age group is more susceptible to infectious diseases, especially of the respiratory tract. Older adults should receive influenza vaccine annually. They should receive a single dose of pneumococcal pneumonia vaccine, with revaccination every 6 years.
- Revaccination for tetanus and diphtheria should be given every 10 years.

Prenatal Screening

- Screen for rubella. Defer rubella vaccination until after delivery.
- If the prenatal patient has not received the hepatitis B vaccine, there is no contraindication to giving it during the pregnancy.

Table 2–3 provides a listing of adult immunizations, as does the Appendix.

Health Promotion Recommmendations

EXERCISE

Regular exercise helps to develop a healthy lifestyle. Fitness describes the positive changes in cardiovascular endurance, muscle strength, coordination, and flexibility produced by exercise.

The goal of most exercise programs is to obtain cardiovascular fitness that permits sustained activity over a period of time. Optimally, aerobic activity should be performed for at least 30 minutes three to four times per week. The goal of such exercise is to reach and maintain a specific heart rate over a period of time. By utilizing this method, each exercise session can be monitored to reach the goal.

TARGET HEART RATE

HR(220 − age) × (60 to 80%). The resulting number is the target range.

Sample: 220 − 48 (age in years) × 70% = 172 × 0.70 = 120 beats per minute

---

Each exercise program should have at least a 5-minute warm-up to prevent muscle injury and a 5- to 15-minute cool-down period after exercise to allow for recovery to normal resting heart rate.

Coordination, balance, and flexibility also improve as a result of an exercise program. As muscles work together, they become efficient as a group. However, any level of conditioning is reversible, making a long-term commitment to exercise necessary.

Exercise can reduce and maintain weight. Weight programs that are combined with exercise are more effective than diet alone.

For any muscle to strengthen, it must work repetitively against fixed resistance, which causes the fibers to hypertrophy. For muscle strength to occur, you must develop a program for a specific muscle group. Depending on the type of program, some cardiovascular fitness effect may also occur. For example, circuit training, a very popular exercise program, develops muscular strength and cardiovascular fitness simultaneously.

Bone density can also increase in women involved in an active exercise program. Pressure on the bones results in increased calcium deposition as a result of increased osteoblastic activity. Exercise designed to prevent osteoporosis involves the use of large muscles attached to the long bones. *Any weight-bearing exercise such as walking helps prevent osteoporosis.*

Exercise should be a regular part of every woman's daily activity. For example, brisk walking benefits the cardiovascular system and prevents osteoporosis. Any athletic program will have long-term benefits for women and will contribute to a healthy life-style.

STRESS MANAGEMENT

The physical reaction to stress is the same regardless of the stressor. Dr. Seyle, the father of discussion about stress, taught us that stress creates a physiologic response that he describes in phases or stages. The first stage is alarm—your body recognizes the stressor and prepares for "fight or flight." The body increases heart rate, respiration, and blood sugar levels. The person perspires, pupils dilate, and digestion slows. A person then chooses whether to use these physiologic responses to run or stay and fight. After fight or flight, the body repairs any damage from the stress. If the stressor is not removed, repairs cannot be made and the body enters an exhaustion stage, in which it becomes susceptible to diseases of stress such as headache and irritable bowel.

Teaching women to deal with stress involves two components. The first is the recognition of stressors. If the woman does not perceive the stress as a stressor, she will not enter into fight or flight (Fig. 2–1). Self-talk becomes important here. She must convince herself that the potential stressor is not a stressor at all, rather it is a

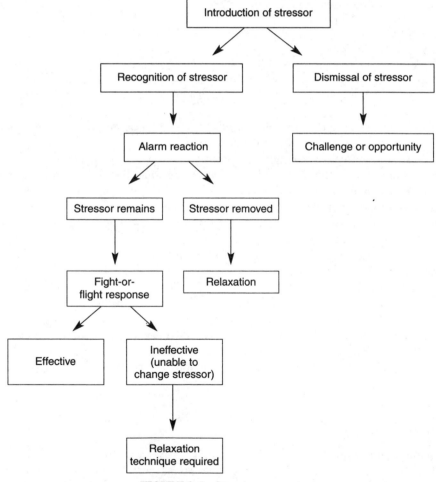

FIGURE 2–1 Stress management.

challenge or an opportunity. The second component involves stress management techniques. A simple but effective technique for stress management is deep breathing. Relaxation techniques reduce chronic stress response. These include such techniques as progressive relaxation and meditation.

In progressive relaxation, you concentrate on relaxing body parts in sequence—relax your right arm, your left arm, your shoulders, your jaw, etc. The hope is that as the muscles of the body relax, the mind will follow and relax as well. With the use of meditation, you concentrate on eliminating all thoughts except thoughts about relaxing. In this case, the mind becomes relaxed and the body follows. Imagery commonly used with relaxation techniques involves thinking about relaxing with images such as warm and heavy, going down in an elevator, or lying on a warm beach.

Women in the 1990s identify stress as a major factor in their lives. Women who are working while fulfilling the roles of wife and mother find their organizational skills taxed and their ability to deal with stress challenged.

Health prevention and promotion are important aspects of NP care. The complex lives of modern women in American culture require that NPs work to assist women in maintaining their health and in preventing future illness. Women look to NPs to provide accurate information regarding the health aspects of their lives. Every NP should be prepared to discuss methods that prevent disease and activities that promote wellness with every client. The first goal is to help women stay healthy by educating and counseling them about general health strategies. The next goal is to involve them in screening programs so that identification of disease at an early stage will allow effective intervention and treatment (see Appendix).

BIBLIOGRAPHY

Association of Women's Health Obstetric and Neonatal Nursing, Washington, D.C.

American College of Obstetricians and Gynecologists, Washington, D.C.

American Cancer Society, Atlanta, GA.

American Heart Association, Dallas, TX.

American Medical Association, Chicago.

Byny, R, and Speroff, L: A Clinical Guide for Care of the Older Woman. Williams and Wilkins, Baltimore, 1990.

Duffy, M: Determinants of health promotion in midlife women. Nurs Res 37:358–362, 1988.

Kannel, W, and Sorlie, P: Some health benefits of physical activity: The Framingham Study. Arch Intern Med 139:857–861, 1979.

Manderino, M, and Brown, M: A practical step by step approach to stress management for women. Nurse Pract 17(7):18–28, 1992.

Murray, R, and Zentner, J: Nursing Assessment and Health Promotion, (5th ed). Appleton and Lange, Norwalk, CT, 1993.

National Center for Health Statistics, United States Department of Health and Human Services: Public Health Service, Washington, D.C.

National Institutes of Health, Department of Health and Human Services: Public Health Service, Washington, D.C.

CHAPTER **3**

NUTRITION

Introduction

The body does not require particular foods or food combinations for health. The human race exists on a wide variety of foods that depend upon what is available to eat and what the culture dictates. Known essential nutrients contained in food are carbohydrates, fats and proteins, vitamins and minerals, and water. Nutrients interact to maintain the human body by providing energy, building and rebuilding tissue, and regulating metabolic processes.

Diet Recommendations

INFANT NUTRITION

At birth, a full-term infant weighs approximately 7 lb. During the first year of life, the infant grows rapidly from this average birth weight to approximately 20 lb. Growth rate, is, therefore, tremendous during that first year. The ideal food for infants, human milk, has all the requirements necessary for growth in the first year of life. Breast milk is produced under the stimulating influence of the hormone prolactin, which is produced in the anterior pituitary. The milk is formed by clusters of secretory cells and is carried through lactiferous ducts to the ampullae under the nipple. Oxytocin stimulates the expression of milk from the ducts and releases it to the baby. This is commonly called the letdown reflex. The newborn's sucking stimulates this reflex.

The mother should follow the baby's lead with what is called a demand schedule of feeding. Diet and rest are important factors in establishing lactation. A balanced diet is needed to support ample milk production. Lactating women require seven servings from the protein group, three from the milk group, and seven from the breads and cereals group daily. One serving with vitamin C, one with vitamin A, three other fruits and vegetables, and three unsaturated fat servings per day are required as well. Natural thirst guides adequate fluid intake.

Mothers should not be discouraged by the naturally slow weight loss after delivery. They should not curtail their diet to encourage weight loss. A nutritionally adequate diet is necessary for the lactating mother. Weight loss will occur in a slow, but natural fashion.

Formula feeding may be preferred by some mothers. A variety of commercial formulas are available. Standards for the levels of nutrition required in infant formulas are based on recommendations from the American Academy of Pediatrics.

No nutritional need exists for introducing solid foods to infants earlier than 4–6 months. Nutritional authorities agree that for the first 6 months of life, the optimum single food for the infant is human milk. Until that time, the infant does not require any additional food and may not be able to handle new foods. Allergy can be a concern with early introduction of food. Solid food should be introduced as the infant reaches the developmental stage, in which desire for and interest in food is communicated. Single foods are given first, one at a time, in small amounts so that adverse reactions can be identified. For most infants, transition foods are fortified infant cereal, followed by fruits, vegetables, egg, potato, and finally meat. Small amounts are given at first, followed by the milk feeding. Over time, the baby will learn to eat and enjoy a wide variety of foods. By the time infants are approximately 8 or 9 months of age, they should be able to eat family foods—chopped, cooked foods that are simply seasoned (see Appendix).

ADOLESCENT NUTRITION

Healthy adolescents often have irregular eating patterns. The gold standard for evaluating eating patterns, the 24-hour dietary intake, may not be sufficient for adolescents. Many skip breakfast and snack excessively. Teens rarely follow a three-meal-a-day plan. Their day-to-day intake can vary dramatically. Adolescent dietary review requires a multiple-day evaluation. When an eating pattern is examined over time, adolescents often achieve adequate overall nutrition.

Weight consciousness pervades American society. Appropriate exercise and diet are important for individuals of all ages. Although the adolescent's concern about prevention of obesity is important, fascination with slimness that often begins in teen years can be problematic. Lack of appropriate amounts of body fat can lead to a delayed onset of puberty and secondary amenorrhea.

Extreme forms of diet control, anorexia and bulimia, are seen most commonly in adolescent girls. Screening for anorexia nervosa, bulimia, and obesity should be routine in the development of a profile of care for adolescent girls (see Chapter 13).

ADULT NUTRITION FOR WOMEN

Probably the most familiar food guide is the *Basic Four Food Groups Guide* developed by the U.S. Department of Agriculture. A revised edition released in 1991 reflects current national nutritional goals for increasing carbohydrate intake and limiting fat consumption (Fig. 3–1). For adult women, the daily recommendations include the following:

A Guide to Daily Food Choices

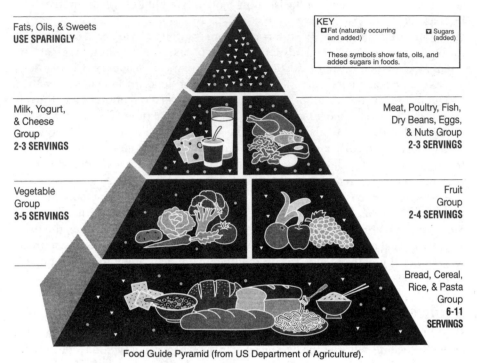

Food Guide Pyramid (from US Department of Agriculture).

FIGURE 3-1 The Food Pyramid

- 6–11 servings of breads, cereals, rice, or pasta
- 3–5 servings of vegetables
- 2–4 servings of fruit
- 2 servings of milk, yogurt, or cheese
- 2–3 servings of meat, poultry, fish, dry beans, nuts, and eggs
- Fats, oils, and seeds to be consumed sparingly and not to replace other foods.

The American Heart Association has outlined modifications of the American diet that will reduce factors related to heart disease. The recommendations are called the "prudent" diet. The recommendations include the following:

- Adjust calories to maintain an ideal body weight.
- Reduce dietary fat intake to 30%–35% of the total calories, with saturated fat contributing no more than 10%.
- Carbohydrates should constitute 50%–55% of the total calories, with complex carbohydrates contributing the majority of the calories.
- Simple carbohydrates (sugar) should constitute no more than 10% of the calories.
- Protein should be 12%–20% of the diet's total calories.

- Dietary cholesterol should be limited to 300 mg or less per day.
- The use of salt and salty food should be limited to no more than 2 or 3 g per day.

The National Cancer Institute has published dietary guidelines intended to reduce the incidence of cancer. The recommendations are as follows:

- Reduce fat intake to 30% of the diet's total calories.
- Increase dietary fiber by increased consumption of fruits, vegetables, and whole-grain cereals.
- Limit the use of foods preserved by salt, pickling, smoking, or nitrite curing.
- Avoid food contaminated with carcinogens.
- Use alcohol in moderation.
- Include foods rich in vitamins A and C.
- Include cruciferous vegetables in your diet.

VITAMINS

Vitamin A, a fat-soluble vitamin important for epithelial tissue bone growth and vision, is found primarily in fruits and vegetables. The recommended amount of vitamin A for women is 800 μg daily. The liver can store large amounts of vitamin A, making consumption of toxic levels possible. Hypervitaminosis of A is potentially teratogenic and should, therefore, be avoided, particularly during pregnancy.

Vitamin D, a fat-soluble vitamin important for the development and maintenance of bones, is found in dairy products. The recommended daily amount for women is 5 μg. Milk, supplemented with vitamin D, also contains calcium and phosphorus.

Vitamin E, a fat-soluble vitamin, is a potent antioxidant found in vegetable oils; the recommended daily amount for women is 8 mg.

Vitamin C, a water-soluble vitamin found in fruits and vegetables, has a recommended daily intake for women of 60 mg daily. Vitamin C is an antioxidant that builds and maintains body tissue in general. Vitamin C plays a role in growth periods of infants and children, in fever and infection, in wound healing, and during times of body stress from injury or illness.

Eight B vitamins have been identified as having partners with key cell enzymes in energy metabolism and tissue building. B vitamins can be found in both plant and animal sources. The following are the recommended amounts of daily intake for the B vitamins:

- Thiamin, 1.0 mg
- Riboflavin, 1.2 mg
- Niacin, 13 mg
- Pantothenic acid, 4–7 mg
- Folate, 200 μg
- Pyridoxine, 1.6 mg
- Biotin, 30–100 μg
- Cobalamin, 2 μg

MINERALS

Major minerals requiring an intake of more than 100 mg daily are calcium, phosphorus, magnesium, sodium, potassium, chloride, and sulfur. The essential minerals required at less than 100 mg daily are iron, iodine, zinc, copper, manganese, chromium, cobalt, selenium, molybdenum, and fluoride.

Of particular importance to women are calcium and iron. Calcium absorption can be enhanced by consumption of vitamin D and a diet rich in protein. Calcium absorption can be decreased with a diet high in fat and excessive in fiber. In a healthy state, the body maintains a constant turnover of calcium in the bone, which is the major source of calcium storage.

The recommended dietary intake of calcium for young women 11–24 years old is 1200 mg/day. Peak bone mass is attained by age 25. Menopausal women require 1500–2000 mg/day of calcium to help preserve bone mass.

Iron stores vary widely, being only about 300 mg in menstruating women. Women require 15 mg/day of iron to maintain adequate reserves. Iron is found in meats, eggs, vegetables, and cereals. Iron is poorly absorbed in the duodenum. Absorption is enhanced by vitamin C and adequate amounts of calcium.

NUTRITION DURING PREGNANCY

Folklore has surrounded pregnancy and nutrition for centuries. Examples are the following: Eating less will produce smaller babies; whatever the fetus needs, it will draw from the mother, regardless of her diet; and whatever the fetus needs, the mother will crave and consume. Clinical observations and research have provided direction for healthier pregnancies. Guidelines for the nutritional care of the pregnant woman have been issued by the American College of Obstetrics and Gynecology and the American Dietetic Association (see Appendix).

Throughout the pregnancy, the need for all the basic nutrients increases. Calories must be sufficient to supply increased energy and nutritional demands. A minimum of 36 kcal/kg of body weight is required for efficient use of protein during pregnancy. Based on the current recommended daily allowances (RDAs), this is an additional 300 kcal/day. This level would be inadequate for women who are large, very active, or nutritionally deficient prior to the pregnancy. Appropriate weight gain during pregnancy is used as an indicator of whether or not sufficient calories are being consumed.

The total amount of protein intake recommended for the pregnant woman is about 60 g/day. Protein is a nutrient basic to tissue growth. More protein is needed to meet tissue demands imposed by the rapid growth of the fetus and the enlargement of the uterus, mammary glands, and placenta, as well as the increasing maternal circulation. Stores will be formed for the woman to utilize during labor and delivery and during lactation. Milk, egg, cheese, and meat are complete proteins. Additional protein may be obtained from legumes and whole grains and to a lesser degree from some plant sources.

Calcium needs are 1200 mg/day. Dairy products are a primary source of calcium.

The pregnant woman needs 30 mg of iron per day. The iron cost of pregnancy is high. If the woman is anemic at conception, larger amounts of iron are needed. During pregnancy, the mother's circulating blood volume increases by 50%. Maternal iron is needed to meet this demand, to meet the fetal needs, and to create a supply that will fortify the woman against loss at labor and delivery. The major food source of iron is liver. Other food sources are meat, legumes, dried fruit, green vegetables, eggs, and enriched bread and cereals.

During pregnancy there is an increased need for folate, to a level more than twice the adult need. An additional amount of 400 µg/day (0.04 mg/day) is recommended.

There is an increased need for vitamin C; the RDA is 70 mg/day for pregnant women.

A variety of foods supply the mother's need for nutrients. A general daily food pattern that meets basic nutritional needs and incorporates the increases required by the pregnancy is recommended. Specific nutrients are required during pregnancy, not specific foods. Diet can be planned around the likes and dislikes of the pregnant woman. The pregnant woman should be encouraged to eat sufficient quantities, to eat regularly, and to avoid skipping meals.

Factors that affect nutritional needs of the pregnant woman are age and parity. The teenage pregnant woman adds her own growth needs to those of the pregnancy. The number of pregnancies and the time intervals between them greatly influence the mother's nutrient reserve. Consultation with a specialist in nutrition should be solicited in each of these situations.

Nutritional Status of Women

Individual nutritional status depends on availability of food and health. Adequate nutrition is demonstrated by a well-developed body, ideal weight for height and body composition, and good muscle development and tone. Skin should be clear and smooth, hair glossy, and eyes clear and bright. Appetite, digestion, and elimination should be within normal limits. Well-nourished women are alert both physically and mentally. Healthy teeth and gums are a sign of good nutritional status.

Women with "borderline" nutritional status meet their day-to-day needs but have little reserve. Illness, injury, or pregnancy require nutritional stores these women do not have. Stress increases the need for B vitamins, iron, and at times sugar and protein. Low-income women, women who live in stressful situations, or women who have poor dietary habits can be found to be "borderline" nutritionally. Dietary surveys indicate that one-third of the people living in the United States are in this category.

Malnutrition appears when nutritional reserves are completely depleted (Fig. 3–2). Nutrient and energy intake are insufficient to meet day-to-day needs. A large number of women living in poverty are malnourished. Poverty especially influences infants, children, pregnant women, and elderly women. Infant mortality rates con-

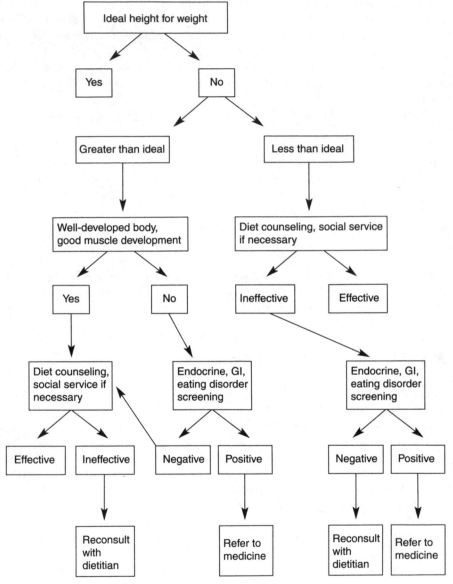

FIGURE 3–2   Malnutrition.

tinue to be high among the poor. One out of four young children in the United States lives in poverty and suffers deficiency diseases such as anemia. These children have lowered resistance to infection and disease. Prenatal care for poor women is often minimal. A relationship exists between low socioeconomic status and malnutrition in elderly females. There is widespread hunger and malnutrition among the nation's growing number of homeless women (see Appendix).

BIBLIOGRAPHY

American College of Obstetricians and Gynecologists, Washington, D.C.

American Heart Association, Dallas, TX.

Gizis, F: Nutrition in women across the lifespan. Nurs Clin North Am 27:272–982, 1992.

National Cancer Institute, Washington, D.C.

National Health and Nutrition Examination Survey, Department of Health and Human Services, Public Health Service, Washington, D.C.

United States Department of Agriculture, Washington, D.C.

UNIT **II**

ASSESSMENT

CHAPTER **4**

HISTORY TAKING

Assessment of a woman's health status involves two major components. The first is interview (history taking), and the second is physical examination. Interview, which precedes physical examination, serves as a guide for emphasis during the examination process. This chapter discusses the interview process, including interviewing skills, a history-taking format, and the importance of cultural considerations in interviewing. Women's work is discussed with an emphasis on occupational hazards. Assessing sexuality during the interview closes the chapter.

Interviewing the Client

A number of studies have revealed that a good interviewer possesses three basic qualities. (1) A good interviewer is appropriately nurturant. This means that the interviewer is helpful and supportive so that the patient grows from the experience. However, too much nurturance can leave the woman unempowered and unable to problem solve. On the other hand, inadequate nurturance can lead to nonresolution of the problem. (2) A good interviewer is a good teacher. In a good interview there is meaningful illustration and explanation. (3) A good interviewer is a facilitator who involves the woman in the problem-solving process. The woman becomes increasingly responsible for giving the data, seeking solutions, and following directions that lead to an agreed upon plan of action.

In the minds of most women, competence and interest are inseparable. It is not satisfactory simply to be competent; interest in the woman must be displayed in order for an interview to be successful. Skill and time are two components of a successful interview. As skill level increases, the time needed for the interview decreases. The nurse practitioner (NP) must be sufficiently skilled to be able to interview in brief time periods in an unhurried and interested manner. The woman must feel like she is receiving the nurse's undivided attention and energy throughout the interview.

A good interview is the path to understanding the woman's concerns. A careful, detailed history that is properly interpreted can lead the interviewer to an accurate diagnosis. Laboratory testing and physical examination will confirm the diagnosis made by taking the history. In addition, the interview can establish a therapeutic relationship.

The interview should be directed to areas of information relevant to the purpose of the woman's visit. Each topic should be fully explored until all of the relevant information is obtained. Jumping from topic to topic makes the flow of information difficult to manage. The NP fully investigates each topic of concern while reassuring, interpreting, and providing information. Reassurance, empathy, support, reflection, interpretation, summation, and touch are some of the techniques used to make an interview meaningful.

Health History

Interviewing a woman includes taking the traditional health history, including her past and current health history as well as the history of her present illness or concern. Family history helps to assess the woman's risk status. Psychosocial history may reveal factors that contribute to the woman's current complaint or concern. In an attempt to identify current or potential problems, a review of systems includes asking questions concerning each of the body's major systems. Each health history must include information about allergies, particularly drug allergies, immunization history, and previous screening tests.

The history must include the following questions (if age-appropriate):

- Age at menarche
- Frequency and duration of menses
- Amount of menstrual flow
- Last menstrual period
- Age at menopause
- Presence and amount of bleeding in between periods
- Presence and level of dysmenorrhea
- Birth control method
- Number of pregnancies and deliveries
- Complications of pregnancy
- Number of abortions
- Sexual preference
- Interest in, and satisfaction with, sexual relations
- History of sexually transmitted diseases
- Use of medication, including prescription drugs, over-the-counter drugs, vitamin supplementation, and home remedies
- Any problems or concerns

See Appendix for a sample history form.

Cultural Diversity

To accurately assess and diagnose a woman's health-care concerns, she needs to be assessed through her cultural lens. Culture is a pattern of learned behaviors and values that are shared among members of a designated group. The technical-economic component of culture refers to how people adapt to their environment, how they prepare food, how they dress, and what they choose for shelter. The social component of culture refers to behavior between and among people. How the culture works, worships, and learns are examples of the social component of culture. The ideology of a culture refers to concepts and relationships within a culture. These ideologies include folklore, myths, ethical codes, and philosophies.

Appreciating each woman's culture is important. Cultural orientation affects attitudes toward aging, family, diet, substance abuse, work and religious habits, and other areas that directly and indirectly affect health.

Women's Work

Women's participation in the world of paid employment has steadily increased during the past three decades. Women now make up 46% of the total work force, with an expectation that by the year 2000, the number will be 50%. Today's working woman can be found in virtually all areas of the economy, performing jobs at every skill level.

Most women, including those with jobs and careers, are also wives and mothers. Those who leave the work force in order to assume primary responsibility for child care risk losing out on new skills, opportunities, and promotions. Men spend an average of 2% of their potential work years out of the work force; women spend 23% of these years unemployed. The major reason for this difference is women taking time off to raise children.

The Family and Medical Leave Act of 1993 mandated that, if they request it, workers of either gender must be granted up to 12 weeks of unpaid leave each year as time off for the birth or adoption of a child, personal sickness, or a serious illness in the family. Employers must continue the health insurance coverage of employees on leave and assure employees that their jobs will be available when they return. However, the act applies only to businesses with 50 or more workers, which translates into 40% of the work force.

Women who work outside of the home also work inside of it. Employed mothers devote substantially more time to caring for their children and their homes than employed fathers do. Mothers use significantly more of their sick time to care for children's illnesses than fathers do. The responsibilities of home and children fall to the employed mother. Role overload, the necessity to fulfill many responsibilities associated with home life and employment, is clearly greater for married women than it is for married men.

Despite the reported experience of problems associated with trying to balance work outside the home with work inside the home, research on the effects of role overload does not support a conclusion of negative consequences for the married and employed woman. She is productive at work and satisfied at home. She copes and rises to the challenge; there does not appear to be any harm to the family unit.

As a group, working women differ little from working men in turnover, absenteeism, and illness. Both groups report similar levels of job satisfaction. In fact, it has been reported that women find work outside of the home a "buffer against other anxieties." Women who work outside of the home report better physical and emotional health then do women who are full-time homemakers. Working women have significantly lower rates of heart disease and lower levels of cholesterol and blood sugar (see Appendix).

Occupational Hazards for Women

Until recently, based on the assumption that every woman who worked would bear children, women's occupational hazards were considered in light of the fetus. Currently, the focus is broadening to include women's occupational hazards that are not related to childbirth. Worker health, safety, and rights are supported by federal and state legislation. All states have workers' compensation laws to cover worker illness and disability. Hazards to worker safety and health are dealt with by the Environmental Protection Agency (EPA) and the Occupational Safety and Health Administration (OSHA).

Environmental health is considered one of the key health issues of the 1990s. Common occupational hazards can be classified as biological, physical, chemical, or accidental.

Bacteria, viruses, and yeast can be transmitted in various work settings. Contact with contaminated objects and interpersonal contact can lead to the transmission of infection. Water supply and ventilation systems can be sources of infection. Infectious disease is a hazard for all workers but is especially hazardous for health-care workers and for those who work with small children, laundry, and food. Methods of protection are hand washing, sanitary procedures, use of protective equipment, and decontamination of dishes and laundry.

Physical hazards that arise from the environment include factors such as noise, temperature and humidity, radiation, and accidents. Excessive noise can cause temporary or permanent hearing loss. Harmful exposure can be reduced by isolating machines, building noise shields around machines, or wearing personal protection equipment. Hearing-monitoring programs can reduce and prevent the harmful effects of noise exposure.

Air quality includes the composition of the air as well as temperature and humidity. Lack of humidity contributes to dryness of the skin and mucous membranes, resulting in irritation. Heat in the absence of humidity leads to headaches, nausea, irritability, and lessened job performance. Ventilation systems must be designed to meet occupational needs.

Radiation in the health-care field accounts for 90% of all man-made radiation exposure. Nonhospital workers at risk include those in dentistry, research, and the nuclear power and weapons industries. Nonionized radiation exposure results in retinal or lens injury or dermal assault.

To what degree a hazard or hazards affect the working woman depends on the type of hazard, the duration of exposure, the level or dose of the exposure, the route of entry, the health of the woman, and the interaction with the hazardous substances. Assessing women for exposure to hazards requires physical evaluation and questioning regarding past and present exposures to hazardous substances.

The occupational health history is the principal clinical tool for diagnosing occupational disease. Basic occupational history questions include the following:

- What is your current occupation?
- What were your longest-held jobs?
- Are you now, or have you ever been, exposed to chemical pesticides, solvents, extreme hot or cold, metals, heavy lifting, fumes, dust, noise, radiation, infectious diseases, body fluids, emotional stress, or other hazards?

Accidents are common in women's occupations. Each year, 10 million traumatic work-related injuries occur; 3 million of them are considered severe. Falls are the most common accident. Women can also be injured by machines. Specifying proper procedures for machine use and redesigning faulty equipment to include guards and warning signals help prevent mechanical injury. Lifting and moving heavy objects place women at risk for strain on the musculoskeletal system. First-aid procedures, equipment, and personnel should be available for the prompt treatment of injured women.

Women who spend a great deal of time standing—for example, women in retail sales and hairdressers—develop circulatory and skeletal pressures, especially in the lower legs and feet. Clerical workers sit for extended periods of time, putting pressure on the musculoskeletal and circulatory systems. Varicosities and hemorrhoids are common among women who sit or stand for long periods of time. Solutions to discomforts related to prolonged sitting and standing include redefining the job, walking at regular intervals, and wearing nonrestrictive clothing.

Sleep deprivation can result in impaired work performance. Shift workers have a variety of sleep problems, excessive gastrointestinal disturbances, and, at times, altered menstrual cycles.

Although exposure to chemicals is pervasive throughout society, the greatest number of specific exposures occurs in the workplace. Several hundred chemicals to which women are exposed in the workplace are known or suspected to be hazardous. The long-range effects of chronic, low-level exposure to hazardous substances have recently come to the attention of workers, which has resulted in legislative action. In the occupational setting, prevention includes adherence to safety and use procedures, use of protective clothing and equipment, adequate ventilation, appropriate storage, and substitution of a less-damaging agent, when possible. (See Appendix for a list of relevant agencies to contact.)

Assessing Sexuality

Sexuality is an aspect of human identity that is expressed in daily interaction as well as in private expressions of love. Sexuality is not limited by age, attractiveness, partner participation, or sexual orientation.

According to the World Health Association, sexual health is "the integration of the somatic, emotional, intellectual, and social aspects of sexual beings in ways that are positively enriching and that enhance personality, communication and love." While being careful not to be biased or judgmental, NPs can design strategies to assist women in achieving sexual health. The purpose of the sexual history is to identify the woman's problems, risks, and concerns regarding sex and sexuality. A sex history should include the following:

- Database: Family background, childhood sexual experiences, sources of sex education, and medical history
- Relationship history: Characteristics of current and past sexual relationships, quality of relationships, issues and conflicts within relationships
- Sexual attitudes, desires, practices: Autosexual practices, level of desire, sexual fears, sexual performance and satisfaction with, arousal, orgasm
- Obstetric and gynecologic information: Children, menstrual patterns, contraceptives

An assessment of sexual disorders should include a consideration of physical, psychologic, and interactional context. The sexual concern or difficulty may lie in the desire phase, arousal phase, or orgasmic phase. The PLISSIT model provides a framework for sexual counseling.

- P = permission giving. The woman is given permission to discuss her concerns or raise questions.
- LI = limited information. Basic information about sexuality is given.
- SS = specific suggestions. Suggestions are given to the woman to assist her is resolving the problem or concern.
- IT = intensive therapy. By performing a sexual assessment, one can identify sexual difficulties that require referral for intensive therapy.

Any information concerning sex and sexuality should be held in the strictest confidence. Sharing information should occur only with the patient's permission.

The importance of intake information at every woman's visit to a NP cannot be underestimated. The intake interview not only guides the physical examination, but it also provides important information about health-related behaviors. The NP is both an educator and a counselor who must have adequate information to provide guidance for teaching, advising, and advocacy. Only with excellent interviewing and listening skills can the NP begin to understand each woman's particular health issues. Only expressed health-related behavior can be addressed. Empowering women to pursue health-promoting behavior is an essential element of NP practice (see Appendix).

BIBLIOGRAPHY

Bates, B: A Guide to Physical Examination and History Taking, 6th ed. Lippincott, Philadelphia, 1995.

Gant, N, and Cunningham, F: Basic Gynecology and Obstetrics. Appleton and Lange, Norwalk, CT, 1993.

Kaplan, H: The New Sex Therapy. Bruner/Mazel, New York, 1974.

Keleher, K: Occupational health: How work environments can affect reproductive capacity and outcome. Nurse Pract 16(1):23–37, 1991.

Masters W, and Johnson V: Human Sexual Response Cycle. Little, Brown, Boston, 1996.

McBride, A: Mental health effects on women's multiple roles. Image 20(1):41–47, 1988.

Moen, P: Women's Two Roles: A Contemporary Dilemma. Auburn House, New York, 1992.

Paul, M: Occupational and Environmental Reproductive Hazards: A guide for clinicians. Williams and Wilkins, Baltimore, 1993.

CHAPTER 5

REVIEW OF SYSTEMS

Perform a comprehensive physical examination in the following manner.

General Review

- Include general state of health, weight, and development. Note posture and gait. Note personal hygiene. Note affect and orientation. Listen to the woman's speech. Vital signs should be taken.
- Skin: Observe the skin and note its characteristics. Note any lesions or discolorations. Inspect and palpate the hair and nails. Assess the exposed skin on areas such as hands. Inspect skin on other areas as they are exposed to evaluate other systems.
- Head: Examine the hair, scalp, skull, and face.
- Eyes: Check visual acuity and visual fields. Observe the eyelids, and inspect the sclera and conjunctiva of each eye. Using a light source, inspect the cornea, iris, and lens. Test pupillary reaction to light. With the ophthalmoscope, inspect the eye.
- Ears: Inspect the auricles, canals, and eardrums. Estimate hearing acuity. Perform Weber and Rinne tests.
- Mouth, throat, and neck: Examine the external nose. With a light source, examine the nasal mucus and septum. Palpate sinuses for tenderness. Inspect the lips, oral mucosa, gums, teeth, tongue, and pharynx. Inspect and palpate the cervical lymph node chains. Note any masses in the neck. Inspect and palpate the thyroid gland.
- Chest: Inspect, palpate, and percuss the chest. Identify the level of diaphragmatic dullness on both sides. Listen and evaluate breath sounds with a stethoscope. Inspect and palpate the carotid pulsations. Listen for bruits. Observe for jugular vein distention. Note location, amplitude, and duration of apical impulse. With the stethoscope, listen at each cardiac auscultatory area.

- Clinical breast examination: With the woman in a sitting position, inspect both breasts, noting the appearance of the skin, particularly color and any thickening. Note the contour of the breasts. Look for masses, dimpling, or flattening. Note any rashes, ulcerations, or discharge from either nipple. Ask the woman to raise her arms over her head and again inspect the breasts, looking for dimpling or retraction. Ask her to press her hands against her hips and again inspect the breasts. With the woman lying down, place a small pillow under her shoulder on the side that is being examined and have her place her arm under her head. With the examiner's fingers flat on the breast, compress the tissue in a rotary fashion, pressing the tissue against the chest wall. Proceed systematically until all of the breast tissue, including the area in the areola, has been palpated. Concentric circles or parallel lines can be used to ensure covering the entire breast. Note the consistency of the tissue. The normal female breast may be soft but also may be somewhat nodular. The nodular texture should be bilateral and may be throughout the breast or may be confined to parts of the breast. Nodularity increases premenstrually and during pregnancy. Feel for any lump or mass that is different from the rest of the breast tissue. If a mass is palpated, note location, size, shape, consistency, tenderness, and motility. Palpate each nipple. Compress the nipple and areola gently between thumb and index finger. Note the color, consistency, and amount of any discharge retrieved. Every woman should be instructed to perform a self breast examination on a monthly basis (Fig. 5–1).
- Peripheral vascular system: Note any swelling, discoloration, or ulcers. Palpate for edema. Note peripheral pulses. Palpate inguinal lymph nodes.
- Abdomen: Inspect, palpate, and percuss the abdomen. Palpate the liver, kidneys, and spleen.
- Musculoskeletal system: Examine the alignment of the spine and its range of motion. Palpate the joints and evaluate range of motion. Evaluate muscle tone, strength, and coordination.
- Nervous system: Observe the patient's gait and ability to walk heel to toe, walk on toes, walk on heels, hop in place, and do shallow knee bends. Perform the Romberg test. Assess strength of grip. Check deep tendon and plantar reflexes. Assess sensory function by testing for pain and vibration in the hands and feet. Evaluate the cranial nerves (see Appendix).

The Pelvic Examination

GENERAL RULES

- The woman should empty her bladder before the examination.
- Hands and speculum should be warm.
- Explain each part of the examination before performing the examination.

■ WHY DO THE BREAST SELF-EXAM?

There are many good reasons for doing a breast self-exam each month. One reason is that it is easy to do and the more you do it, the better you will get at it. When you get to know how your breasts normally feel, you will quickly be able to feel any change, and early detection is the key to successful treatment and cure.

Remember: A breast self-exam could save your breast—and save your life. Most breast lumps are found by women themselves, but, in fact, most lumps in the breast are not cancer. Be safe, be sure.

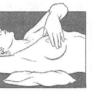

Finger Pads

■ WHEN TO DO BREAST SELF-EXAM

The best time to do breast self-exam is right after your period, when breasts are not tender or swollen. If you do not have regular periods or sometimes skip a month, do it on the same day every month.

■ NOW, HOW TO DO BREAST SELF-EXAM

1. Lie down and put a pillow under your right shoulder. Place your right arm behind your head.

2. Use the finger pads of your three middle fingers on your left hand to feel for lumps or thickening. Your finger pads are the top third of each finger.

3. Press firmly enough to know how your breast feels. If you're not sure how hard to press, ask your health care provider. Or try to copy the way your health care provider uses the finger pads during a breast exam. Learn what your breast feels like most of the time. A firm ridge in the lower curve of each breast is normal.

4. Move around the breast in a set way. You can choose either the circle (A), the up and down line (B), or the wedge (C). Do it the same way every time. It will help you to make sure that you've gone over the entire breast area, and to remember how your breast feels.

5. Now examine your left breast using right hand finger pads.

6. If you find any changes, see your doctor right away.

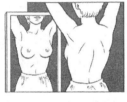

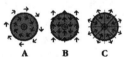

A   B   C

■ FOR ADDED SAFETY:

You should also check your breasts while standing in front of a mirror right after you do your breast self-exam each month. See if there are any changes in the way your breasts look: dimpling of the skin, changes in the nipple, or redness or swelling.

You might also want to do a breast self-exam while you're in the shower. Your soapy hands will glide over the wet skin making it easy to check how your breasts feel.

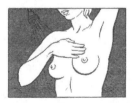

FIGURE 5–1   Breast self-examination.

- Position the woman with her head and shoulders slightly elevated to relax her abdominal muscles and to be sure that her face can be observed during the examination. The woman's arms should be placed at her sides.
- Drape the woman to preserve modesty.

EXTERNAL EXAMINATION

Using a good light source, examine external genitalia. Assess the sexual maturity of the adolescent patient using the guidelines in Table 5–1. Inspect the external genitalia, including the labia, clitoris, urethral orifice, and introitus. Note any inflammation, ulceration, discharge, swelling, or nodules. If there are any lesions, palpate them. Check Bartholin's glands. If urethritis is suspected, milk the urethral glands.

INTERNAL EXAMINATION

The internal examination is performed with the patient in the lithotomy position. The examiner begins in a seated position with an excellent light source. Insert the appropriate speculum lubricated with warm water. Inspect the cervix for lesions, ectropia, or presence of infection. If discharge obscures the view, wipe it away with a large cotton swab. Secure the speculum and obtain a Papanicolaou (Pap) smear and cultures such as for gonorrhea and *Chlamydia*. Inspect the vagina as the speculum is being removed. Close the blades after the cervix is cleared and just prior to the point at which the speculum is emerging from the introitus. After removal of the speculum and with the labia separated for better visualization, ask the woman to strain down and note any bulges of the vaginal walls.

From a standing position and with lubricated index and middle fingers, perform a bimanual examination. Note any tenderness in the vaginal wall, including the urethra and bladder anteriorly. Palpate the cervix. Place the opposite examining hand on the abdomen between the umbilicus and the symphysis pubis. While elevating the cervix and uterus with the pelvic hand, press the abdominal hand in and down until the uterus is palpated. In order to assist the abdominal hand with feeling the uterus, the fingers of the pelvic hand can slide into the anterior or posterior vaginal fornix. Placing the abdominal hand on the right and left lower quadrants, respectively, assists in moving the adnexal structures toward the pelvic hand. Moving both the hand on the abdomen and the fingers in the vagina allows for palpation of the adnexa. Assessing the strength of the vaginal muscles is accomplished by asking the patient to squeeze her vaginal muscles as hard as she can around the examiner's two fingers in the vagina.

If clinically relevant, a rectovaginal examination may be performed at this point. For example, postpartum examinations require rectovaginal examinations to rule out fistulas and ensure adequate healing of lacerations.

A rectal examination is performed while the woman remains in a lithotomy position. This position allows for visualization of the perianal area. Prevent contamination of the rectum with vaginal secretions by changing gloves prior to the rectal

TABLE 5-1   STAGES OF PUBERTAL DEVELOPMENT
AS DEFINED BY TANNER

Girls		
Growth of Breasts	**Mean Age (years)**	**Range (years)**
I. Prepubertal.		
II. Subuareolar tissue forms a breast bud—a mound of tissue limited to the areola; areola widens; papilla is erect.	11.2	9.0–13.3
III. Breast tissue enlarges beyond areola, but there is no separation of their contours.	12.2	10.0–14.3
IV. Areola and papilla form a second mound above the plane of the enlarging breast tissue.	13.1	10.8–15.3
V. Adult breast; areola and breast tissue return to the same plane; papilla is erect.	15.3	11.9–18.8

Growth of Pubic Hair	**Mean Age (years)**	**Range (years)**
I. Prepubertal; no pubic hair.		
II. Coarser, curly, pigmented hair on each side of mons veneris or labia majora.	11.7	9.3–14.1
III. Coarse, curly hair spread across pubis.	11.7	10.2–14.6
IV. Abundant adult pubic hair, but limited to the pubis.	12.4	10.8–15.1
V. Pubic hair present on medial aspects of thighs.	13.0	12.2–16.7
VI. Menarche.	14.4	11.4–15.5
	13.5	

Boys		
Growth of Genitalia	**Mean Age (years)**	**Range (years)**
I. Prepubertal.		
II. Scrotum and testes enlarge; scrotum thins and becomes pigmented.	11.6	9.0–14
III. Phallus grows: Further enlargement of testes and scrotum.	12.9	10.3–15
IV. Further enlargement of genitalia.	13.8	11.2–16
V. Adult size and shape of genitalia.	14.9	12.2–17

Growth of Pubic Hair	**Mean Age (years)**	**Range (years)**
I. Prepubertal; no pubic hair.		
II. Coarser, curly, pigmented hair on each side of penile base.	13.4	10.8–16
III. Coarse, curly hair spread across pubis.	13.9	11.4–16
IV. Abundant adult public hair, but limited to pubis.	14.4	11.7–17
V. Pubic hair present on medial aspects of thighs.	15.2	12.5–17

TABLE 5-1—*Continued*

	Nipple Diameter (mm)	
Pubertal Stage	**Cross-Sectional Data (Mean ± SD)**	**Longitudinal Data (Mean ± SD)**
Breast		
1	2.89 ± 0.81	3.0 ± 0.77
2	3.28 ± 0.89	3.37 ± 0.96
3	4.07 ± 1.32	4.72 ± 1.40
4	7.74 ± 1.64	7.25 ± 1.46
5	9.94 ± 1.38	9.41 ± 1.45
Pubic Hair		
1	2.95 ± 1.02	3.14 ± 1.31
2	3.32 ± 0.91	3.69 ± 1.34
3	4.11 ± 1.54	4.44 ± 1.17
4	7.15 ± 1.81	6.54 ± 1.47
5	9.66 ± 1.59	8.98 ± 1.56

Nipple Diameter Related to Breast and Pubic Hair Stage in Longitudinal and Cross-Sectional Studies

examination. The cervix may be felt through the anterior rectal wall. A retroverted uterus is also palpable through rectal examination.

PAP SMEAR

The Pap smear is a screening tool for detecting atypical cells of the cervix. It helps to identify neoplastic and preneoplastic changes in the cervix as well as infection of the cervix. False-negatives and false-positives vary widely with the laboratory reading the tests. It is essential to be familiar with the reliability of the laboratory reading Pap smears.

To obtain a good Pap smear specimen, good visualization of the entire cervix is essential. An endocervical brush and plastic spatula can be used. The endocervical brush obtains endocervical cells, and the spatula retrieves cells from the ectocervix and squamous columnar junction. Both the brush and the spatula must be rotated 360 degrees. Roll the cells onto a slide. Spray the slide or slides within 10 seconds of application of the cells. Label the specimen correctly.

Pap smears can also be done with a broom that is inserted into the cervix, swept 360 degrees to obtain cells that are sent to the laboratory in a solution. This method is called "thin prep." Many providers also use an endocervical brush with this method. Many providers prefer not to use a brush with pregnant women.

The Bethesda system is the current format for reporting Pap smear results. (see Appendix). Classes have been eliminated, and the following phrases, which describe the findings, have been substituted:

- "Atypical cells of undetermined significance"
- "Squamous intraepithelial lesion"
- "Low grade squamous intraepithelial lesion (SIL) includes human papilloma virus (HPV) changes"
- "Carcinoma in situ"
- "High grade SIL with moderate or severe dysplasia"

An abnormal Pap smear requires a consultation with a physician to determine procedure for follow-up. A repeated Pap smear and a colposcopy are common methods for following up an abnormal Pap smear (Table 5–2).

TABLE 5–2   MANAGEMENT OF ABNORMAL PAP SMEAR RESULTS

Result	Interpretation
Satisfactory but limited by	No endocervical component; should be repeated in 6 weeks.
Unsatisfactory for evaluation	Repeat smear in 6 weeks.
Fungus consistent with *Candida*	*Candida* colonization is not dangerous to women or their partners. If no complaints are offered by the woman or she has been treated, the Pap smear should be repeated at the regular interval.
Trichomonas vaginalis	Treat on the basis of the Pap smear finding.
Predominance of coccobacilli consistent with shift in vaginal flora	This finding suggests bacterial vaginosis. Treat or further evaluate for treatment with wet mount.
Bacteria morphologically consistent with *Actinomyces*	This result refers to anerobic bacteria that may cause pelvic inflammatory disease (PID). This finding requires evaluation of the woman.
Reactive cellular changes associated with inflammation	This result dictates benign metaplasia, irritation, post-traumatic repair, *Chlamydia* or gonorrhea, viral infection, or cervical cancer. Presistent presentation of this finding leads to colposcopic referral.
Atrophy with inflammation	This result suggests estrogen deficiency. Treatment is necessary only if the woman is symptomatic.
Atypical squamous cells of undetermined significance (ASCUS)	Abnormal, yet not consistent with SIL. ASCUS has two categories: "Reactive changes" and "premalignant process is favored." Reactive changes probably represent a benign process, making repeat Pap in 4–6 months necessary for evaluation. Premalignant process should be treated as low-grade SIL described below.
Low-grade SIL	This result indicates HPV and cervical intraepithelial lesion (CINI). Colposcopy is indicated.
High-grade SIL	Refer for colposcopy.
Endometrial cells, cytologically benign in a postmemopausal woman	Refer for endometrial sampling.
Atypical glandular cells of undetermined significance (CAGCUS)	This result indicates bacterial or HPV infection or adenocarcinoma. Refer for colposcopy.

Diagnostic Testing

Diagnostic testing is often essential to patient care. Although history and physical examination remain the foundation of diagnosis and treatment, diagnostic testing adds additional knowledge. Diagnostic tests can confirm a diagnosis, identify a patient with subclinical disease, and also provide prognostic information.

Upon completion of the history and physical examination, diagnosis and differential diagnoses are formulated. Laboratory testing can confirm the diagnosis and rule out differential diagnoses, or confirm a differential diagnosis and rule out the more likely diagnosis.

Interpreting diagnostic testing is based partially on understanding the terminology used with testing. *Accuracy* is the degree of closeness by which the measurement comes to the true value, as measured by a "gold standard." *Precision* is the test's ability to give nearly the same result in repeated determinations. *Sensitivity* is the probability that a test will be positive when it is applied to a person who actually has the disease. *Specificity* is the probability that the test will be negative when it is applied to a person who actually does not have the disease.

Nurse practitioners (NPs) must choose among tests with imperfect specificity and sensitivity. A new test, for example, may offer more specificity but less sensitivity. Costs, both in patient inconvenience and invasiveness and in dollars, factor into the choice of testing. Low false-negative rates should be favored when effective treatment for the disease exists. Low false-positive rates are most important when a positive diagnosis does not influence therapy but does create a burden for the patient. Testing should be ordered with the prognostic and therapeutic implications of the diagnosis kept in mind.

Women with Mental and Physical Disabilities

Evaluating women who are disabled involves more than altering examination rooms and arranging for additional personnel. Evaluation should consider positioning, creative orientation to the examination, and careful consideration of contraception and pregnancy risks.

Alternative positions for pelvic examination can be utilized with disabled women. The knee-chest position can be used with the woman lying on her side with both knees bent and her top leg brought closer to her chest. An assistant should provide support for the woman while she is on the examination table. A diamond-shaped position can be used in which the woman lies on her back with her knees bent and her heels together at the foot of the table. The assistant can assist the woman in holding her feet together while she supports her during the examination. The speculum must be inserted with the handle up. An M shape can be used, in which the woman lies on her back, knees bent and apart and her feet resting on the examination table close to the buttocks. The assistant should support the knees and feet. The speculum must be inserted with the handle up. A V shape can be used with the woman on her back with her legs straightened and spread wide apart. The legs must be supported by the assistant or assistants. Obstetric stirrups can be used.

Women who are visually impaired may assume a foot-stirrup position for examination. During the examination, the woman may feel more at ease with constant tactile and verbal communication. Assistants should remember to identify themselves as they enter the room. Some visually impaired women will ask to be oriented to their surroundings and instrumentation used during the examination. Staff should verbally describe where the furnishings are and where the patient should put her clothing and belongings. If the woman is accompanied by a dog, she will ask the NP not to pet or distract the dog while the dog is accompanying her.

The hearing-impaired woman may assume the foot-stirrup position. Her head should be elevated so that she can see the NP. She may wish to examine the instruments prior to the examination. The woman may choose sign language, an interpreter, lip reading or writing, or a combination of these methods for communicating during the examination. She may choose not to have the interpreter in the room during the examination. When using an interpreter, it is difficult to address the patient and not the interpreter, but it is very important to look at and speak to the patient.

The NP should review transfer techniques from basic nursing before caring for women with physical disabilities. Transfers include the pivot and two-person transfer. Spasms may be a common aspect of a woman's disability. Spasms may occur during transfer or during the examination. If a spasm occurs, gently support the area in spasm and allow the spasm to resolve before continuing with the examination.

Women with mental disabilities require patient explanation of pelvic examination. Instrumentation to be used should be explained at a level at which the woman can understand. The purpose and procedure for examination must be thoroughly explained to the patient. Contraceptive issues must be clearly explained to the mentally disabled woman. Visual family planning aides can be helpful. Informed consent must be obtained before a method of contraception is agreed on.

Because of relative circulatory status, oral contraceptives and progestin are contraindicated in spinal cord–injured patients. Intrauterine devices are also contraindicated in spinal cord–injured woman because of the inability of these women to sense complications such as infection and ectopic pregnancy. Women with arthritis may have difficulty using barrier methods if their hands are affected by the disease.

Women who are disabled and pregnant require evaluation of how the pregnancy is affecting the disability and how the disability is affecting the pregnancy. Creativity is required in coordinating the care of disabled and pregnant women. Modifications must be made to enhance the woman's health prior to delivery. Effects of the disability on labor and delivery must be considered. Family adjustments that might be necessary prior to delivery and after delivery must be considered. The effect of medication on the fetus must be considered. Numerous resources within the health-care community must be employed for pregnant and disabled women. Working with pregnant women with disabilities is always done using a team approach with a NP as an important member of the team.

BIBLIOGRAPHY

Bates, B: A Guide to Physical Examination and History Taking, 6th ed. Lippincott, Philadelphia, 1995.
Gant, N, and Cunningham, F: Basic Gynecology and Obstetrics. Appleton and Lange, Norwalk, CT, 1993.

TREATING

ILLNESS

CHAPTER 6

INTEGUMENT AND

LYMPHATICS

Patients frequently request women's health nurse practitioners (NPs) to evaluate affected skin. Symptoms associated with skin located in the genital, groin, buttocks, and breast regions prompt the need for a clinical examination.

Overall screening of women includes examination of the skin for possible pathology. The practitioner can diagnose malignant melanoma, condyloma, and folliculitis based on observation with or without a patient complaint.

This chapter begins with a brief discussion of dermatologic disorders (for a more complete discussion, consult a dermatologic text) and ends with a more detailed discussion of skin disorders most commonly presented to women's health practitioners (Fig. 6–1).

Skin Infections

BACTERIAL INFECTIONS

Impetigo, the most common bacterial infection of the skin, is caused by gram-positive bacteria such as *Staphylococcus* or *Streptococcus*. The lesions appear as thin-walled vesicles or pustules on erythematous bases. The lesions most commonly present on exposed areas of the skin and rupture easily, leaving a serous exudate. Treatment includes systemic antibiotics and local care.

Ecthyma is a deeper infection of the skin caused by *Streptococcus*. The lesions resemble impetigo, but deeper ulcers also occur in the skin. Standard treatment is antibiotic therapy.

Erysipelas is produced by streptococci. Clinical manifestations include fever,

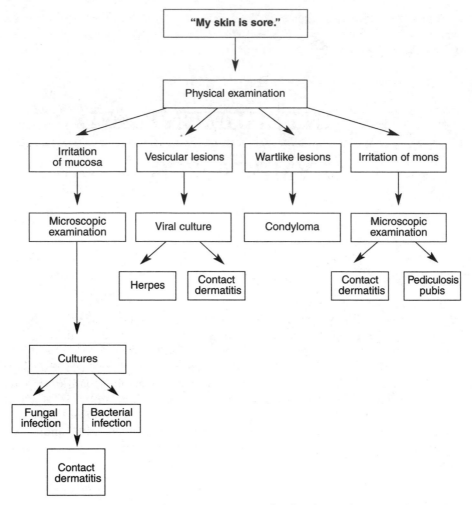

FIGURE 6–1 Diagnosing skin disorders.

malaise, and skin erythema and tenderness. Erysipelas, seen frequently in the elderly, is treated with antibiotics.

Cellulitis, a complication of localized infection, is caused by streptococci or staphylococci.

Folliculitis develops in traumatized skin. Bacterial folliculitis is characterized by inflammation surrounding a hair follicle. Folliculitis can occur without infection in areas traumatized by rubbing or scratching.

Furunculosis and carbuncles, painful, hot erythematous nodules containing pus, are treated with incision and drainage and systemic antibiotics.

Toxic shock syndrome is associated with *Staphylococcus aureus*. Prolonged tampon use may support bacterial growth and thus precipitate this syndrome. The syndrome begins with a sudden high fever, headache, myalgia, vomiting, diarrhea, skin eruption, and hypotension. Treatment includes hospitalization, volume expanders, and appropriate antibiotic therapy.

FUNGAL OR YEAST INFECTIONS

Dermatophyte infection is a common superficial cutaneous infection that occurs in skin, hair, and nails. Any scaling eruption in these areas should be scraped, sampled, and examined using potassium hydroxide (KOH) to exclude or include fungal infection.

Candidiasis is a common cutaneous infection. *Candida albicans* resides in the intestinal tract and on mucosal surfaces and thrives on damaged skin and in moist alkaline environments. Candidiasis commonly flares with antibiotic usage, especially in persons who are immunosuppressed. Iron deficiency anemia and diabetes also promote candidiasis.

Common Drug Reactions

Eruptions may occur on the skin and on mucous membranes following systematically administered drugs. The eruption is usually not related to the therapeutic effect of the drug. A drug eruption may resemble many other skin diseases and may produce one or more types of lesions. Urticaria is a common drug eruption.

Many chemicals and drugs can combine with components of the skin, allowing the skin to respond excessively to ultraviolet light. This can result in photosensitivity and sunburn.

Contact Dermatitis

Contact with an antigen or an irritant can produce dermatitis in any individual. The eczematous response in contact dermatitis is vesicles at the site of exposure. Poison ivy is an example of an irritant that causes contact dermatitis. Other common causes include nickel, potassium dichromate, formalin, rubber compounds, soap, laundry detergent, and clothes dryer softening sheets. Treatment includes removal of the allergen and topical corticosteroids. Antihistamines may be used for relief of itching.

Urticaria

Some agents produce urticaria directly through histamine release and others through mast cell mediators. Examples of agents that may produce urticaria include foods such as strawberries, tomatoes, shellfish, and chocolate. The primary lesion is a wheal or red swelling accompanied by itching, stinging, or slight burning as the primary symptoms.

Hair Loss

The hair matrix can be destroyed by physical agents and by infections or inflammation. Hair loss may occur as a result of metabolic disease or drug therapy. Physiologic alterations, such as those that occur during pregnancy, can also produce hair loss by altering the relationship between the follicles' resting phases and growing phases. Pharmacologic agents such as oral contraceptives can also change the relationship of resting and growing hair follicles. Hair loss should be differentiated from hair breakage, which results from physical or chemical stress to the shaft.

Tumors of the Skin

Most tumors of the skin are benign and include skin tags or skin polyps, keloids, fibromas, lipomas, and hemangiomas. Malignant tumors include squamous cell and basal cell carcinoma and melanoma.

Squamous cell carcinoma, a malignant epithelial tumor with a potential for invasion and metastasis, is commonly located on the face, scalp, or lip. This form of carcinoma is usually related to chronic exposure to the sun and is highly variable in appearance. Some squamous cell carcinomas are hyperkeratotic, some are nodular, and others form papules or plaques. Ulcer formation can occur. Treatment requires surgical excision.

Basal cell carcinoma, the most prevalent of cutaneous malignancies, is an epithelial tumor that may cause local skin destruction and invasion but rarely extends beyond the skin.

Malignant melanoma arises from the melanocytes in the skin. Although it can occur anywhere on the skin, in the eye, and in the vagina, it is most commonly seen on the head, neck, back, and lower extremities. The major risk factors for melanoma are family history, personal history, and an atypical mole.

Herpes Infection

Herpes is a virus infection that affects men, women, and children. Genital herpes infection is a lifelong disease that may result in painful recurrent lesions that may have psychosocial effects. Genital herpes can produce serious negative outcomes in neonates born to women infected at the time of delivery.

Etiology: The cutaneous lesions of herpes simplex virus (HSV) infections are produced by HSV 1 (most commonly oral) and HSV 2 (commonly associated with genital infection). Each of these viral types can infect any skin area. Recurrence in the genital area from type 1 is less common than from type 2. Many women seek clinical assistance to confirm the herpes infection they suspect or to reduce frequently recurring symptoms.

Occurrence: Unknown.

Age: Genital herpes occurs in sexually active women.

Ethnicity: Not significant.

Contributing Factors: Sexual activity. Reactivation of the latent herpes virus can be stimulated by sunlight, trauma, or immunosuppression.

Signs and Symptoms: Primary HSV 1 usually presents as severe pharyngitis or gingivostomatitis with fever and lymphadenopathy. Primary HSV 2 presents as painful vulvovaginitis with ulcerations and lymph node enlargement. Fever and malaise also occur in the majority of women. Small, maculopapular-vesicular blisters occur 12–24 hours after contact with a herpes virus. Eventually there is re-epithelialization of the skin, usually without scarring.

During the initial 3–4 days of primary infection, some woman autoinoculate themselves to other areas (commonly mouth to genitalia), but secondary infections are usually mild, brief, self-limiting, and incapable of establishing disease in other areas.

After acute infection, the virus lies dormant in the dorsal root ganglion and circulates to the skin when there is a breakdown in host defenses. The result is a localized, self-limiting form of the illness. It may begin with tingling or discomfort. Most women experience the maculopapular-vesicular rash. Recurrent infections can occur in different distributions, but along the same ganglia.

Diagnostic Tests: In most cases, the diagnosis is a clinical one. Viral culture with DNA probe can be used to diagnose this disorder.

Differential Diagnosis: Contact dermatitis, condyloma acuminata, chancroid, excoriation, bacterial infection.

Treatment: The goals of therapy are to speed healing and reduce symptoms, reduce the frequency and severity of recurrences, and decrease the risk for complications. Acyclovir, the mainstay of treatment, is effective against both types. It shortens viral shedding time and reduces the time to heal. The earlier the treatment begins, the better. Treat symptomatic lesions with oral acyclovir, 200 mg five times daily. Titrate the dosage depending on the patient response. Acyclovir can be given in 800-mg doses two to four times daily.

Chronic acyclovir prophylaxis can be given to women who experience more than six outbreaks per year. Use the smallest dose of acyclovir that will prevent infection. Good local skin care and the use of a drying agent help speed the transition from acute vesicle to crusting.

Follow-up: Follow all herpes genital infections closely during pregnancy. Primary infection should be followed closely for resolution.

Sequelae: Secondary bacterial infection can occur. Chronic pain associated with this disease has been identified. One can have post-herpetic neuralgia without evidence of skin lesions. Both hemorrhagic cystitis and dyspareunia can occur as a result of this disease. HSV has been associated with retina necrosis. Secondary infection can occur.

Prevention/Prophylaxis: Herpes infection is a risk associated with sexual activity. Using condoms can reduce the risk but does not always prevent transmission of the disease.

Referral: Refer all infected women who are also pregnant to an obstetrician. Women with suspected eye involvement should be referred to an ophthalmologist.

Education: Herpes has acquired an unjustifiable reputation from the media. The only substantial risk with HSV is during childbirth. Risk of infection to the fetus can be reduced by culturing any possibly herpetic lesions and performing cesarean birth if necessary. The stigma associated with the disease must be reduced. Reassuring a frightened patient is important therapy.

Women must be educated about transmission. The risk of transmission is greatest during the first 96 hours after the appearance of the lesions. Silent shedding must be explained, as should the fact that condoms reduce the probability of infecting others with the disease.

Human Papillomaviruses

Warts result from skin infection with the human papillomavirus (HPV).

Etiology: HPV, a DNA virus with more than 60 types identified, causes tumors of the epidermis. At least five types are potentially oncogenic, with two implicated in cervical carcinoma and three in squamous cell carcinoma. Warts can be transmitted by direct contact or autoinoculation.

Occurrence: Unknown.

Age: During the sexually active years.

Ethnicity: Not significant.

Contributing Factors: Sexual activity.

Signs and Symptoms: Anogenital warts and condyloma acuminata, which result from sexual transmission of HPV, grow on mucous membrane. They range in size and are often asymptomatic.

Diagnostic Tests: Appearance is generally sufficient for diagnosis. Acetic acid in a 5% solution can be used to enhance visualization of small condylomata. The colposcope can provide magnification. HPV can appear as a diagnosis on a Pap smear.

Differential Diagnosis: Condyloma lata of syphilis, squamous cell carcinoma, molluscum contagiosum, lipomas.

Treatment: Trichloracetic acid (TCA) in solution can be applied to external condylomata. TCA does not require removal. TCA should be applied carefully in order to protect unaffected areas. Petroleum or KY jelly can be applied to the unaffected area surrounding the condylomata during TCA application.

Podofilox 0.5% (Condylox) can be applied to external lesions by the women infected with the disease. The manufacturer's directions and restrictions must be followed carefully.

A carbon dioxide laser can be used for extensive external disease and for HPV of the cervix.

Liquid nitrogen can be applied to resistant external lesions.

Follow-up: Lesions can become numerous and large, requiring more extensive treatment. The woman with this disease should be examined at least every 4 weeks for evaluation until resolution of the disease. A Pap smear should be performed every 6 months in women treated for external condylomata for at least 2 years.

Sequelae: Recurrences occur in one-third of women.

Prevention/Prophylaxis: Prevention entails avoiding others with warts and removing condylomata so that the viral reserve is reduced.

Referral: A Pap smear showing cervical dysplasia and the evidence of HPV requires referral. Women with extensive condylomata may require referral for possible laser treatment or use of liquid nitrogen.

Education: Condylomata may disappear spontaneously. For some women, the treatment is lengthy, time-consuming, and expensive. Bolstering the immune system with adequate sleep and rest, excellent nutrition, and vitamin therapy may reduce the viral reserve. When a diagnosis is made, sexual partners should be examined for the disease.

Pediculosis Pubis

Human lice are wingless, blood-sucking insects of two types: *Pediculus humanus,* which infests the head and body, and *Phthirus pubis,* which infests the pubic area. These insects are elongated or rounded and 3–4 mm in length or diameter.

Etiology: Transmission is by contact with infested clothing or bedding, and/or by sexual transmission. The adult louse lives and lays eggs in clothing, often in the seams, and travels onto the skin for feeding. The second and third pairs of legs serve as claws that clasp hair tightly. The nits hatch and evolve into adults in 2–3 weeks. Lice live approximately 1 month. *Phthirus* affects primarily the pubic hairs; however, the eyelashes and axillary, chest, and thigh hair can be involved.

Occurrence: Unknown.

Age: Lice can be transmitted to a woman of any age.

Ethnicity: Not significant.

Contributing Factors: Close contact with lice through clothing, bedding, or sexual activity.

Signs and Symptoms: Itching, which is the cardinal symptom, is caused by the lice injecting saliva, digestive juices, and feces into the skin.

Diagnosis: Diagnosis is made by direct examination of egg cases in the involved area. They are usually visible to the naked eye, but a hand lens and light may help. Microscopic examination of nits or adult lice is also diagnostic.

Differential Diagnosis: Contact dermatitis, bacterial infection, viral infection.

Treatment: Lindane 1% shampoo used for 4 minutes and washed off, followed by permethrin 1% cream used for 10 minutes and then rinsed off. Lindane should not be used during pregnancy or lactation.

To prevent reinfestation, treat asymptomatic close contacts simultaneously. Wash bed sheets and clothing worn in the last few days in hot soapy water or dry-clean any nonwashable items.

Treat eyelashes by applying occlusive ophthalmic ointment to the eyelids twice daily for 10 days.

Follow-up: Evaluate patients in 1 week. Treatment can be repeated if the parasites are still present.

Sequelae: Secondary infection can occur. Reactions to medicated shampoo can occur.

Prevention/Prophylaxis: Avoidance of the parasites.

Referral: Treatment failure should be referred. Coexisting dermatologic conditions should be referred.

Education: Tell sexual partners that they must be treated simultaneously to prevent reinfestation. Family and household members who are infected should also be treated simultaneously.

Summary

Examination of the skin is an important part of the screening examination for each woman. Women frequently present to NPs with complaints related to skin disorders, particularly if the affected area is on the breasts or genitalia.

Every NP should be familiar with common skin ailments and their treatment as well as with skin disorders that are life-threatening, such as malignancies.

BIBLIOGRAPHY

Barton, SE, Munday, PE, and Patel, RJ: Asymptomatic shedding of herpes simplex virus from the genital tract. Int J STD & AIDS 7 (4):229–232, 1996.

Brown, S, Becher, J, and Brady W: Treatment of ectoparasitic infection: Review of English language literature. Clin Infect Dis 20(Suppl 1):104–109, 1995.

Brugha, R, et al: Genital herpes infection: A review. Int J Epidemiol 26(4):698–709, 1997.

Goroll, A, May, L, and Mulley, A. Primary Care Medicine. JB Lippincott, Philadelphia, 1995.

Roberts, SW, et al: Genital herpes during pregnancy: No lesions, no cesarean. Obstet Gynecol 85(2): 261–264, 1995.

Shelley, WB, and Slehhey, ED: Stat single dose of acyclovir for prevention of herpes simplex. Cutis 57(6):453, 1996.

CHAPTER 7

CHEST

Evaluation of the chest plays an important role in women's health examinations. Breast cancer is associated with high rates of morbidity and mortality for women. A combination of breast self-examination, practitioner examination, and screening tests enhances early detection and therefore reduces mortality. Physical examination detects early disease and provides an excellent opportunity for teaching breast self-examination and discussing the importance of mammography.

Depending on the definition used, 15%–25% of adult Americans have hypertension. Every woman should have a blood pressure check at every clinical visit.

Cardiovascular disease is by far the leading cause of death among women in the United States. More women die of cardiovascular disease than from all other causes combined. The responsibility for screening and intervention lies with all practitioners. In any practice setting, efforts should focus on the prevention of cardiovascular disease through risk reduction and on early identification of cardiovascular disease in patients with symptoms.

This chapter discusses prevention, diagnosis, and treatment for benign and malignant breast disease and screening and prevention of cardiovascular disease.

Cardiac Disease

Cardiovascular disease, specifically coronary heart disease (CHD), is the leading cause of death in women in the United States. In women, deaths from cardiac disease total more than twice the number of deaths from cancer. Gender differences exist in both the diagnosis and the treatment of CHD. Morbidity from cardiac disease is also higher in women than it is in men. There is a growing body of knowledge related to preventive strategies, diagnostic testing, responses to medical and surgical therapies, and other aspects of cardiovascular disease in women, but current information is still insufficient. Because of the underrepresentation of women in previous clinical trials, few comparisons of long-term outcomes between men and women with CHD have been made.

Etiology: The major cause of heart disease in women is coronary artery disease (CAD). Although other forms of heart disease exist in women, including valvular disease and heart disease during pregnancy, the incidence is less and therefore these diseases will not be discussed in this chapter.

Occurrence: Cardiovascular disease hospitalizes 2.5 million women per year and claims the lives of 500,000 annually. These numbers exceed those of men. Cardiovascular disease accounts for 37% of the deaths in all women and 50% of the deaths in postmenopausal women. CAD remains the leading cause of mortality in women, accounting for 28% of deaths. Morbidity from cardiovascular disease is higher in women than in men. Women's higher morbidity and mortality rates can be partially explained by the tendency for women to be older, sicker, and to have more advanced disease at diagnosis.

Age: Increased incidence of CHD in women occurs after age 54. In women 55 years of age and older, there is a tenfold increase in CHD. The increased risk for men in the same age group is 4.6. This change in risk in women is thought to be largely related to the onset of menopause.

Ethnicity: Black women have the highest mortality rate—48%—4 years after myocardial infarction.

Contributing Factors: Family history may predispose women to heart disease. Of significance is any first-order relative, male or female, with a history of heart disease. Blood pressure is a more common risk factor in women than it is in men. Hypertension affects an estimated 70% of women over 65 years of age. Smoking has well-established deleterious health effects. Concerns for women include the antiestrogenic effect of smoking, earlier onset of menopause in smokers, and interaction with oral contraceptives. Women smokers taking oral contraceptives have a 20-fold increase in myocardial infarction because of the enhanced risk of thrombosis. This risk increases for women who are both perimenopausal and smokers.

Hyperlipidemia is an important risk factor in women. Levels of high-density lipoprotein (HDL), which are inversely associated with CHD, are higher throughout a woman's life than a man's. After menopause, however, HDL levels drop slightly, whereas the risk for CHD rises. The risk for CHD in women increases when the HDL level falls to less than 45 mg/dL and in men at under 35 mg/dL. Levels of low-density lipoproteins (LDL) rise after menopause, surpassing those of men, whose LDL levels tend to plateau at age 50.

Diabetes presents a very unfavorable risk factor for women, who in general experience a twofold greater risk for CHD than diabetic men. In addition, mortality from myocardial infarction and congestive heart failure is two times higher for diabetic women than for diabetic men.

Obesity, with incumbent higher waist-size-to-hip-size ratios, has been shown to increase the risk for CHD in women (see Appendix).

Signs and Symptoms: Gender plays an important role in manifestation of CHD. In men, the three major presentations include angina, sudden death, and myocardial infarction. In women, angina appears to be the most common manifestation. Women are twice as likely as men to present with angina and less likely to present with sudden death or infarction. Acutely, women are more likely than men to have heart failure and cardiogenic shock associated with infarction, perhaps in part because women present with an infarction on an average of 5 hours later than men.

Women have a higher mortality rate than men during hospitalization and at 6 weeks and 1 year after infarction. Four years after infarction, mortality rates were 36% for women and 21% for men.

Diagnostic Tests: Chest pain compatible with angina warrants evaluation for coronary disease in both men and women. The higher prevalence of angina as the presenting symptom places a greater burden on diagnostic strategies than the more easily recognized myocardial infarction. History is important for diagnosis. In one study, women who had typical anginal pain had a 70% incidence of angiographically documented CAD as compared to 2%–7% of those with atypical chest pain (Oettgen & Douglas, 1994).

The exercise electrocardiogram (ECG) is poor at detecting or excluding CAD in asymptomatic women. Instead, there is a greater risk of CAD in women with poor exercise tolerance. Stress ECG, sensitive for 98% of men, decreases to 75% sensitivity in women. When you combine exercise ECG with thallium scintigraphy, the sensitivity in women increases from 75% to 85%.

Women with suspected CAD are referred less frequently for coronary angiography and coronary bypass surgery. Male patients are 6.5 times more likely to be referred for catheterization than female patients. This seems paradoxical in light of the fact that the noninvasive tests are less accurate in women and the need for a gold standard such as angiography would be more desirable in women to define the presence or absence of disease.

Differential Diagnoses: Muscular disorders, including muscle spasm or strain. Skeletal disorders, including costochondritis, rib fracture, and metastatic disease. Neurologic disorders, including herpes zoster and nerve root compression. Pleuropulmonary disorders, including pneumothorax, pulmonary embolism, and bronchospasm. Esophageal disorders, including spasm and reflux, cholecystitis, and peptic ulcer disease. Psychogenic disorders, including anxiety and depression.

Treatment: Invasive diagnostic and therapeutic procedures are underutilized in women. Over 80,000 men and women hospitalized for CAD in Massachusetts and Maryland were evaluated for referral for coronary angiography or a revascularization process. After correction for age, occurrence of myocardial infarction (MI), presence of diabetes, and race, men were twice as likely to be referred than women (Villablanca, 1996); 55% of eligible women versus 72% of eligible men received thrombolytic therapy, even though thrombolytic therapy for acute

MI has equal benefit for both men and women. Use of pharmacologic agents in women with CHD is being investigated.

Follow-up: Exercise rehabilitation benefits both men and women. Physicians refer fewer women with CAD than men for exercise rehabilitation.

Sequelae: Women have higher operative mortality rates and they are twice as likely as men to have continued symptoms after coronary angioplasty.

Prevention/Prophylaxis
Smoking cessation
Weight reduction
Physical exercise
Excellent control of hypertension
Good control of diabetes
Reduced dietary intake of fat
Early diagnosis of rheumatic heart disease
Hormone replacement therapy

Referral: Any indicator for heart disease warrants a referral for evaluation.

Education: Inform the patient that:

The risk of CHD can be reduced in women by 14% within 2 years of stopping smoking.
Postmenopausal use of hormones reduces the risk of heart disease.
Weight gained after the age of 18 years is associated with increased risk.
There is an inverse relationship between minimal alcohol use and CHD.
A correlation exists between the intake of vitamin E and protection against CHD.
One to six aspirin per day reduces the risk of CHD.

Carcinoma of the Breast

Breast cancer is the leading cause of death in women aged 35 through 54. More than 150,000 women develop beast cancer each year in the United States. Of these, 50,000 will die of the disease. The lifetime probability that an American woman will develop breast cancer is 10%. Four out of five women have a relative or acquaintance who has developed breast cancer. Despite advances, mortality from breast cancer has changed very little over the past 30 years.

Etiology: Unknown.

Occurrence: Breast cancer accounts for 32% of all cancers in women and 18% of all cancer deaths in women.

Age: The risk of developing breast cancer increases with age. Women under 40 years of age account for 20 percent of breast cancer cases. The median age at the time of diagnosis is 54 years, whereas 45% of the cases occur after age 65 years. Half of breast cancer deaths are in women over 65.

Ethnicity: Breast cancer is more common in white women over the age of 45 than in black women in this age group.

Contributing Factors: A number of factors have been associated with increased risk of breast cancer, including:

Personal or family history of breast cancer. The risk for women who have a first-degree relative with breast cancer is two to three times higher than in the general population.
Biopsy positive for hyperplasia
Nulliparity and delayed childbearing
Early menarche
Late natural menopause

Breast feeding may decrease the risk for breast cancer, and the use of oral contraceptives does not affect the risk of developing breast cancer. The effect of adding progestin to estrogen supplementation has not been shown to be protective against the development of breast cancer.

Other factors that may be associated with breast cancer, but about which the literature is still inconclusive, are diet, exogenous hormones, alcohol consumption, breast trauma, viral infection, higher socioeconomic status, and obesity.

Signs and Symptoms: Breast examination is an integral part of a woman's health care (see Fig. 5–1). Every woman should be taught to perform breast self-examination. A diagnostic evaluation for breast cancer begins with physical examination and history. Any firm mass suggests malignancy. Fixation to the skin, skin edema, nipple retraction, or deep fixation are further evidence of carcinoma. When a mass is suspected or detected, history should be recorded, with particular emphasis on date of onset, size, and exact location (Fig. 7–1).

Diagnostic Tests: Mammograms detect more than 90% of breast cancers. A general agreement exists about the effectiveness of annual screening among women over the age of 50 years, but there is some difference of opinion about the efficacy of screening mammograms for women under the age of 50. Mortality rates in women ages 40–49 who were screened for breast cancer with mammography have been compared to rates in women in the same age group who were not screened for breast cancer. Results have been conflicting. The improved safety of mammography, not evidence of its efficacy, in women under the age of 50 is what inspired the American Cancer Society to recommend screening for women in this age group.

Mammography can serve as a diagnostic aide for breast masses. Biopsy is required to confirm the diagnosis, but mammography is a useful adjunct to palpation of a breast mass.

Nonpalpable lesions presenting as asymptomatic clusters of microcalcifications require repeat mammography or biopsy. Although most of these lesions are benign, 15%–20% represent early cancer. Consultation with a radiologist is essential to determine the significance of this finding.

Cytologic detection by biopsy is most useful in the diagnosis of breast can-

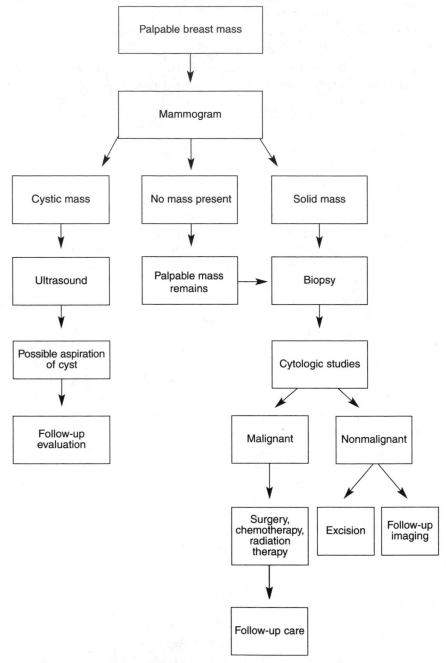

FIGURE 7–1   Lump in breast.

cer. A malignant cytologic finding permits immediate planning of treatment and discussion of treatment alternatives. Open biopsy can be performed, as can needle biopsy under radiologic guidance.

Differential Diagnosis: Nonmalignant breast mass.

Treatment: Clinical staging determines the therapy for breast cancer. The woman's wishes, the size and histology of the lesion, the size of the breast, and the skill and experience of the oncology team determine the course of surgical treatment. The use of radiation and/or chemotherapy is determined based upon the staging of the disease.

Follow-up: Follow-up depends on the course of therapy. Women may have courses of chemotherapy or radiation therapy before or after surgery. After therapy women are seen at regular intervals. One regime involves clinical evaluation every 3 months with annual pelvic examination, mammogram, chest x-ray, and liver function tests. This program continues for 2 years, with an increase to 4-month intervals in the third and fourth years, and every 6 months thereafter.

Sequelae: The 10-year survival rate for early-stage lesions (up to 2 cm and no node involvement) is 75%–85%. This figure drops to 40% survival if there is node involvement. Recurrent disease occurs most often in the first 2 years following treatment, but because women continue to die of breast cancer for periods exceeding 15–20 years following treatment, follow-up must continue indefinitely.

Prevention/Prophylaxis: The combination of breast self-examination, physical examination by a health-care provider, and a mammogram provides the most effective means of screening for breast cancer.

A publication of the Public Health Service entitled *Healthy People 2000* recommends, in objective number 5, increased efforts to screen older women for breast cancer.

Referral: All palpable masses that do not resolve after menses should be referred for further evaluation. Women with palpable findings should be referred for evaluation regardless of mammogram results. Breast tissue is considerably denser in young women, making a negative mammogram result not always negative for malignancy.

Education: Teach breast self-examination to all women. Menstruating women should perform breast self-examination approximately 7 days after the onset of menses. For women who do not experience menses, a day of the month should be chosen for breast self-examination.

Many women in the United States have breast implants. Examination of the augmented breast should include examination of the natural tissues as well as evaluation of the implant. During the examination, the implant is displaced with one hand and the breast tissue palpated with the other. Integrity of the implant is evaluated.

Nonmalignant Conditions of the Breast

The nurse practitioner is in a favorable position to educate, screen, counsel, and treat women with breast disease. Every woman should be taught breast self-examination. Any and all symptoms of breast disease must follow a protocol to rule out carcinoma. When a benign condition is diagnosed, treatment should be within the realm of the nurse practitioner's expertise.

Etiology

Breast pain can be caused by edema, ductal dilation, and/or inflammation response.

Cystic change refers to dilatation of the ducts. Most common is the development of microcysts (2 mm or less), but 20%–40% of microcysts progress to form palpable macrocysts. Macrocysts may regress with menses, may persist, or may disappear and reappear.

Fibrous change, occurring in the menstrual years, is characterized by a firm, palpable mass usually located in the upper quadrant of the breast that develops following an inflammatory response to ductal irritation.

Hyperplasia, a layering of cells, is associated with a fivefold increase in the risk of breast cancer.

Adenosis is related to changes in the acini in the distal mammary lobule. These small ducts become surrounded by a firm, hard, plaquelike material. This is most commonly seen in women in their 30s and 40s.

Papilloma is a lesion seen in later menstrual years. It creates a small palpable mass adjacent to the areola, accompanied by serosanguineous nipple discharge.

Ductal ectasia is the presence of dilated, distended terminal collecting ducts.

Subareolar abscesses are seen most commonly in younger women. This condition is not related to mastitis.

Fat necrosis is associated with trauma to the breast and usually presents as a hard, tender mass.

Occurrence: Fibrocystic change, the most common benign condition of the breast, occurs in approximately 10% of women under the age of 21, but becomes much more common in the premenopausal period. There is usually a regression of some of the signs of fibrocystic change during menopause.

Age: Depends on diagnosis.

Contributing Factors: Caffeine ingestion has been associated with fibrocystic changes of the breast.

Signs and Symptoms: The common symptoms of fibrocystic change are pain and tenderness, usually bilaterally, and most often in the upper outer quadrants of the breasts. Premenstrual pain is most often noted. Solid painless masses in the breast are detected with breast self-examination. Ductal ectasia presents as a

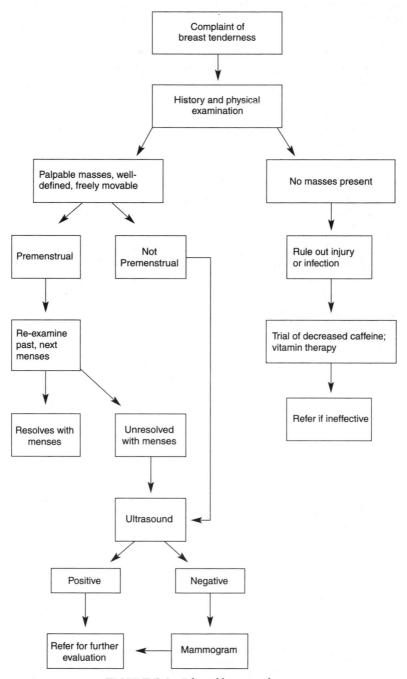

FIGURE 7–2   Bilateral breast tenderness.

mass near the areola with burning and itching. There may be a greenish to black nipple discharge. Subareolar abscess presents with pain and inflammation (see Appendix).

Diagnostic Testing: Breast examination may reveal skin changes and/or the presence of a mass. Nipple discharge can be detected.

Mammograms can be used for both screening and diagnostic purposes. Significant findings consist of alterations in the density of the breast tissue, calcifications, thickening of the skin, fibrous streaking, and nipple changes. Any of these may indicate early carcinoma and may warrant further evaluation. Mammography can also aid in the identification of fibroadenoma, lymph nodes, galactocele, or fat necrosis.

If a cystic mass is seen on mammogram, ultrasound can characterize it with greater accuracy than mammography (Fig. 7–2).

Excisional biopsy and needle aspiration are useful for both diagnosis and treatment of benign breast disease. Cytologic evaluation should be performed. Biopsy is required if any of the following findings are present: bloody fluid on aspiration, failure of the mass to disappear after aspiration, recurrence of a cyst after two aspirations, solid mass not diagnosed as a fibroadenoma, bloody nipple discharge, nipple ulceration, and the presence of skin edema or erythema.

Differential Diagnosis: Breast cancer

Treatment: Dietary modifications may be helpful, particularly reduction in caffeine for cystic changes. Administration of vitamins A and E has been shown to reduce the discomfort of cystic formation in breasts. Oral contraceptives suppress symptoms of fibrocystic changes in 70%–90% of women (see Appendix).

Macrocysts can be drained of fluid to confirm diagnosis and decrease discomfort. Fibroadenoma, hyperplasia, adenosis, and papilloma, which require biopsy for diagnosis, may require excision for therapy.

Ductal ectasia is treated with excisional biopsy, and subareolar abscess is treated with antibiotics and at times incision and drainage.

Follow-up: Depends upon diagnosis and treatment.

Prevention/Prophylaxis: A combination of breast self-examination, examination by a health-care provider, and mammography screening.

Referral: Any suspicion of breast cancer demands referral.

Education: Teach all women breast self-examination.

BIBLIOGRAPHY

Cardiac Disease

Major Findings from the Nurse's Health Study, 1976–1994.
Binder, E, et al: Effects of endurance exercise and hormone replacement therapy on serum lipids in older women. J Am Geriatr Soc 44:231, 1996.
Oettgen, P, and Douglas, P: Coronary artery disease in women: Diagnosis and prevention. Adv Int Med 39:467, 1994.

Villablanca, A: Coronary heart disease in women. Postgrad Med 100(3):191, 1996

Wenger, N. et al: Cardiovascular health and disease in women. N Engl J Med, 329(4):247, 1993.

Breast Cancer

American College of Obstetricians and Gynecologists: Carcinoma of the Breast. ACOG, Washington, DC, 1997.

NIH Consensus Statement on Breast Cancer Screening 1997.

Public Health Service, United States Department of Health and Human Services. 1991. Healthy People 2000: National Health Promotion and Disease Prevention Objectives. United States Printing Office, Washington, D.C., DHHS PUB No. 91-50212.

Carty, N, et al: Management of fibroadenoma of the breast. Ann Royal Coll Surg Engl 77(2):127, 1995.

Dahlbeck, S, Donnelly J, and Thieriault, R: Differentiating inflammatory breast cancer from acute mastitis. Am Fam Physician 52(3):929, 1995.

Shapiro, TJ and Clark, P: Breast cancer: What the primary care provider needs to know. Nurse Practitioner 20(3):36, 1995.

Nonmalignant Conditions of the Breast

American College of Obstetricians and Gynecologists: Nonmalignant Conditions of the Breast. ACOG, Washington, DC, 1997.

Deschamps, M, et al: Clinical determinants of mammographic dysplasia patterns. Cancer Detect Prev 20(6): 610, 1996.

Dixon, J, et al: Assessment of the acceptability of conservative management of fibroadenoma of the breast. Br J Surg 83(2):264, 1996.

Issacs, J: Benign tumors of the breast. Obstet Gynecol Clin North Am 21(3):487, 1994.

Levi, F, and Randimbison, L: Incidence of breast cancer in women with fibroadenoma. Int J Cancer, 57(5):681, 1994.

CHAPTER **8**

REPRODUCTIVE

Many adolescent females enter the health-care system with a reproductive concern. Young women often leave the pediatrician and enter the realm of women's health with a concern related to reproduction. Many adult women who left the health-care system re-enter via a reproductive health concern. Unfortunately, women commonly leave the system after the birth of their last child and do not return until they have a reproductive symptom or symptoms. Need for contraception or an unwanted pregnancy is a common reason for entry into the system. Abnormal vaginal bleeding, amenorrhea, infertility, symptoms of endometriosis, and symptoms of infection are all common reasons for establishing a relationship with a women's health nurse practitioner.

This chapter discusses reproductive concerns for women, including infections, benign and malignant diseases of the genital tract, as well as pelvic relaxation and abnormal bleeding. Contraception and infertility are also discussed. Assessment of the reproductive tract is discussed in Chapters 4 and 5.

Entry into women's health care means entry into a holistic environment. Entry may be via a reproductive concern, but all aspects of a woman's health must be considered. Nurse practitioners (NPs) are skilled at providing treatment and encouraging prevention, but they are also aware of the importance of referral. The NP needs an adequate referral system. He or she refers when medical or surgical intervention is required and consults with any appropriate member of the health-care, social service, or community team in order to provide comprehensive care for women who seek assistance.

Unwanted pregnancy is an example of entry into a woman's health-care setting in which the NP provides care, but the NP also counsels and refers to a variety of resources.

Unwanted Pregnancy

Pregnancy can be unwanted for financial, social, educational, health-related or genetic reasons, or for reasons of abuse. Diagnosis of pregnancy is made with a human chorionic gonadotrophin (hCG) urine slide test done at the office or with a urine or serum laboratory pregnancy test. Pregnancy is confirmed during an office visit with a physical examination and a repeat pregnancy test if the initial test was conducted at home. Examination should be performed in a nonjudgmental manner followed by a full exploration of the thoughts and feelings of the woman and discussion of options for resolution. Options for unwanted pregnancy are therapeutic abortion, adoption, and keeping the child.

Therapeutic abortion, when performed properly, is safe. There is less than 1 death per 100,000 procedures reported in first-trimester abortions. First-trimester abortions are performed at 12 weeks or less, on an outpatient basis, and as a 1-day procedure. Second-trimester termination is a hospital-based procedure that may take several days to complete. (Dilation is required prior to the procedure itself.) A mortality rate of 7 deaths per 100,000 procedures has been reported. Complications of second-trimester terminations are affected by gestational age, method of procedure, and by a coexisting complicating illness. In the United States, no conclusive evidence indicates serious psychologic sequelae after termination.

Adoption is an option for women who do not wish to raise the child but also do not wish to terminate the pregnancy. Adoption can be accomplished through a state or local agency. Open adoption, that is, the birth mother and the child keeping in contact, is becoming more common.

Keeping the child is an option. Identification of social supports, such as extended family and community agencies, may assist the pregnant woman in selecting this option.

Follow-up visits are planned according to the woman's decision. It may take more than one visit with the NP for a decision to be reached. Abortion requires referral to an appropriate medical center. Adoption and keeping the child require referral for prenatal care and social services. Every woman experiencing an unwanted pregnancy requires contraceptive counseling.

Infections

The genital tract in women is a route of entry for organisms. Infections may occur in or on the vulva, the vagina, the cervix, or the uterus. An organism may ascend further and infect the tubes and ovaries. Infection entering via the genital tract may become systemic. Examples of this are pelvic inflammatory disease (PID) and syphilis. Human immunodeficiency virus (HIV), discussed in Chapter 15, and hepatitis B, discussed in Chapter 10, are also systemic diseases that may enter the body via the genital tract.

Assessment

The vagina is not a sterile cavity. The normal flora of the vagina contains bacterial organisms, with lactobacilli being predominant. Both aerobes and anaerobes can be found in the vagina. Group B β-hemolytic streptococci can be cultured from the vaginas of approximately 20% of women.

Infections of the vagina are common, causing considerable discomfort for many women. Overall factors contributing to vaginal infection are lifetime number of sexual partners, coitus on first date, and previous sexually transmitted disease(s).

History taken prior to examination for vaginal infection should include:

- Onset of discharge, its appearance and odor
- Exposure to a sexually transmitted disease
- Previous infection
- Allergies
- Presence of symptoms such as dysuria, pruritus, pain, dyspareunia, rash
- Partner's symptoms
- History of diabetes
- Recent use of antibiotics
- Use of over-the-counter medications for relief of symptoms

Physical examination must include:

- Careful inspection of the external genitalia
- Noting the presence and appearance of discharge
- Inspection of the vagina
- Wet mount, culture, and Papanicolaou (Pap) smear
- Noting tenderness on bimanual examination

The three most commonly seen types of vaginal infection—bacterial vaginosis, *Candida* infection, and trichomoniasis—will be discussed, followed by *Chlamydia* infection and lymphogranuloma, along with systemic infections that enter via the vagina—that is, PID, gonorrhea, syphilis, and toxic shock syndrome.

Bacterial Vaginosis

Bacterial vaginosis is a bacterial infection of the vagina.

Etiology: Overgrowth of anaerobes, *Gardnerella* and *Mycoplasma hominis,* is the core of bacterial vaginosis (BV).

Occurrence: BV is the most common vaginitis in women of childbearing age. BV causes 40%–50% of symptomatic vaginal infections. Up to 50% of women who are asymptomatic for vaginitis will culture positive for the organisms that cause BV.

Age: Sexually active women ages 15–44.

Ethnicity: Three times more black women than white women present with a symptomatic BV infection.

Contributing Factors: The number of sexual partners.

Symptoms: Of women infected with BV, 50% have no symptoms upon infection or mild discomfort as the only symptom; 50% of women report increase in vaginal discharge that is foul-smelling. They also report swelling, burning, and itching (Table 8–1).

Diagnostic Tests
- pH > 4.5
- Presence of thin, gray, milky homogeneous discharge
- Positive whiff test (add 10% potassium hydroxide [KOH] to secretions on a glass slide)
- Clue cells present on wet mount (clue cells are epithelial cells coated with bacteria)

Differential Diagnosis: Gonorrhea, *Chlamydia* infection, herpes, condyloma, allergy (soaps, sprays, contraceptive foam, cream, or jelly), foreign body (lost tampons, condoms), atrophic vaginitis.

Treatment: The organisms that create BV can be present in culture without symptoms. BV is treated if symptoms are present. If the woman is pregnant, BV is treated with or without symptoms. Treatment includes:
- Metronidazole 2 g stat (85% effective) or metronidazole 500 mg bid for 7 days (recommended during pregnancy after first trimester)
- Oral clindamycin 300 mg bid for 7 days or clindamycin cream h.s. for 7 days
- Metronidazole gel (Metrogel) 0.75% intravaginally twice daily for 5 days

Follow-up: Recurrent BV dictates partner needs treatment.

Sequelae: Infection following abortion, infection following hysterectomy, preterm labor, and PID. *Mycoplasma* infection is associated with endometritis, low-birth-weight infants, habitual abortion, and infertility.

TABLE 8–1 VAGINITIS

	Bacterial Vaginosis	**Candidiasis**	**Trichomoniasis**
Source	Bacterial infection	Yeast infection	Parasitic infection
Symptoms	Asymptomatic or foul-smelling discharge	White vaginal discharge; vaginal itching and burning	Yellow-green discharge; vaginal itching and irritation
Findings	pH > 4.5; gray discharge; positive "whiff" test and clue cells on wet mount	pH < 4.5; thick, white discharge; erythema, edema, and excoriation; hyphae and spores on wet mount	pH between 5 and 7; yellow-green discharge; "strawberry" cervix; motile trichomonads and leukocytes on wet mount
Treatment	Antibiotic; treat partner(s)	Antifungal medication; partner(s) need not be treated	Antibiotics; treat partner(s)

Prevention/Prophylaxis: Use of condoms.

Referral: Consultation is required for ineffective therapy and recurrent infection.

Education: Encourage proper use of medication. Recommend follow-up examination if symptoms do not resolve after therapy. Instruct the patient not to consume alcohol with metronidazole. Metronidazole should not be taken in the first trimester of pregnancy. The results of clinical trials indicate that a woman's response to therapy and the possibility of relapse or recurrence are not affected by treatment of her sex partner; therefore, routine treatment of the woman's partner is not recommended.

Candidiasis

Candida infection, commonly called a "yeast" infection, is a fungal infection that frequently occurs in the vagina.

Etiology: *Candida albicans* is responsible for 80%–90% of all *Candida* infections. The remaining infections are related to *C. glabrata* and *C. tropicalis.*

Occurrence: Many women report at least one episode of *Candida* infection; 20%–25% of all symptomatic vaginal infections are related to *Candida.*

Age: After menarche and prior to menopause.

Ethnicity: Not significant.

Contributing Factors: Depressed immunity, high blood glucose level, administration of antibiotics, use of oral contraceptives, low pH prior to menses.

Signs and Symptoms: Itching; burning; dysuria; dyspareunia; and thick, white vaginal discharge (see Table 8–1).

Diagnostic Tests
- pH of 4.5 or below
- Presence of thick, white adherent discharge
- Erythema, edema, and excoriation of the vulva
- Positive yeast culture
- Hyphae and spores on wet mount (visualization can be enhanced with 10% KOH)

Differential Diagnosis: Hypersensitivity, allergic or chemical reaction, and contact dermatitis.

Treatment: Clotrimazole, miconazole, butoconazole, tioconazole, or terconazole in cream form used for 3–7 days h.s. is 80% effective. Nystatin may also be used. Oral fluconazole can be used for recurrent infections if the woman is not pregnant.

Follow-up: Follow-up appointments are necessary only if infection is not resolved with treatment. No need to treat partners.

Sequelae: Recurrent candidiasis.

Prevention/Prophylaxis: Use of antibiotics only as appropriate, good control of diabetes.

Referral: Consultation is needed for unresolved vaginitis.

Education: Instruct the patient to complete the medication regime prescribed. Teach the patient to dry the vaginal area as completely as possible after bathing and before dressing. Loose underwear that permits airflow decreases the incidence of recurrent candidiasis.

| Chlamydia

Chlamydia infection is a parasitic disease of the mucous membranes of the genital and urinary tracts.

Etiology: *Chlamydia trachomatis* (CT) is the causative organism. Transmission is by sexual contact.

Occurrence: CT is responsible for close to 4 million cases of genital and urinary tract infections in the United States per year.

Age: Adolescents and young women.

Ethnicity: CT is seen more often in black women than in Hispanic or white women.

Contributing Factors: Age under 21 years, new sexual partner, multiple partners, partner with multiple partners; 30%–50% of the time gonorrhea is present with CT.

Signs and Symptoms: Symptoms depend on area of infection; 75% of infected women have cervical infection; in 50% the urethra is infected, and in 33% the endometrium is infected. Infected women may be asymptomatic; they may have mucopurulent discharge, postcoital bleeding, and/or dyspareunia, lower abdominal discomfort, vaginal bleeding, and dysuria.

Diagnostic Tests
- Culture of the endocervix with a DNA probe
- Urine-based testing—urinary ligase chain reaction
- Presence of mucopurulent discharge
- Cervical ectropy and/or edema
- Friability of the cervix
- Uterine or adnexal tenderness

Differential Diagnosis: Gonorrhea, cystitis, PID.

Treatment: Doxycyline 100 mg bid for 7 days or azithromycin 1 g orally in a single dose. Treatment of partners prevents reinfection. Frequent coinfection with gonorrhea guides treatment of both diseases simultaneously. Sexual partners with exposure 60 days prior to diagnosis should be evaluated, tested, and treated.

Follow-up: Women do not need to be retested for chlamydial infection after finishing therapy unless symptoms persist or you suspect reinfection.

Sequelae: PID, ectopic pregnancy, and infertility.

Prevention/Prophylaxis: All sexually active teenage women and women 20–24 years of age should be routinely screened for CT.

Referral: Consultation is recommended for unresolved infection.

Education: Reinforce the importance of completing the medication regimen. Inform the patient that douching should be avoided in all women with CT because it increases the incidence of PID. Partners should be referred for treatment. Advise the woman to abstain from intercourse until she completes the therapy.

Gonorrhea

Gonorrhea is a sexually transmitted bacterial infection.

Etiology: *Neisseria gonorrhoeae,* a gram-negative diplococcus, is transmitted sexually by direct contact with infected mucosa to the cervix and endocervix, the urethra, the Bartholin's glands, the Skene's glands, the rectum, or the pharynx. The most common site of infection is the cervix.

Occurrence: 600,000 cases of gonorrhea are reported to the Centers for Disease Control (CDC) each year.

Age: The most common ages for women who develop gonorrhea are 15–29.

Ethnicity: Gonorrhea is diagnosed more often in black than in white women.

Contributing Factors: Multiple sexual partners.

Signs and Symptoms: The woman can be asymptomatic. She may present with vaginal discharge, dysuria, dysmenorrhea, pelvic pain, dyspareunia, menorrhagia, intermenstrual bleeding, fever, chills, or abdominal pain. Vaginal discharge may be apparent on examination. Adnexa may be tender on bimanual examination.

Diagnostic Tests: Culture with a DNA probe—one swab is used in the cervix for both CT and gonorrhea.

Differential Diagnosis: CT, BV, trichomoniasis, and candidiasis.

Treatment: Ceftriaxone 125 mg IM or ciprofloxacin 500 mg PO once, or ofloxacin 400 mg PO once *and* doxycycline 100 mg bid for 7 days. Ceftriaxone is recommended for pharyngeal gonorrhea. Doxycycline is recommended to eliminate CT that often occurs simultaneously with gonorrhea. All sexual partners within the last 30 days of diagnosis require evaluation and treatment.

Follow-up: Depends on the severity of the disease; follow-up can be within 24–72 hours. Culture should be repeated following completion of therapy.

Sequelae: PID, infertility, increased rate of ectopic pregnancy.

Prevention/Prophylaxis: Use of condoms.

Education: Stress the need for all women infected with gonorrhea to be tested for HIV and syphilis. Stress the importance of the patient's taking all of the medication. Inform the patient that all partners should be treated. Advise the patient to abstain from intercourse until therapy is completed.

Lymphogranuloma Venereum

Lymphogranuloma is a sexually transmitted disease characterized by localized lymphatic infection.

Etiology: Chlamydia endemic to tropical areas.

Occurrence: Unknown.

Age: Any sexually active female.

Ethnicity: Lymphogranuloma is a disease from tropical areas of the world.

Signs and Symptoms
- Lymphogranuloma has an incubation period of 5–7 days. The first sign of infection is a pustule or papule on the vaginal wall, vulva, or cervix that ulcerates and then heals spontaneously.
- A bubo, that is, a tender, firm, infected lymph node that resolves spontaneously, follows the pustule or papule.
- The third stage is fibrosis of the lymphatic tissue.

Diagnostic Tests: Serologic complement fixation test confirms the diagnosis.

Differential Diagnosis: Syphilis, Hodgkin's disease, lymphoma, cat scratch fever, and lymphadenitis.

Treatment: Doxycycline 100 mg bid for 21 days.

Follow-up: Follow-up is necessary at 1- and 2-week intervals until resolution of symptoms. A 6-month follow-up visit should be scheduled after successful treatment.

Sequelae: Scar formation, fistula formation, and suppuration of lymphatic vessels.

Prevention/Prophylaxis: Use of condoms. Avoid intercourse with partners who have open lesions.

Referral: Consultation with a physician for confirmation of diagnosis and treatment.

Education: Instruct the patient that she must complete the full course of medication. Inform the patient that her partner should have an examination. Stress importance of follow-up visits.

Pelvic Inflammatory Disease

Pelvic inflammatory disease (PID) is a spectrum of diseases that includes endometritis, salpingitis, oophoritis, tubo-ovarian abscess, and pelvic peritonitis.

Etiology: The two most common organisms causing PID are *Neisseria gonorrhoeae* and *Chlamydia trachomatis*. Other possible organisms causing infection are *Escherichia coli*, streptococci, *Haemophilus influenzae, Mycoplasma* and *Ureaplasma* species.

Occurrence: One million women per year in the United States are reported to have PID.

Age: Adolescents have the highest incidence of any age group for PID; 70% of all cases of PID are diagnosed in women under 25 years of age.

Ethnicity: Not significant.

Contributing Factors: PID is related to a sexually transmitted disease 60% of the time. Multiple sex partners, previous sexually transmitted disease, recent insertion of an intrauterine device (IUD), douching, and cigarette smoking are all contributing factors.

Signs and Symptoms: Symptoms range from almost completely asymptomatic to life-threatening. Symptoms include bilateral lower abdominal pain, bleeding, abnormal discharge, fever, nausea and vomiting, dysmenorrhea, and dyspareunia (Fig. 8–1).

Diagnostic Tests: Physical examination revealing adnexal tenderness, cervical motion tenderness, fever, and abnormal discharge. Complete blood count (CBC) reveals elevated erythrocyte levels. Culture for gonorrhea and CT organisms may be positive. Transvaginal ultrasound will show thickening of the tubes with or without free pelvic fluid or tubo-ovarian complex. Laparoscopy can confirm PID.

Differential Diagnosis: Ectopic pregnancy, appendicitis, bowel disease, endometriosis, ovarian torsion, and bleeding from a corpus luteum.

Treatment: No currently available data compare the efficacy of parenteral versus oral therapy. Parenteral therapy can be administered on an outpatient or inpatient basis. The decision to hospitalize is made by the providers. Hospitalization is recommended if the woman is pregnant, does not respond to therapy, is severely ill, has an tubo-ovarian abscess, or is HIV-positive. If medical management is on an outpatient basis, follow-up is essential.

Treatment of PID should be initiated in sexually active young women if the following are present: lower abdominal tenderness, adnexal tenderness, and cervical motion tenderness. Additional criteria that support a diagnosis of PID according to the CDC are temperature greater than 101°F, abnormal cervical or vaginal discharge, elevated erythrocyte sedimentation rate, elevated C-reactive protein level, and laboratory documentation of infection. Any of these symptoms require treatment for PID.

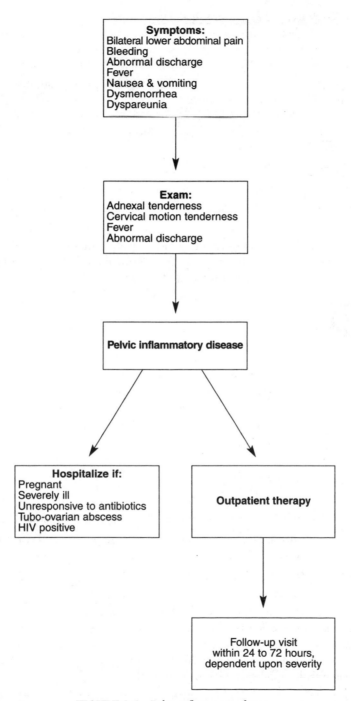

FIGURE 8–1 Pelvic inflammatory disease.

Medications used for therapy include a parenteral regime such as cefotetan 2 g IV every 12 hours or cefoxitin 2 g IV q 6 hr plus doxycycline 100 mg IV or orally q 12 hr. An oral regime such as ofloxacin 400 mg orally twice daily for 14 days plus metronidazole 500 mg orally twice daily for 14 days can be utilized.

Follow-up: The first follow-up visit is within 24–72 hours depending upon severity. Women who do not demonstrate improvement within 3 days after initiation of therapy usually require additional intervention. Sexual partner(s) exposed within 60 days of diagnosis should be treated simultaneously with the woman. Cultures should be repeated in 4–6 weeks.

Sequelae: Chronic pelvic pain, recurrent disease, ectopic pregnancy, and infertility.

Prevention/Prophylaxis: Screening cultures for at-risk populations, use of condoms.

Referral: A diagnosis of PID always requires a medical consultation.

Education: Stress the importance of partner(s) being examined and treated. Discuss the need for decreased activity and adequate diet and fluid intake during therapy. Emphasize the importance of completing medical therapy. Suggest that the patient use condoms. Recommend HIV testing.

Syphilis

Syphilis, a sexually transmitted disease that can affect any tissue, has a wide range of signs and symptoms ranging from none to neurologic impairment. Syphilis has periods of active disease and periods of latency.

Etiology: *Treponema pallidum,* a sexually transmitted spirochete.

Occurrence: 50,000 cases of syphilis are reported to the CDC per year, 2.9 per 100,000 women.

Age: The most common age group for this disease is 20–25 years.

Ethnicity: Syphilis is seen more commonly in Hispanics and blacks and inner-city residents. Rates have remained highest in the South and lowest in the West.

Contributing Factors: Gonorrhea infection, HIV infection, and drug abuse are contributing factors.

Signs and Symptoms: Syphilis occurs in stages.

- Primary syphilis. After contact, a chancre, a painless firm ulcer with raised edges, appears in 10–90 days and heals within 3–8 weeks.
- Secondary syphilis. Multiple skin lesions appear that last 3–12 weeks.
- Latent syphilis. Syphilis for more than 1 year or of unknown duration.
- Tertiary syphilis. Latent syphilis for many years; 20%–30% of untreated people with syphilis develop tertiary syphilis.

Diagnostic Tests: Rapid plasma reagin (RPR) or Venereal Disease Research Laboratories (VDRL) are the two screening tests for syphilis. These tests are 80%–90%

accurate in making a diagnosis. A positive RPR or VDRL result must be confirmed with a fluorescent treponemal antibody absorption test (FTA-ABS).

Differential Diagnosis: Herpes, condyloma, lymphogranuloma venereum, granuloma inguinale, and chancroid (*Haemophilus*-created ulceration).

Treatment: Primary and secondary syphilis are treated with penicillin 2.4 million units IM. Latent and tertiary syphilis are treated with three doses of penicillin 2.4 million units IM at 1-week intervals. All confirmed cases of syphilis must be reported to the health department for follow-up. Sexual partners exposed to the disease within 90 days of diagnosis should be treated.

Follow-up: Titers should be repeated and the woman should be re-examined at 1 month, 3 months, 6 months, and 12 months after diagnosis and treatment.

Sequelae: Cardiovascular syphilis, neurosyphilis, congenital syphilis (transplacental transmission occurs during the second and third trimesters).

Prevention/Prophylaxis: Use of condoms.

Referral: All cases of latent and tertiary syphilis require consultation with a physician. Pregnant women with syphilis require consultation. HIV-positive women with syphilis require consultation.

Education: Emphasize the need for treatment of partner(s). Explain the disease process to the woman. Stress the importance of follow-up visits. Recommend HIV testing.

Toxic Shock

Toxic shock is a syndrome in which bacterial growth, plus a toxin that acts as a superantigen, creates a serious systemic infection.

Etiology: Infection with a bacteriophage, a specific strain of *Staphylococcus aureus,* creates a toxin. The toxin plus enterotoxin B cause clinical symptoms.

Occurrence: Unknown.

Age: One of the variables predictive of toxic shock is advancing age. Host factors are important determinants for the development of the disease. Toxic shock can occur in both menstruating and nonmenstruating women.

Ethnicity: Not significant.

Contributing Factors: Menses, use of tampons, vaginal infections, vaginal delivery or cesarean birth, or spontaneous abortion.

Signs and Symptoms: Temperature $> 102°F$, erythematous rash, hypotension, vomiting, and myalgia.

Diagnostic Tests: Bacterial culture of the cervix and vagina, platelet count, blood urea nitrogen (BUN), and serum glutamic pyruvic transaminase (SGPT).

Differential Diagnosis: Shock from another origin.

Treatment: Hospitalization.

Follow-up: After hospitalization follow-up requires close monitoring for resolution of symptoms. Medication management is required.

Sequelae: Of menses-related cases of toxic shock syndrome, 30% have reoccurrence.

Prevention/Prophylaxis: Appropriate use of tampons.

Referral: All cases of toxic shock syndrome require medical consultation.

Education: Inform the patient that following diagnosis of toxic shock, she should discontinue the use of tampons.

| Trichomoniasis

Trichomoniasis is a vaginal infection caused by the organism *Trichomonas vaginalis*.

Etiology: *T. vaginalis,* a flagellated protozoan, acts in a parasitic relationship with the vaginal mucus. Transmission is by sexual contact.

Occurrence: Of all symptomatic vaginal infections, 15%–20% are related to *Trichomonas*. *Trichomonas* organisms may also be found in the urethra.

Age: After puberty and before menarche.

Ethnicity: Not significant.

Contributing Factors: Number of sexual partners.

Signs and Symptoms: Dysuria, yellow-green vaginal discharge, itching, dyspareunia, and vaginal and/or vulvar irritation (see Table 8–1).

Diagnostic Tests

- Presence of thin, yellow-green vaginal discharge
- pH between 5 and 7
- Vulvar irritation and edema
- Strawberry cervix—petechial hemorrhages on the cervix
- Motile trichomonads and leukocytes seen in saline wet mount (50%–60% sensitive)
- Vaginal or cervical culture (90% sensitive)
- Pap smear (60%–70% sensitive)

Differential Diagnosis: BV, gonorrhea, *Chlamydia* infection, herpes, condyloma, foreign body, and allergies.

Treatment

- Metronidazole 2 g stat (80%–88% effective).
- Metronidazole 500 mg bid for 7 days (95% effective).
- Partner(s) must be treated simultaneously (30%–70% of partners are also infected by trichomonads).

Follow-up: For unresolved infection.

Sequelae: Premature rupture of membranes and post-hysterectomy cellulitis have been associated with trichomoniasis.

Prevention/Prophylaxis: Use of condoms.

Referral: Consultation is required for unresolved infection.

Education: Instruct patient to complete the medication regimen. Inform the patient that all partners must be treated. Intercourse should be avoided until the woman and her partner(s) have been treated. Instruct the patient to avoid alcohol when taking metronidazole. Instruct the patient not to take metronidazole in the first trimester of pregnancy.

Benign Diseases of the Reproductive Tract

This section discusses the benign diseases of the reproductive tract: endometriosis, adenomyosis, and leiomyomas. A history of pelvic pain or abnormal vaginal bleeding may indicate these disorders. The pelvic exam may reveal uterine enlargement, pelvic mass, or tenderness. For more information about the history interview, see Chapter 4. See Chapter 5 for more information about performing a physical examination.

Endometriosis and Adenomyosis

Endometriosis is extrauterine growth of the endometrial glands or stroma.

Etiology: Believed to occur through retrograde menstruation or differentiation of "totipotential" cells, or both. Adenomyosis is endometriosis interna. The normal endometrial lining invades the myometrium.

Occurrence: Of women of reproductive age, 5%–15% have endometriosis. The most common sites for endometriosis are within the pelvis. Rarely does endometriosis occur outside of the pelvis.

Age: The most common age for the diagnosis of endometriosis is the late 20s. Adenomyosis occurs most commonly in women aged 40–50.

Ethnicity: Not significant.

Contributing Factors: Factors leading to endometriosis are unknown. The risk for endometriosis appears to be related to increased exposure to menstruation— shorter cycle length, increase in flow, and reduced parity. Contributing factors for adenomyosis include increased parity, previous cesarean birth, induced abortions, dysmenorrhea, abnormal uterine bleeding, and late menarche.

Signs and Symptoms: Common sites for implantation are ovaries, serosal surfaces of uterus, bladder, bowel, and rectovagina. An endometrioma is an ovarian cyst that has formed as a result of endometriosis.

Symptoms are related to the site of implantation. Symptoms may include dysmenorrhea, pelvic pain, infertility, dark vaginal "spotting" before menses, or referred back pain. Sites of implantation bleed during menses and create symptoms in two-thirds of the women with endometriosis. One-third of women with the disease have no symptoms. The degree of pain is not directly related to the level of involvement in this disease. A woman may have minimal endometriosis and extreme pain with menses, or she may have minimal pain but extensive disease.

In adenomyosis, during menses the lining grows and develops but cannot shed. This causes bleeding into the myometrium and thus pain occurs during menses. Adenomyosis can cause abnormal vaginal bleeding.

Diagnostic Tests

- Pelvic tenderness on examination.
- In adenomyosis, the uterus is enlarged, tender, and boggy.
- Ultrasound of the pelvis.
- Magnetic resonance imaging (MRI) of the pelvis.
- Laparoscopy is the gold standard for diagnosis of endometriosis.
- Adenomyosis is frequently diagnosed on a pathology report following hysterectomy.

Differential Diagnosis: PID, adhesions, pregnancy, fibroids, ovarian neoplasms, diverticulitis, and irritable bowel syndrome.

Treatment: Symptoms can be treated with nonsteroidal anti-inflammatory medications. Oral contraceptives on a continuous regimen can be utilized to suppress menstruation. Gonadotropin-releasing hormone (GnRH) agonists can be utilized to suppress menses. Surgical therapy to eliminate implantation sites can be utilized. Hysterectomy can be prescribed for adenomyosis.

Follow-up: Close follow-up for either medical or surgical therapy is indicated.

Sequelae: Infertility from direct tubal damage, immunologic factors, and increased prostaglandin levels.

Prevention/Prophylaxis: None.

Referral: Every woman with a possible diagnosis of endometriosis or adenomyosis requires consultation with a physician.

Education: Endometriosis is treated with a combination of therapies. Explanations of the disease process and various therapies are an important part of the treatment.

Leiomyomas (Fibroids)

Leiomyomas are benign tumors of the reproductive tract in women.

Etiology: Leiomyomas arise from the uterine musculature, grow slowly, and diminish rapidly at menopause.

Occurrence: Fibroids are a common condition of the female genital tract. They are usually found in the uterus but may appear in the vulva or vagina. One in five women will be diagnosed with a fibroid tumor.

Age: Fibroids are less common in adolescents than they are in adult women.

Ethnicity: One out of three women of African-American descent will be diagnosed with leiomyomas. When risk factors are controlled, there is a higher rate of fibroids in premenopausal black women. The average age at diagnosis for black women is 37.5 years. For white women, the average age is 41.6 years.

Contributing Factors: Age at first birth, history of infertility.

Signs and Symptoms: Menometorrhagia, lower abdominal pain, anemia, and constipation. Symptoms can increase in the perimenopausal period. Symptoms decrease with menopause.

Diagnostic Tests
- Pelvic examination.
- Ultrasound of the pelvis is used to differentiate leiomyomas from neoplasms.
- Endometrial biopsy and hysteroscopy can assist in diagnosis.
- MRI can confirm the diagnosis.

Differential Diagnosis: The vast majority of smooth muscle tumors are leiomyomas. The occurrence of leiomyosarcomas is very infrequent. Great care must be taken to differentiate between the two at the time of diagnosis.

Treatment: Medical treatment consists of progesterone and GnRH agonists. When medical treatment fails, surgical treatment—myomectomy or hysterectomy—is performed.

Follow-up: Fibroids are generally asymptomatic and do not require intervention. Careful monitoring for growth is recommended. Medical therapy requires follow-up for resolution of symptoms. Surgical therapy requires follow-up.

Sequelae: Fibroids require special management in cases of infertility, pregnancy, and menopause.

Prevention/Prophylaxis: None.

Referral: Diagnosis of fibroid requires consultation with a physician.

Education: Stress the benign nature of fibroid "tumors." Inform the patient that uterine myomas are frequent tumors that require treatment only if they are symptomatic. Explain about the possible therapies if appropriate.

Cancer of the Genital Tract

Assessment

Cancer is one of the leading causes of morbidity and mortality in women of any age. This section discusses cancers of the cervix, endometrium, ovaries, and vulva, with emphasis on diagnosis and referral. Refer to Table 8–2 for an overall comparison

TABLE 8–2   CANCER OF THE GENITAL TRACT

Type of Cancer	Most Common Type	Most Common Stage	Most Common Symptom	Screening
Vulvar	Squamous	I	Vulvar lesions; changes in pigmentation or thickness	Visualization by provider; vulvar self-examination
Vaginal	Squamous	Rare	None	Pap smear
Cervical	Squamous	I	Intermenstrual bleeding	Pap smear
Endometrial	Adenocarcinoma	I	Postmenopausal bleeding	None
Ovarian	Epithelial	III	Asymptomatic or pelvic pressure; bloating; dull pelvic pain	None

of malignancies of the genital tract and to Fig. 8–2 for evaluation of a pelvic mass found on examination. (Breast cancer is discussed in Chapter 7.)

Careful history taking can identify women at risk for carcinoma of the genital tract. Attention to risk factors guides screening for cancer. Pelvic exams and Pap smears performed at regular intervals help to ensure early detection of carcinoma. See Chapter 2 for further discussion of screening for cancer. Refer to Chapters 4 and 5 for a complete discussion of the history and physical examination.

Cervical Cancer

In virtually all cases, intraepithelial neoplastic changes precede invasive squamous cervical cancer. These changes have been called dysplasia, cervical intraepithelial neoplasia (CIN), squamous intraepithelial lesion (SIL), and carcinoma in situ. Cells in the cervical epithelium develop the capacity to divide repeatedly rather than mature in a controlled fashion.

Etiology: A specific agent likely to be responsible for cervical cancer is human papilloma virus (HPV), the cause of most venereal warts. HPV of genotypes 16 and 18 shows a significant presence in women with cervical cancer.

Occurrence: In the United States the annual incidence of invasive cervical cancer is 13,550, with an annual mortality of 6,000. For any American woman, the lifetime probability of developing cervical cancer is 0.7%. The incidence of carcinoma in situ is more than three times that of invasive disease.

Age: The overall incidence of cervical cancer for any age group is 4 per 100,000. Carcinoma in situ can occur in women aged 25–29. However, a peak in incidence occurs in women aged 30–45, with 6 per 1,000 women developing carcinoma in

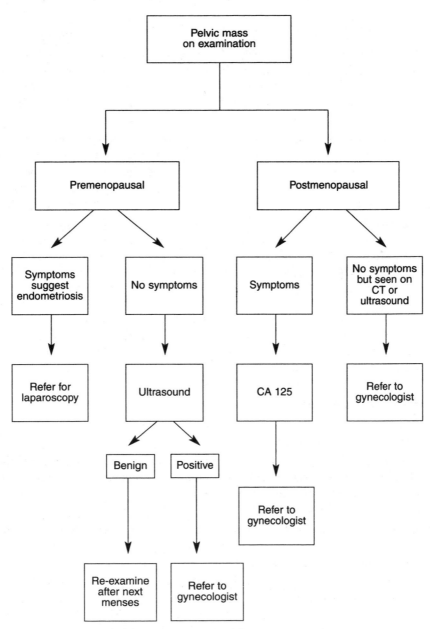

FIGURE 8–2 Pelvic mass.

situ. Another peak occurs in women older than 60, with 5 per 1,000 developing carcinoma in situ. Prevalence of invasive carcinoma is highest in older age groups, rising precipitously after age 50.

Ethnicity: Racial and ethnic disparities in the incidence of cervical cancer are reduced or eliminated when socioeconomic status is overlooked.

Contributing Factors: Onset of intercourse before age 20, multiple sex partners, sexual partner who has multiple partners, history of HPV or sexually transmitted disease, smoking, exposure to diethylstilbestrol (DES) in utero, lack of barrier contraception, immunosuppression, and lack of screening.

Signs and Symptoms: The classic symptom of cervical cancer is intermenstrual bleeding following intercourse or douching. This symptom occurs late in the course of the disease. The mean duration of a detectable asymptomatic period is approximately 10 years for carcinoma is situ and approximately 5 years for invasive carcinoma.

Diagnostic Tests: Early detection of this disease improves prognosis. The Pap smear is a screening device for cervical cancer. All women who are or have been sexually active or who have reached the age of 18 years should have an annual Pap smear and pelvic examination. After a woman has had three consecutive satisfactory normal evaluations, she may have Pap tests less frequently at the discretion of her health-care provider.

Women with any risk factors associated with cervical cancer should have annual Pap smears. Women who have been exposed to DES should have their first Pap smear at the onset of menstruation, a baseline colposcopy at first intercourse, and Pap smears every 6–12 months until age 30 and annually thereafter (see Table 5–2).

Differential Diagnosis: Cervical infection, dysfunctional uterine bleeding, and atrophy.

Treatment: Surgical excision.

Follow-up: Depends on treatment. If hysterectomy is performed, the woman should have a Pap smear every 3 months for 2 years, every 6 months for 3 years, and yearly thereafter.

Sequelae: The most important factor affecting prognosis is stage of the disease. Histologic type influences outcome. Lymph node metastasis reduces the 5-year cure rate.

Prevention/Prophylaxis: None.

Referral: All cases of cervical carcinoma require referral to a gynecologist for evaluation and treatment.

Education: The Pap smear is a simple, painless, and cost-effective tool that screens for cervical cancer. Since its inception, the number of deaths from cervical cancer has decreased. Women who adhere to the recommended screening intervals have a survival rate of 95% related to early detection. New technology has been introduced to reduce the Pap smear false-negative rate. Encourage all women to have regular Pap smear screening.

Endometrial Cancer

Cancer of the endometrium is the most common invasive pelvic malignancy of women in the United States.

Etiology: Adenocarcinoma of the endometrium of the uterus has a histologic precursor of atypical endometrial hyperplasia.

Occurrence: Endometrial cancer, which is three times more prevalent than cervical cancer, represents 10% of all cancers in women. There are approximately 40,000 new cases diagnosed each year in America and 4,000 deaths per year. The lifetime probability of developing endometrial cancer for all American women is 3%.

Age: Advancing age is the most important risk factor for endometrial cancer; 5% of tumors occur before age 40. Most tumors occur in the sixth and seventh decades of life.

Ethnicity: Not significant.

Contributing Factors: Obesity and glucose intolerance have been correlated with endometrial carcinoma. Strong evidence exists that estrogen, endogenous or exogenous, has a role in the development of endometrial cancer. There is a high incidence of this cancer in women with polycystic ovarian syndrome. An association exists between menstrual abnormalities and infertility and endometrial cancer. Of women with endometrial cancer, 20%–30% are nulliparous. The use of estrogen after menopause substantially increases the risk of endometrial cancer. A program of estrogen plus progesterone for postmenopausal therapy has not been associated with endometrial cancer. Low parity, late menopause, and hypertension have been associated with endometrial carcinoma.

Signs and Symptoms: Postmenopausal bleeding is by far the most common symptom associated with endometrial carcinoma.

Diagnostic Tests: There is no screening tool for endometrial carcinoma. Detection requires diligent attention to risk factors and history. Endometrial biopsy and pelvic ultrasound assist with diagnosis. Transvaginal ultrasound measures the endometrial thickness and suggests the need for endometrial biopsy. Dilation and curettage (D&C) hysteroscopy is required to verify a diagnosis of endometrial cancer.

Differential Diagnosis: Infection, atrophy.

Treatment: Surgical excision.

Follow-up: Operative and histologic findings assign the risk for recurrence. Radiation therapy is used for women with intermediate or high risk. Hormonal therapy and chemotherapy may be used for advanced disease.

Sequelae: Various factors influence the prognosis, including histologic differentiation, depth of invasion, and lymph node metastases. Histologic type also influences the outcome.

Prevention/Prophylaxis: None.

Referral: All cases of suspected endometrial cancer must be referred to a gynecologist for evaluation and treatment. Endometrial sampling should be discussed with a gynecologist for those women at risk for endometrial cancer.

Education: Explain the significance of postmenopausal bleeding to every woman at the time of menopause. Estrogen should not be taken without progesterone in the postmenopausal period.

| Ovarian Cancer

Cancer of the ovary is the most lethal of pelvic malignancies in women. Late diagnosis is the primary reason for the poor prognosis. Reliable screening for this disease had not yet been developed.

Etiology: Unknown.

Occurrence: Each year in the United States, more than 20,000 new cases of ovarian cancer are diagnosed and more than 12,000 women die of the disease. The lifetime probability of developing the disease is 1 in 70 for American women.

Age: The annual incidence in women aged 30–50 is 20 per 100,000. In women aged 50–75, the incidence is 40 per 100,000.

Contributing Factors: Increasing age and family history are the most important risk factors for ovarian cancer. Family history is present in 7% of women with the disease. A clustering of related cancers—ovarian, breast, endometrial, or colorectal—may suggest a hereditary form of the disease. In some families an autosomal dominant pattern of inheritance is thought to exist, making the risk for ovarian cancer higher. This dominant pattern is thought to occur in 1% of ovarian cancer victims.

    Use of the oral contraceptive pill reduces the risk of ovarian cancer by 35%–50%. Any pregnancy reduces the risk by 50%; increasing the number of pregnancies further reduces the risk. Tubal ligation and possibly hysterectomy appear to reduce the risk of ovarian cancer.

Signs and Symptoms: Ovarian cancer may be totally asymptomatic. The woman may experience pelvic pressure, bloating, dull pelvic pain, or bladder pressure. Ovarian cancer may be related to ovarian enlargement.

Diagnostic Tests: Annual pelvic examination is recommended past age 18 for all sexually active women. Rectovaginal examination may be necessary to detect ovarian enlargement. Ovarian enlargement cannot always be palpated, making pelvic examination a limited diagnostic test. Transvaginal ultrasonography with the use of color Doppler images improves the sensitivity for diagnosis of ovarian cancer. Laparoscopy is the gold standard tool for diagnosis of ovarian cancer. There is a great deal of interest in cancer antigen (CA) 125 as a diagnostic tool. Sensitivity of the test currently is between 9% and 96%. Specificity is higher in postmenopausal women and lower in women who have not yet experienced menopause. Many women screened for ovarian cancer with this testing methodology receive false positives. CA 125 level fluctuates with the menstrual cycle and is elevated in ovarian cysts, fibroid tumors, pregnancy, endometriosis, and PID.

Differential Diagnosis: Stool-filled sigmoid colon, distended bladder, pelvic kidney, diverticular abscess, cysts (dermoid, functional, cystadenoma), tubo-ovarian abscess.

Treatment: Surgical excision.

Follow-up: Frequently chemotherapy and radiation therapy follow surgery. Bone marrow transplants are recommended in selected cases.

Sequelae: On diagnosis, three out of four cases of ovarian carcinoma have spread beyond the ovary. Ovarian cancer is less common than breast cancer and other gynecologic malignancies but has the highest case-fatality rate.

Prevention/Prophylaxis: None.

Referral: Women with a significant family history of ovarian cancer should be referred for screening with CA 125 and ultrasound.

Education: Routine screening for women without family history of ovarian cancer is not currently recommended. Stress the importance of an annual pelvic examination for all women.

Vulvar Cancer

The most common premalignant condition of the vulva is vulvar intraepithelial neoplasia (VIN).

Etiology: VIN has been associated with HPV. The vulva can develop carcinoma with the potential to become invasive.

Occurrence: Vulvar cancer comprises 5% of all cancers of the genital tract.

Age: VIN is most commonly associated with women in the 20–30 age group. Squamous cell carcinoma occurs in women more than 45 years of age. Granular cell carcinoma occurs in women aged 30–40. Basal cell carcinoma occurs in women older than 70.

Ethnicity: Granular cell carcinoma occurs more often in African-American women.

Contributing Factors: VIN is associated with immunocompromised women, smoking, and HPV.

Signs and Symptoms: Changes in pigmentation, thickness, or symmetry of the vulva can indicate carcinoma. Mild whitening of the epithelium can be noted, but lesions that are tan or brown can also indicate cancer.

Diagnostic Tests: Colposcopy can reveal some of the features of carcinoma of the vulva. Any suspicious mass of the vulva should be biopsied.

Differential Diagnosis: Condyloma, infection.

Treatment: Surgical excision.

Follow-up: After surgery, vulvar cancer is followed every 3 months for the first year and every 6 months for the second year.

Sequelae: Depends on the extension of the excision.

Prevention/Prophylaxis: Treatment of HPV, avoiding cigarette smoke.

Referral: Any suspicious lesion on the vulva should be referred to a physician for biopsy.

Education: Encourage vulvar self-examination.

Other Reproductive Disorders

This section discusses secondary amenorrhea, abnormal breast discharge, infertility, pelvic relaxation, and abnormal vaginal bleeding. Careful history taking and physical examination guides assessment for these disorders. Refer to Chapters 4 and 5 for further discussion of taking a history and performing a physical examination.

Secondary Amenorrhea

Primary amenorrhea is defined as failure to menstruate at puberty. This will be discussed in Chapter 13. Secondary amenorrhea is defined as the cessation of menses after it has been established, that is, an interruption in normal menstruation.

Etiology: Reasons for lack of menses include pregnancy, menopause, insufficient body fat, use of hormones for contraceptive reasons, thyroid disease, pituitary tumor, polycystic ovarian syndrome, premature ovarian failure, and Asherman's syndrome.

Occurrence: The incidence of secondary amenorrhea is 3.3% in the population of menstruating American women.

Age: Secondary amenorrhea can occur in any woman after menses have been established during puberty.

Contributing Factors: Situational stress, dieting, concurrent illness, increased exercise, and drugs.

Signs and Symptoms: Cessation of menses for 3 or more months in a woman with formerly regular menses.

Diagnostic Tests: Menstrual history must be taken carefully. Information must be obtained on contraceptive history and medications. Physical examination must include weight and general appearance, including hirsutism and virilization (see Chapter 13), palpation of the thyroid, and breast examination (particularly for

---

CAUSES OF AMENORRHEA
- Hypothalmic dysfunction
  - Mild—related to stress, dieting, exercise, drugs
  - Severe—related to anorexia nervosa; concurrent illness; excess androgen; prolactin, or cortisol
- Pituitary disease
- Ovarian
  - Menopause
  - Premature ovarian failure
  - Polycystic ovarian syndrome
- Uterine
  - Asherman's syndrome
  - Cervical scarring
- Endocrine disease
  - Thyroid
  - Cushing's
- Pregnancy

---

evidence of discharge). Speculum examination should be performed, noting atrophy, and bimanual examination, noting enlarged uterus or adnexa. Lab data must include serum HCG, serum prolactin, and thyroid-stimulating hormone (TSH) levels and Pap smear.

After pregnancy has been ruled out, giving the patient a trial of progesterone is a common diagnostic test. The woman is given 10 mg of medroxyprogesterone (Provera) daily for 5 days. She will or will not have withdrawal bleeding after the completion of the progesterone trial (Fig. 8–3).

Differential Diagnosis: See etiology.

Treatment: Hormone replacement, bromocriptine, and surgery are possible treatments for secondary amenorrhea. Treatment depends on diagnosis.

Follow-up: Medical or surgical therapy requires close follow-up for evaluation of menstrual patterns.

Prevention/Prophylaxis: Avoidance of excessive dieting and exercise.

Sequelae: Secondary amenorrhea can be treated successfully in most cases by a gynecologist. Reproductive endocrinology consultation is required for serious disease.

Referral: Consultation with a reproductive endocrinologist is necessary for secondary amenorrhea related to hypothalamic, pituitary, or ovarian dysfunction, as well as for thyroid disorders.

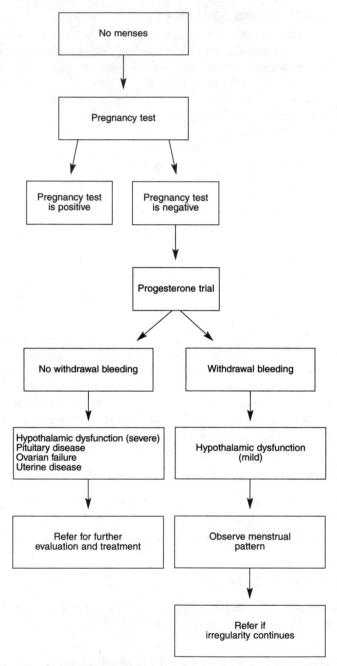

FIGURE 8–3   Secondary amenorrhea.

Education: Reassure any women with amenorrhea following the use of oral contraceptives about future fertility. If the desire for pregnancy is not immediate, advise the patient regarding methods of contraception because spontaneous ovulation can and does occur. Stress the importance of proper evaluation and treatment in women who require referral.

Abnormal Breast Discharge

The third most common symptom of breast disease is fluid emission from the mammary nipple. Discharge is symptomatic of disease in only 8%–10% of evaluated women.

Etiology: Pregnancy, stimulation of the breast, trauma to the chest, exercise, and stress can all cause breast discharge. Many medications cause breast discharge, including antipsychotic medications, oral contraceptives, and antiemetics. Tumors of the breast, pituitary, or hypothalamus can cause breast discharge. Infections cause discharge.

Occurrence: Of all women with breast symptoms, 5%–8% report discharge.

Age: Breast discharge can occur at any age.

Contributing Factors: Sexual activity, exercise programs, thyroid disease.

Signs and Symptoms: Breast discharge can be unilateral or bilateral, clear or cloudy, dark or light, or bloody. Watery and bloody discharge can be associated with carcinoma. The woman will report that she is not pregnant, not lactating, pain-free, and has not experienced trauma.

Diagnostic Tests: Pap smear of the breast discharge and microscopic inspection aid in diagnosis. Serum prolactin level should be measured to rule out pituitary tumor. Careful history of medication use, last menstrual period, sexual activity, birth control method, methods of exercise, and recent trauma or illness must be obtained. Physical examination of both breasts should be performed. Mammogram may be indicated.

Differential Diagnosis: Thyroid disease, drug-induced galactorrhea, pituitary tumor, intraductal papilloma, intraductal carcinoma, and galactocele.

Treatment: Bromocriptine, a medication that inhibits the secretion of prolactin, can be given. Pituitary tumors are surgically removed, as are intraductal papillomas and carcinomas. Galactocele can be aspirated.

Follow-up: Bromocriptine treatment requires a follow-up visit every 2–3 months. Surgical therapy is followed up at the discretion of the surgeon.

Prevention/Prophylaxis: None.

Sequelae: Resolution can be achieved for all benign reasons for breast discharge.

Referral: Consultation with a physician is required for breast discharge related to medication, tumor, or infection.

Education: Inform the patient that breast discharge in nonlactating women should be reported to a health-care provider for diagnosis and treatment.

| Infertility

The definition of infertility is unprotected sexual intercourse for 1 year without conception. The 1-year length is related to the rate of conception in fertile couples of 50% in 3 months, 75% in 9 months, and 90% in 1 year.

Etiology: The etiology of infertility is discussed in terms of male and female. Male factor relates to azoospermia or oligospermia. Etiology can be gonadal, gonadotropic, obstructive, or functional. Female infertility is emphasized in this chapter, including:

- Disorders of ovulation, accounting for 20%–40% of female factors. Hypothalamic dysfunction, polycystic ovarian syndrome, premature ovarian failure, hyperprolactinemia, androgen excess, Turner's syndrome, hypothyroidism, uncontrolled diabetes mellitus, and hypercortisolism can cause lack of ovulation.
- Tubal damage, accounting for 25%–40% of female factors. Tubal damage is caused by pelvic adhesions related to PID or endometriosis.
- Uterine pathology, accounting for 5% of female factors. Uterine pathology is caused by fibroids, endometriosis, septate uterus, duplication of cervix and uterus, exposure to DES, and intrauterine adhesions (Asherman's syndrome).
- Cervical abnormalities, accounting for 3%–5% of female factors. Cervical abnormalities are caused by cervical incompetence, cervical stenosis related to prior surgery on the cervix, or abnormalities of cervical mucus.
- Vaginal factors, such as an intact hymen, a vaginal septum, or vaginal infection.
- Luteal phase defect as defined by decreased progesterone secretion.
- Recurrent fetal loss (three or more spontaneous abortions) is classified as infertility.

Both partners can contribute to infertility. For example, infection with *Mycoplasma* in either or both partners can influence fertility. Some women produce an antisperm antibody that prevents conception.

Occurrence: In the United States, 10%–15% of couples are diagnosed as infertile.

- One-third of infertility is related to male factor.
- One-third of infertility is related to female factor.
- One-third of infertility is related to both male and female or cause is unknown.

Age: Childbearing age. Infertility increases with age, most significantly from the late 30s forward.

Contributing Factors: Aging, reduced frequency of intercourse, timing of intercourse, use of lubricants with spermicidal properties, douching, exposure to occupational hazards (chemicals, radiation), exposure to environmental hazards (heat, smoking, alcohol, drug abuse), excessive weight loss, psychologic stress.

Signs and Symptoms: Pregnancy does not occur after 1 year of unprotected regular intercourse.

Diagnostic Tests (Fig. 8–4)

- Male history and physical examination:
  - Semen analysis (Table 8–3)
- Female history with emphasis on menstrual and reproductive history:

History for woman with infertility
- Age
- Menstrual history (irregular menstrual bleeding, hypothermia, amenorrhea)
- Obstetric history
- Previous contraceptive methods
- Symptoms of ovulation
- Dysmenorrhea
- Dyspareunia
- Premenstrual spotting
- Frequency of intercourse
- Medical history (PID)
- Surgical history
- Family history
- Drug use
- Galactorrhea
- Hirsutism
- Heat and cold intolerance
- Medication history
- Alcohol or cigarette use

- Female physical examination with emphasis on thyroid gland, secondary sex characteristics, obesity, and hirsutism. Pelvic examination to rule out lack of mobility, pelvic masses, enlargement, thickening, or tenderness.
- Pap smear to rule out cervical cancer or infection.
- Pregnancy test.
- Ovulation prediction kit and basal body temperature chart to determine ovulation.

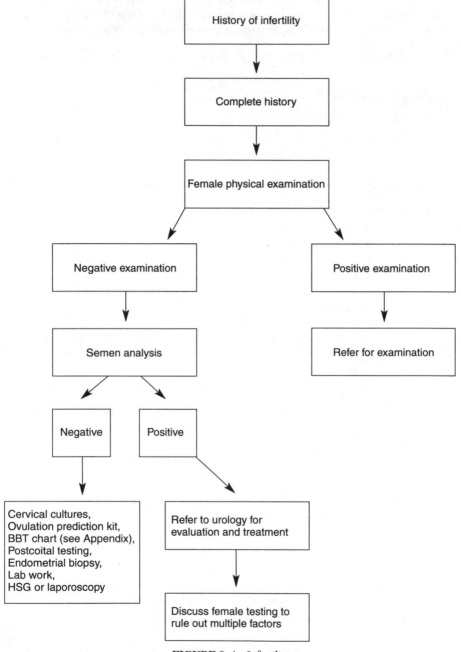

FIGURE 8–4   Infertility.

TABLE 8–3   NORMAL SEMEN ANALYSIS

Characteristic	Results
Volume	2–6 mL
Concentration	> 20 million/mL
Viscosity	Liquefaction in < 30 min
pH	7.2–7.8
Motility	> 50%
Morphology	> 50% normal
Leukocytes	< 1 million/mL

- Endometrial biopsy, performed late in the cycle following a pregnancy test, to verify ovulation and rule out luteal phase defect.
- Vaginal and cervical cultures for gonorrhea, *Chlamydia, Mycoplasma,* and *Ureaplasma* organisms.
- Urine culture.
- Serum prolactin; follicle-stimulating hormone (FSH); luteinizing hormone (LH); serum progesterone (days 21–23); TSH; and T_3, T_4, and T_7 levels.
- Postcoital test to assess cervical mucus for sperm, ferning, and spinnbarkeit at ovulation.
- Hysterosalpingogram, an injection of dye through the cervix, performed in radiology to rule out tubal obstruction or abnormalities of the uterine cavity.
- Hysteroscopy, an injection of dye through the cervix, performed in the operating room.
- Laparoscopic surgery to diagnose and treat adhesions, endometriosis, fibroids, or polycystic ovaries. The surgery is performed early in the cycle on an outpatient basis under general anesthesia. (Hysteroscopy and laparoscopy can be performed simultaneously.)

Differential Diagnosis: Anorexia nervosa, bulimia, and psychiatric disorders.

Treatment: Infertility can be treated medically or surgically. Ovulation can be induced medically. Tubal disorders and uterine pathology are usually treated surgically. Multiple therapies can be implemented. Both partners may require treatment.

Follow-up: Infertility evaluation and treatment are often lengthy and require commitment of time, energy, and finances.

Prevention/Prophylaxis: Prevention of PID would reduce the incidence of infertility.

Sequelae: Successful diagnosis and treatment of infertility result in pregnancy.

Referral: Of couples diagnosed with infertility, 44%–96% go on to conceive without treatment. The reason for infertility may resolve itself. Watchful waiting is in many cases a reasonable suggestion to couples. Referral, if indicated, should be to a reproductive endocrinologist.

Education: Counseling for infertility is necessary no matter what the cause. Resolution or adaptation must be facilitated. Infertile couples may choose to wait and watch, treat, adopt, employ a surrogate, or live without children. Couples who choose waiting should be educated about the timing of ovulation, the findings of their infertility "workup," and the prevention of sexually transmitted diseases.

Pelvic Relaxation

The pelvic floor is composed of the anterior, middle, and posterior compartments. When there is a disorder in one, there is often a disorder in another. Cystocele is the most frequent disorder of the anterior compartment. Uterine prolapse occurs in the middle compartment, whereas rectocele occurs in the posterior compartment.

Etiology: Most pelvic floor dysfunction relates to childbirth trauma and progresses with age. A small number of pelvic floor dysfunctions are congenital or hereditary.

Occurrence: Unknown.

Age: Over 35 years of age.

Contributing Factors: Childbirth, aging, and atrophy.

Signs and Symptoms: Mild prolapse will create minimal symptoms. Significant prolapse can produce a range of complaints.

- Uterine prolapse:
  - First degree—cervix descends nearly to the introitus.
  - Second degree—cervix descends and protrudes through the introitus.
  - Third degree—total prolapse with evagination of the cervix and uterus.

Uterine prolapse produces low back pain, "pressure," and "aching," premenstrually and during menses; dysmenorrhea; and dyspareunia.

- Cystocele—herniation of posterior bladder into the anterior vagina. The herniation can be minimal, moderate, or large. The primary symptom with cystocele is urinary incontinence.
- Rectocele—outpouching of the anterior rectal wall into the posterior vagina. This outpouching can be minimal, moderate, or large. The primary symptom is inability to evacuate without straining. Some women with rectocele must insert digital pressure onto the posterior vagina in order to evacuate.

Diagnostic Tests: History should include onset of symptoms, frequency of symptoms, conditions under which symptoms occur, and any attempted relief measures. Prolapse is diagnosed by physical examination.

Differential Diagnosis: Urinary tract infection, enterocele, and herniation of the peritoneum into the posterior cul-de-sac.

Treatment: Uterine prolapse can be treated with a pessary. If a pessary is fitted for the woman, she must be able to remove it, clean it, and replace it. Uterine prolapse can also be treated with vaginal hysterectomy. Cystocele and rectocele are treated with Kegel exercises. Both can also be treated with surgery.

Follow-up: Surgical therapy requires follow-up for monitoring of healing and resolution of symptoms. Nonsurgical therapy requires frequent follow-up for resolution of symptoms.

Sequelae: Stasis of the urine in a large cystocele can lead to chronic or recurrent cystitis.

Prevention/Prophylaxis: Kegel exercises to be performed on a daily basis after vaginal delivery.

Referral: Second- and third-degree uterine prolapses and cystocele and rectocele unresponsive to Kegel exercises should be referred to a physician for evaluation and treatment.

Education: Teach Kegel exercises to women with mild cystocele and/or rectocele. When a pessary is prescribed, demonstrate its use.

Abnormal Vaginal Bleeding

Normally in the absence of implantation of a fertilized egg, the ovarian corpus luteum undergoes regression in 9–11 days after ovulation. The normal menstrual cycle ranges from 23–39 days. The menstrual period lasts 2–7 days, with most of the bleeding occurring in the first few days. Normal ovulation may be accompanied by a small amount of midcycle "staining." At times, *mittelschmerz,* pain associated with ovarian follicle rupture and release, accompanies the staining.

Abnormal vaginal bleeding occurs at an inappropriate time or in an excessive amount.

Etiology: Possible causes include malignancy, disturbance in the hypothalamus-pituitary-ovary connection, fibroids, polyps, foreign bodies, pregnancy, and puberty.

- Uterine fibroids are a common cause of abnormal bleeding, representing about one-third of the presenting cases. Fibroids that are submucosal can lead to heavy bleeding. Location of fibroids, not necessarily the size, creates abnormal bleeding.
- Postcoital bleeding and intermenstrual spotting are characteristic of cervical carcinoma.
- Polyps can create intermenstrual spotting, seen especially after intercourse.
- Infection is a common cause of vaginal bleeding. Postcoital, intermenstrual, or heavy menstrual bleeding can be related to cervical or endometrial infection.
- Foreign bodies such as IUDs can cause endometrial irritation and resultant bleeding. Tampons can irritate the vaginal mucosa and create bleeding.
- Ectopic pregnancy can present as a delay in menses followed by spotting and pain. Delayed menses followed by vaginal bleeding and cramping characterize pregnancy loss.
- Oral contraceptives create "breakthrough bleeding," indicating that the balance of estrogen and progesterone is incorrect for this woman.

- Anovulatory cycles are seen in puberty and perimenopause and can create irregular vaginal bleeding.
- Postmenopausal bleeding can indicate endometrial carcinoma.
- Polycystic ovarian syndrome creates chronic anovulation and thus irregular vaginal bleeding (see Chapter 13).
- Hypothalamic dysfunction creates oligomenorrhea or amenorrhea (see Chapter 13).

Occurrence: Depends on etiology.

Age: Abnormal vaginal bleeding can occur in any menstruating female and in postmenopausal women.

Contributing Factors: Situational stress, weight loss, exercise training, iron deficiency anemia, chronic illness.

Signs and Symptoms: Variation from the woman's normal menstrual pattern. Menses occur at an inappropriate time or in an excessive amount.

Diagnostic Tests: History and physical examination are the cornerstones of diagnosis for abnormal vaginal bleeding (Fig. 8–5).

History: A careful and detailed menstrual history must be obtained. The woman's usual menstrual pattern must be identified. Method of contraception, symptoms of pregnancy, presence of premenstrual symptoms, intensity of the bleeding (measured in use of pads and tampons), duration of the bleeding, as well as time in the cycle of the bleeding must be elicited. Presence of vaginal discharge, bleeding related to intercourse, and presence of pain should be described. Recent emotional stress and/or weight loss should be determined. Medication use should be reviewed. In postmenopausal women, any history of bleeding, even minimal bleeding, can be evidence of malignancy.

Physical Examination: Speculum and bimanual examination should be performed, looking for discharge, erosion, polyps, tenderness, and signs of pregnancy. Examination of the postmenopausal woman should note friability of the vaginal mucosa and cervix.

Laboratory Testing: Pregnancy test, CBC, pelvic ultrasound, Pap smear, and cervical culture can be performed to assist in diagnosis. In perimenopausal bleeding, a measurement of FSH level can be confirmatory (a level of more than 40 suggests ovarian failure). Pelvic ultrasound and D&C hysteroscopy are diagnostic for endometrial carcinoma in the postmenopausal woman.

Differential Diagnosis: See Fig. 8–5.

Treatment: The diagnosis determines whether a surgical or medical approach is more appropriate.

Follow-up: Organic pelvic pathology, hormone-related dysfunction, systemic problems, endocrine causes, and disorders of pregnancy all require close follow-up after diagnosis.

Sequelae: Monthly menses should occur after medical therapy.

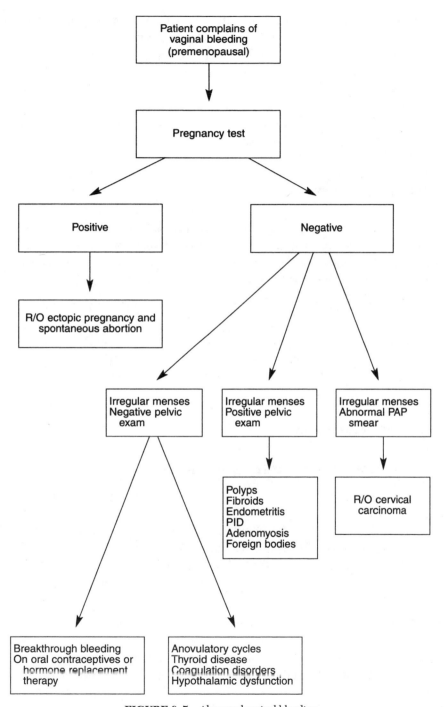

FIGURE 8–5 Abnormal vaginal bleeding.

Prevention/Prophylaxis: Abnormal uterine bleeding is a frequent complaint. Making an accurate diagnosis and ruling out serious causes are essential.

Referral: Consultation with a physician for evaluation and treatment is essential. Prompt referral is necessary in cases of heavy vaginal bleeding or possible ectopic pregnancy.

Education: Inform the patient that abnormal menstrual bleeding can affect a woman at any age. A health-care provider should investigate stress to the patient that causes irregular or heavy vaginal bleeding.

Contraception

No ideal contraceptive exists, since no method is completely safe, effective, inexpensive, acceptable, and available. Choosing a contraceptive is an important decision. The method must be effective, able to prevent unwanted pregnancy, relatively safe for the women, and fit the couple's lifestyle so that it is used correctly and consistently (Table 8–4).

The couple should choose the method together, weighing all the considerations. Knowledge about all of the methods helps in decision making. Many couples change methods of contraception throughout their relationship. Complete explanation of only one method does not permit changing methods. The following discussion of contraception methods generally goes from the simplest to the most complex.

Barrier Methods

Contraceptive Spermicides and Condoms

The use of a condom and spermicide is a barrier method to preventing pregnancy. Condoms are thin sheaths, most commonly made of latex, that prevent the transmission of sperm from the penis to the vagina. Condoms can vary in texture and color. They are available lubricated or nonlubricated and can have spermicide within them. Spermicides contain nonoxynol in various bases such as cream, jelly, foam, or suppositories.

The Food and Drug Administration (FDA) has approved a female condom. The female condom is a polyurethane pouch with a ring that, when inserted like a diaphragm, covers the cervix, and another ring that fits over the labia. The condom can be inserted several minutes or several hours prior to intercourse.

Effectiveness: Approximately 70%–94%, with effectiveness greatly influenced by the users. The use of spermicide with condoms, provided that both methods are used correctly, has an effectiveness rate in the high 90% range. Latex condoms can be considered effective protection against HIV infection.

TABLE 8–4 CONTRACEPTION

Method	Desired Characteristic	Dangers	Side Effects	Benefits (non-contraceptive)
Oral contraceptives	High efficiency	Cardiovascular complications	Nausea, bleeding, headaches, breast tenderness	Protective against some cancers and ovarian cysts; decreased menstrual loss and dysmenorrhea
IUDs	High efficiency	PID, anemia	Increased vaginal bleeding	None
Implants	High efficiency	Infection at site	Menstrual changes	Lactation not disturbed; decreased menstrual loss and dysmenorrhea
Injections	High efficiency	None	Menstrual changes, weight gain	Lactation not disturbed
Sterilization	High efficiency	Infection, anesthesia risk	Subsequent regret	None
Condoms	Limited or no side effects	None	Decreased sensation, allergy	Protects against STDs
Diaphragms	Limited or no side effects	Toxic shock syndrome	Pelvic pressure	Protects somewhat against STDs

Method of Action: Condoms, whether male or female, prevent semen from entering the vagina. Spermicide serves as a backup.

Risks and Benefits

- Some women are allergic to latex and therefore cannot use this method.
- Some women are allergic or sensitive to spermicide.
- The use of condoms necessitates interruption of the love-making process.
- Condoms may decrease tactile sensation.
- Condoms and spermicides decrease the risk for sexually transmitted diseases.
- Neither condoms nor spermicide require a prescription or fitting from a provider.
- The retail cost is low; condoms may be purchased at family planning programs at very low cost.

Contraindications: Allergy to spermicide or latex. (Condoms can be purchased that are not made of latex. However, these condoms do not prevent sexually transmitted diseases or HIV.)

Assessment: None required.

Instructions for Use
- Instructions for use of the spermicide depend on the base in which it is contained. Manufacturer's instructions should be followed.
- The condom must be applied to an erect penis prior to intercourse. About an inch of the condom should not be applied to the penis to act as a reservoir for ejaculatory fluid and to prevent breakage. The open end of the condom should be held tightly during withdrawal to prevent spilling the ejaculatory fluid.
- If the condom has torn or slipped off, immediately insert contraceptive foam or gel into the vagina. Postcoital contraception can be used (two combined estrogen and progesterone pills [50 μg] as soon as possible, and two more 12 hours later).
- Store condoms in a cold, dry, and dark place. Condoms can be stored in a wallet for up to 1 month.
- Condoms should only be used once.
- Oil-based preparations such as mineral oil, baby oil, etc., should not be used with condoms. They damage the latex (see Handouts).

Follow-up: None is required or recommended unless the woman has expressed difficulty with use of this method.

Referral: None.

Cervical Cap

The cervical cap is a barrier method of contraception in which a latex dome fits over the cervix. The cap comes in various sizes.

Effectiveness: The cervical cap, when used consistently, is very effective in preventing pregnancy. It is as effective as a diaphragm and in some users more effective.

Method of Action: The rubber dome fits tightly over the cervix and prevents the entry of sperm into the os.

Risks and Benefits
- Can be used with or without spermicide.
- Can be left in place for several days (last intercourse more than 6 to 8 hours before removal). Cervical caps are comfortable and create less chance of bladder infection.
- Not all women can be fitted with a cap.
- Not all women can be taught to insert and remove the cap.
- There is a lack of practitioners trained to fit cervical caps.
- Cervical caps are imported from England and are issued in sizes 22, 25, 28, and 31.

Contraindications: Abnormal Pap smear, cap cannot be fitted, abnormal appearance of the cervix.

Assessment

- The cervical cap should be fitted when the woman does not have menses.
- The woman must have a history of normal Pap smears, with the most recent Pap smear done on the date of cap fitting according to the FDA.
- A history of toxic shock should be ruled out prior to fitting.
- Previous cervical surgery may interfere with fitting.
- Caps should not be fitted until 6 weeks after vaginal delivery.
- Pelvic examination should include observations for cervical abnormalities and infection.
- The size, shape, position, and length of the cervix should be observed.
- The presence of uterine prolapse, cystocele, or rectocele should be noted on bimanual examination. The presence of pelvic relaxation may interfere with fitting.

Instructions for Use

1. During fitting, place the appropriate cap on the woman's cervix.
2. Evaluate the suction of the cap.
3. Re-evaluate the suction after at least 5 minutes.
4. Assess the coverage of the cap over the cervix.

The woman must practice inserting and removing the cap until she is confident in her ability to do so without the provider. See instructions for cervical cap fitting in the Handouts.

Follow-up: A visit for questions and comments after the cap has been used is encouraged.

Referral: Abnormal pelvic exam or Pap smear requires referral.

Diaphragm

The diaphragm is a barrier contraceptive device made of rubber that, when placed in the vagina, prevents pregnancy by covering the cervix. Diaphragms are made with various types of springs within a flexible rim and are available in various sizes and styles.

Effectiveness: Greatly affected by the woman's ability to use the diaphragm correctly, but the range is 80%–95%.

Method of Action: A diaphragm is held in place by the symphysis pubis and the posterior vaginal fornix. The diaphragm is used with spermicidal cream or jelly. The diaphragm covers the cervix and prevents sperm from entering the os. The spermicide acts as a back up for any penetration of sperm beyond the barrier.

Risks and Benefits

- Barrier methods have minimal side effects.
- Some women cannot be fitted well with a diaphragm and some cannot be taught to correctly insert and remove the diaphragm.

- Diaphragms are associated with an increased incidence of bladder infection because of the pressure of the rim against the urethra.
- Toxic shock syndrome has been reported in women using the diaphragm during menses.
- Women can be sensitive or allergic to spermicide used with a diaphragm.
- A diaphragm is used until signs of wear indicate a need for replacement, the woman gains or loses 20 lb, or delivers a child vaginally.
- Diaphragms are an economical means of birth control. After the initial investment in the diaphragm and the fitting, maintenance involves the purchase of spermicide.

Contraindications: Some women cannot be properly fitted with a diaphragm. Some women are uncomfortable with the idea of insertion and removal of a diaphragm.

Assessment: A diaphragm should fit snugly between the posterior fornix, the pubic symphysis, and the lateral vaginal walls. It should not create pressure or discomfort. The woman should be able to demonstrate proper insertion and removal. A diaphragm must be fitted with the assistance of a health-care provider. A diaphragm should be fitted after confirmation of a normal pelvic examination and Pap smear.

Instructions for Use

1. Insert prior to intercourse and remove no sooner than 6–8 hours after intercourse.
2. The diaphragm should be used with a spermicide designed for use with a diaphragm.
3. The diaphragm should be resized if significant weight loss or gain—more than 20 lb—or vaginal delivery occurs.
4. The diaphragm should be cleaned with soap and water, dried, and kept in a designated container between uses.
5. A new application of spermicide should be used prior to repeated intercourse.
6. The diaphragm should *not* be left in place more than 24 hours.

See instructions for using a diaphram in the Handouts.

Follow-up: A follow-up visit after the woman has used the diaphragm is advised for questions or concerns.

Referral: Abnormal pelvic examination or Pap smear would require referral.

Intrauterine Devices

An intrauterine device (IUD) is a foreign body placed in the uterus to prevent pregnancy by causing a change in the cellular makeup of the endometrium.

Effectiveness: Rate of failure is 0.5%–2.9%.

Method of Action: Exactly how an IUD prevents pregnancy is unknown. Hormonal surveillance for early pregnancy loss has not supported the hypothesis that IUDs act as abortifacients. A scarcity of viable sperm in the fallopian tubes has been noted in IUD users. One of the current IUDs available releases progesterone at a rate of 65 μg per day. The device is designed from a vinyl acetate copolymer with barium sulfate that makes it radiopaque. The progesterone-releasing IUD has a first-year failure rate of 2.9% and must be replaced annually because of depletion of the hormone reserve.

The most recently developed copper IUD is the Paraguard Cu 380A, the only available copper IUD. This device, with a first-year failure rate of 0.5%, has been approved by the FDA for 10 years of use. Other types of IUDs are being investigated.

Risks and Benefits
- Ease of compliance.
- Increased incidence of PID in users of IUDs.
- Uterine perforation at the time of the insertion.
- Increased incidence of second-trimester abortion in women conceiving with an IUD in place.
- Risk of premature delivery, low-birth-weight babies, and stillbirth increases when an IUD is not removed during the first trimester of pregnancy.
- Iron supplementation may be required for women who experience heavy menses.
- The risk of expulsion is 1.2%–7.1%. Most expulsions occur within the first three menstrual cycles.
- Increase in dysmenorrhea associated with the use of an IUD.
- Less expensive per year than hormonal methods.

Absolute Contraindications
- Acute pelvic infection
- Known or suspected pregnancy
- Malignant disease of the cervix or uterus
- Undiagnosed vaginal bleeding

Relative Contraindications
- Multiple sex partners
- History of PID
- History of ectopic pregnancy
- Abnormal uterine bleeding
- Abnormal Pap smear
- Impaired response to infection
- Impaired coagulation response
- Emergency treatment not readily available
- Heart disease (susceptible to bacterial endocarditis)
- Endometriosis

- Fibroids or bicornate uterus
- History of dysmenorrhea or menorrhagia
- Allergy to copper
- Anemia

Assessment
- An IUD should be inserted during menses.
- Complete physical exam is necessary prior to insertion.
- Negative Pap smear is required.
- Negative cervical cultures of gonococcus and CT are required.
- Hemoglobin and hematocrit levels must be within normal range.
- The woman must be at least 6 weeks postpartum.

Instructions for Use: Insertion technique:

1. Bimanual exam is performed to determine position and size of uterus.
2. The vagina and cervix are cleansed with a povidone-iodine (Betadine) solution.
3. The uterus is sounded (must be 6 cm or more).
4. The IUD is inserted per manufacturer's instructions.
5. After insertion, the woman is observed for hypotension and syncope.
6. If the woman has mild cramping, any prostaglandin inhibitor in a dosage from 400–800 mg can be prescribed.
7. The woman is instructed not to have intercourse or use tampons for 7 days after insertion.
8. The woman must learn to feel the string that protrudes into the vagina. She must check for placement of the string frequently in the first few months of use and thereafter, after each menses (see Appendix and Handouts).

Warning Signs: Contact the nurse practitioner if any of the following occur:

P = period late
A = abdominal pain or pain with intercourse
I = infection exposure or abnormal discharge
N = not feeling well, particularly fever and chills
S = string missing

Follow-up: A follow-up appointment is made for 6 weeks after one menstrual cycle to rule out complications and to verify placement of the IUD.

Complications
- During insertion, a severe vasovagal response can occur. A physician must be immediately available. Blood pressure and pulse must be monitored after insertion until the woman is stable. Oxygen can be given as needed. Use of atropine as per physician protocols.
- Excessive bleeding or cramping may indicate perforation. Physician consultation is required for management.
- Missed menses requires elimination of pregnancy as a cause. The IUD must be removed when pregnancy is diagnosed.

- Breakthrough bleeding can occur. The IUD is removed only if hematocrit is less than 30 and/or the IUD is partially expelled, or the woman desires its removal.
- Cramping and pelvic pain can occur. If the IUD is partially expelled, it must be removed.
- PID must be ruled out as a reason for cramping and bleeding. If the woman is infected, she must be treated, cultured, and the IUD removed. The IUD is not to be reinserted for at least 3 months after treatment of infection.
- Spontaneous abortion must be ruled out when cramping and pelvic pain occur.
- Expulsion of the IUD has occurred if it is seen in the cervical os or vagina; if the string is lengthened, indicating partial expulsion; or the string is absent. If the IUD is partially expelled, it can be removed and replaced if the woman desires. Lost IUDs or no visualization of the device or the string requires physician consultation. If the IUD cannot be visualized at all, a physician consultation is required before an IUD can be reinserted.

Referral: Physician availability during insertion is required. Physician consultation for IUD complications is recommended.

Oral Contraception

Oral contraceptives (OCs) combine synthetic estrogen and progesterone to be taken orally to prevent conception. The tablets are consumed daily for 21 days, after which there is withdrawal menstrual bleeding. Women can choose to take an inert pill for the 7 days that the combination of estrogen and progesterone is not taken. There are a few progesterone-only contraceptive pills available.

Effectiveness: If taken as directed, oral contraceptives are almost 100% effective. If taken correctly, only 1 in 1000 women become pregnant.

Method of Action: Suppression of ovulation is the major method of action. Additional factors include altering the endometrium to make it unreceptive to implantation and altering cervical mucus to make penetration by sperm more difficult.

Benefits and Risks: There are numerous research-based noncontraceptive benefits of OCs.

- OCs protect against both ovarian and endometrial cancer. A protective effect (40% reduction) has been observed with as little as 3–6 months of use. Further declines in risk are accompanied by longer periods of use. The protective effect can last up to 15 years after consuming the last pill.
- OCs have a protective effect against benign breast disease, salpingitis, ectopic pregnancy, dysmenorrhea, and iron deficiency anemia.
- Fewer menstrual disorders, for example, menorrhagia, irregular menstrual

bleeding, or intermenstrual bleeding, occur in OC users. OCs also improve primary dysmenorrhea.

- When compared to those who never use OCs, there is no overall increase in risk of developing breast cancer for OC users up to age 55.
- OCs can decrease acne by lowering serum testosterone levels.
- OC use confers little or no risk of cardiovascular disease, particularly among women who are nonsmokers.
- A growing body of evidence suggests that the benefits of OCs for healthy, nonsmoking women over 40 may outweigh the risks. The American College of Obstetricians and Gynecologists states that OCs, particularly low-dose OCs, are safe for nonsmoking women over 35.
- The cost of OCs varies greatly by manufacturer and distributor. The high cost of OCs in many pharmacies may prompt some women to discontinue the method.
- Depression (sometimes severe) and other mood changes may occur in women on OCs.

Contraindications: Personal history—not a family history—of:
- Thrombus or embolus
- Cerebrovascular accident
- Coronary artery disease
- Known or suspected carcinoma of the breast, uterus, cervix, or ovaries
- Disease of the liver (normal liver function studies for at least 1 year after disease process, prior to use of OCs)
- Pregnancy

Relative Contraindications
- Migraine headaches
- Hypertension
- Mononucleosis
- Undiagnosed vaginal bleeding
- Elective surgery planned within first OC cycle
- Major injury to lower extremities
- 40 years of age or older coupled with another risk factor
- 35 years of age coupled with heavy smoking
- Diabetes
- Gallbladder disease
- Sickle cell disease
- Delivery within the past 10–14 days
- Cardiac or renal disease
- Lactation
- Smoking
- Elevated cholesterol

Assessment: Complete physical exam and Pap smear within 1 year of the prescription. In 1993, the FDA voted in favor of giving women an option to delay pelvic examination without being denied a prescription for OCs. Pelvic examination may be performed at follow-up examination.

1. Complete personal and family medical history.
2. Laboratory profile should include a lipid screen in women who have an immediate family member with hypertension under age 40 on medication, or with a family history of vascular disease or myocardial infarction (MI).
3. Fasting blood sugar should be considered if a family member is diabetic.
4. Liver profile should be considered if the woman has a history of hepatitis or other liver disease or she has a history of drug or alcohol abuse.

Instructions for Use
1. Begin oral contraceptives at onset of menses. One tablet is taken daily for 21 days at approximately the same time of day. Following the 21 days, no tablets or one inert tablet daily is consumed for 7 days. OCs are resumed on a daily basis after the 7 days of rest or inert tablets.
2. A backup method should be utilized if the woman runs out of pills, forgets to take a pill, discontinues the pill, and/or desires protection from sexually transmitted diseases.
3. There is a high rate of discontinuation of OCs. No more than 50%–75% of women who start using OCs are still using them after 1 year. Many women become pregnant after discontinuing OCs. Women who discontinue usually do so for nonmedical reasons. For this reason, teaching a second method of birth control at the time of teaching about OCs is recommended.
4. If one pill is missed, take the tablet as soon as remembered. If two or three pills are missed, a backup method must be employed.
5. If the woman smokes, she should stop smoking.

Early Warning Signs: Contact the NP if any of these occur:

A = abdominal pain—severe
C = chest pain
H = headache (severe)
E = eye problems
S = severe leg pain

Follow-up: After two or three cycles of OCs, blood pressure and weight should be taken and side effects and symptoms reviewed with the patient. Menstrual history on OCs should be reviewed.

Complications
- Amenorrhea can occur with the use of OCs. If this occurs, pregnancy should be ruled out. When pregnancy is ruled out, reassurance can be provided or a change of OCs considered.
- Breakthrough bleeding on the first or second package of OCs is a common occurrence. If the bleeding persists longer than the first or second package or the breakthrough bleeding is significant in amount and frequency, a change in OCs is indicated. Breakthrough bleeding should be diagnosed after infection and pregnancy have been ruled out.

Referral: Physician consultation is required for the following:
- Change in vision
- Numbness
- Chest pain
- Possible phlebitis
- Severe recurrent headaches or new headaches
- Increase in blood pressure with a diastolic pressure of more than 90 mm Hg
- Severe fluid retention
- Depression
- Scheduled surgery
- Development of any of the contraindications to taking the OC

Trends: Today, the most widely used preparations are low-dose pills containing 35 μg of estrogen or less combined with lower doses of progestins. The FDA recommends that women use pills containing the lowest effective amount of estrogen. Most recent clinical trials of 20 μg of estrogen OCs show a pregnancy rate that is no different than with 35-μg pills. This is because of the synergistic effect of estrogen with progesterone. Using 20-μg pills requires diligence in taking OCs at the same time each day. Benefits of 20-μg pills and incidence and management of side effects are under investigation.

Myths
- Weight gain. Studies show that as many young women lose weight as gain weight on OCs.
- Taking a rest. There is no evidence to support the idea that women need a "rest" from OCs. "Taking a break" may lead to unwanted pregnancy and an increase in side effects.
- Infertility. There is no evidence that OCs cause permanent infertility. There may be a temporary delay in conception after the use of oral contraceptives.

Drug Interaction: Drugs that may reduce OC efficacy are antituberculosis medications, antifungals, anticonvulsants, and antibiotics. Drugs whose activities may be modified by OC use include analgesics, anticoagulants, antidepressants, tranquilizers, anti-inflammatories, bronchodilators, antihypertensives, and antibiotics. If a woman is on any of these medications concurrently with OCs, consultation is suggested.

Injectable Contraception

Depo-medroxyprogesterone (DMPA) is progesterone that prevents ovulation by suppressing FSH and LH levels and eliminating the LH surge. This drug must be injected every 3 months IM. Women in whom estrogen is contraindicated can use DMPA, approved for contraception by the FDA in 1992.

Effectiveness: Failure rate is 0.3% This method of contraception requires compliance once every 13 weeks.

Method of Action: DMPA, a long-acting injectable progesteronal contraceptive, is delivered in microcrystals suspended in an aqueous solution that slowly dissolves and releases the drug into the body. Contraceptive levels of progesterone are maintained for up to 4 months following injection. In women using DMPA, circulating levels of progestogen block the LH surge; thus, the method works by suppressing ovulation. Secondary mechanisms of action include thickening the cervical mucus and altering the endometrium.

Benefits and Risks
- No overall relative risk for breast cancer among users of DMPA.
- Lack of estrogen risks and side effects.
- Requires an office visit for injection every 3 months.
- Cost of DMPA equals that of oral contraceptives.
- No demonstrated drug interaction between DMPA and antibiotics.
- No adverse effect on lactation.
- Can be started 1–4 days postpartum
- Menstrual cycle disturbance occurs with any progesterone-only method of contraception.

Contraindications
- Known or suspected pregnancy
- Unexplained vaginal bleeding

Relative contraindications
- Pregnancy planned in the near future
- Concern over weight gain
- Concern over irregular menstrual flow

Assessment
- Pap and pelvic examination should be completed prior to injection of DMPA.
- Pregnancy must be ruled out prior to administration.
- DMPA can be administered after delivery.

Instructions for Use: A 150-mg dose is administered IM every 13 weeks. The first dose is given during the first 5 days of a menstrual cycle.

Warning Signs: Contact the NP if any of the following occur:

Weight gain
Headaches
Heavy bleeding
Depression

Follow-up: Every 3 months for injection and evaluation of side effects.

Complications
- Amenorrhea occurs in 30%–50% of women using this medication within the first year and up to 80% of users by the fifth year of use.
- Weight gain, depression, breast tenderness, and menstrual irregularity can

occur using DMPA. These symptoms may persist for 6–8 months after discontinuing the medication.

- Delay in return to fertility can occur for 6 months to 1 year after discontinuing the drug.
- Almost all women using DMPA will experience spotting or irregular or prolonged bleeding, particularly during the first few months of use.

Referral: Management strategies for irregular bleeding can vary from simple reassurance to the use of estrogen. One or two cycles of OCs or a nonsteroidal anti-inflammatory drug other than aspirin can help stabilize the endometrium and stop the bleeding. Ibuprofen 800 mg three times daily for 5 days has been demonstrated to help reduce bleeding in some women. Anaphylactic reactions to DMPA are rare but have occurred immediately following injection. Emergency support measures such as epinephrine, steroids, and diphenhydramine should be available.

Subdermal Implants

A subdermal implant is progesterone (levonorgestrel) contained within non-biodegradable silicone rubber capsules, designed to be placed under the skin of the arm, that release a progestin at a constant rate over 5 years.

Effectiveness: 99% effective for 5 years.

Method of Action: The six capsules that make up the system release progestin on an average of 30 µg daily into the bloodstream. The progesterone suppresses ovulation, thickens the cervical mucus, and alters endometrial proliferation.

Risks and Benefits
- Menstrual irregularities, including prolonged bleeding, spotting, and amenorrhea, can occur. These changes in menses are seen predominantly in the first year of use.
- Weight gain or loss, nausea, and depression have been reported.
- Infection at the implant site is uncommon, as is expulsion of the capsules.
- Fertility promptly returns to preinsertion levels once implants are removed.
- Women users must desire long-term contraception.
- A health-care provider must insert and remove the capsules.
- Initial economic investment is high. The cost over a 5-year period equals other hormonal contraceptives; 76%–90% of women continue to use the method after the first year; 33%–78% complete the 5 years.
- Subdermal implants are immediately reversible.
- Subdermal implants do not affect lactation.

Contraindications
- Thromboembolic disease
- Acute liver disease
- Breast cancer
- Undiagnosed vaginal bleeding
- Pregnancy
- Cardiovascular disease

- Diabetes
- Heavy smoking

Assessment
- History to rule out contraindications
- Physical examination including Pap smear
- Review of risks and benefits
- Explanation of insertion and removal techniques

Instructions for Use: Clinical instruction is required for insertion of subdermal implants). The implants are inserted in the upper arm about 8–10 cm above the elbow (see Appendix and Handouts).

1. An insertion graph is used to guide cleansing with antiseptic solution.
2. The area is anesthetized.
3. Small incisions are made with a scalpel.
4. A trocar is inserted at a shallow angle.
5. The obturator is removed and loaded with a capsule.
6. After all capsules are loaded, the incisions are closed with Steri-Strips.
7. The insertion site is covered with dry compresses and gauze is wrapped around the arm.

The insertion site should be kept dry for 3–5 days. Implants become effective within 24 hours of insertion. Implants do not protect against STDs. Implants must be replaced every 5 years.

Warning Signs: Contact the NP if any of these occur:
- Severe lower abdominal pain
- Heavy vaginal bleeding
- Arm pain
- Pus or bleeding at the insertion site
- Delayed menstrual periods after an interval of regular menses
- Migraine headache

Follow-up: A follow-up visit for evaluation is scheduled at approximately 2 weeks after insertion. A repeat visit is scheduled at 3 months after insertion for evaluation of side effects and problems.

Complications
- Inability to insert or remove implants correctly
- Hypermenorrhea
- Headaches
- Mastalgia
- Galactorrhea
- Acne

Referral: Women diagnosed with the following require consultation prior to insertion: hyperlipidemia, hypertension, migraine headaches, or use of anticonvulsants.

Drug Interaction: Anticonvulsants increase the failure rate of subdermal implants.

Sterilization

Sterilization is surgical intervention to permanently prevent pregnancy. Sterilization can be performed on a man or a woman. For female sterilization, the most common method is access to the tubes by laparoscopy and application of bands or clips to each tube. This method is indicated for women who desire irreversible contraception.

Effectiveness: Failure rate is 1.9%.

Method of Action: Surgical prevention of conception.

Risks and Benefits: In the United States, sterilization is the leading method of contraception chosen by married individuals (both female and male); 26% of American women rely on sterilization for birth control. Between ages 35 and 44, 33% of women use sterilization as their method of birth control.
  - Highly effective permanent method of birth control.
  - Menstrual dysfunction may occur after sterilization, either related to discontinuing birth control pills or to the sterilization process itself. Research has proposed that changes in menstruation can be related to tissue destruction during tubal ligation.
  - Of pregnancies that occur following sterilization, 33% are ectopic.
  - Postpartum sterilization is not performed laparoscopically because of the presence of a large uterine fundus and vascular edematous adnexa. A surgical incision is required for postpartum sterilization. Postpartum sterilization must be discussed at length during pregnancy. Consent forms should be signed during pregnancy. Desire for sterilization should be confirmed with the woman after delivery. Sterilization should be performed only if mother and baby are healthy.
  - Regret after sterilization is primarily associated with the age of the woman at the time of sterilization. Women under 30 are twice as likely to regret sterilization versus those over 40. Regret can also be linked to changes in marital status, death of a child, socioeconomic status, and emotional factors.
  - Sterilization does not prevent sexually transmitted diseases (STDs).
  - Sterilization is cost effective when cost is spread out over time.
  See Appendix and Handouts.

Contraindications: Desire for pregnancy in the future. Medical conditions that prohibit anesthesia and surgery.

Assessment
  - Physical and pelvic examinations are required prior to surgery, including Pap smear and pregnancy test.
  - Laboratory testing, as required by the physician, must be performed prior to the procedure.
  - Counseling for the procedure must include explanation of the permanence of the procedure.
  - Decision making should occur well in advance of the operation, with both

partners included in discussion and the decision. Sterilization should be discussed in the context of all other forms of contraception. Failure rate and risk of ectopic pregnancy should be discussed.

See the sterilization consent form in the Appendix.

Complications: Anesthesia complications, surgical complications such as infection and bleeding, ectopic pregnancy, menstrual dysfunction, and poststerilization regret.

Follow-up: Surgical intervention requires careful follow-up. Sterilization requires a short-term stay and follow-up for signs of bleeding and reversal of anesthesia. Sterilization incision should be examined within 1 week of surgery for signs of infection or bleeding. A pelvic exam to assess healing should be performed 4 to 6 weeks after the surgery.

Referral: Refer women for sterilization after careful discussion of the risks and benefits with the woman and her partner.

BIBLIOGRAPHY

General

American College of Obstetricians and Gynecologists: Guidelines for Women's Health Care. ACOG, Washington, DC, 1996.
Foulks, MJ: The Papanicolaou smear: Its impact on promotion of women's health. JOGNN 27(4):367, 1998.
Youngkin, E, and Davis, M: Women's Health. Appleton & Lange, East Norwalk, CT, 1994.

Cancer

Collins, W, Bourne, T, and Campbell, S: Screening strategies for ovarian cancer. Curr Opin Obstet Gynecol 10(1):33, 1998.
Copas, P, et al: Basal cell carcinoma of the vulva. J Reprod Med 41(4): 283, 1996.
Plaxe, S, and Saltzstein, S: Impact of ethnicity on the incidence of high risk endometrial carcinoma. Gynecol Oncol 65:8, 1997.
Seltzer, V, and Pearse, W: Women's Primary Health Care. McGraw-Hill, New York, 1995.
Simone, J, et al: Granular cell tumor of the vulva. J Louisiana State Med Soc 148(12): 539, 1996.
Mitchell, M, et al: Colposcopy for diagnosis and treatment of squamous intraepithelial lesions: A meta-analysis. Obstet Gynecol 91(4):626, 1998.

Contraception

Fraser, I, et al: Norplant consensus statement and background review. Contraception 57:1.
Goroll, A, May, L, and Mulley, A: Primary Care Medicine. JB Lippincott, Philadelphia, 1995.
Grimes, D, and Wallach, M (eds): Modern Contraception. Emron, Totawa, NJ, 1997.
Hatcher, RA, et al: Contraceptive Technology, ed 16. Irvington Publishers, New York, 1994.
United Nations Development Programme: Long term reversible contraception: Twelve years of experience with the TCu380A and the TCu220C. Contraception 56:341, 1997.

Endometriosis

Arumugam, K, and Lim, J: Menstrual characteristics associated with endometriosis, Br J Obstet Gynecol, 104(8):948, 1997.
Duleba, A: Diagnosis of endometriosis. Obstet Gynecol Clin North Am 24(2):331, 1997.

Eskenazi, B, and Warner, M: Epidemiology of endometriosis. Obstet Gynecol Clin North Am 24(2):235, 1997.

Infections

Blythe, M: Pelvic inflammatory disease in the adolescent population. Semin Pediatr Surg 7(1):43, 1998.

Benaim, J, Pulaski, M, and Coupey, S: Adolescent girls and pelvic inflammatory disease. Arch Pediatr Adolesc Med, 152(5):449, 1998.

Caillouette, J, et al: Vaginal pH as a marker for bacterial pathogens and menopausal status. Am J Obstet Gynecol 176(6):1275, 1997.

Centers for Disease Control and Prevention: 1998 Guidelines for Treatment of Sexually Transmitted Diseases. MMWR, 47.

Jonsson, M, et al: The associations between risk behavior and reported history of sexually transmitted diseases among young women: A population based study. Int J STD AIDS 8(8):501, 1997.

Marrazzo, JM, et al: Community based urine screening for Chlamydia trachomatis with a ligase chain reaction assay. Ann Intern Med 127:796.

Munday, P: Clinical aspects of pelvic inflammatory disease. Hum Reprod 12(11 Suppl):121, 1997.

Oakeshott, P, et al: Opportunistic screening for chlamydial infection at time of cervical smear testing in general practice. Br Med J 31:316, 1998.

Page, D, et al: Bacterial vaginosis and preterm birth, J Nurse Midwifery, 43(2):83, 1998.

Sobel, J: Vaginitis. N Engl J Med 26:(337):1896, 1997.

Thorsen, P, et al: Few microorganisms associated with bacterial vaginosis may constitute the pathologic core. Am J Obstet Gynecol 178(3):580, 1998.

Miscellaneous

Hutchins, F: Uterine fibroids: Diagnosis and indications for treatment. Obstet Gynecol Clin North Am 22(4):659, 1995.

Kjerulkk, K, et al: Uterine leiomyomas. J Reprod Med 41(7):483, 1996.

Parazzini, F, et al: Risk factors for adenomyosis. Hum Reprod 12(6):1275, 1997.

Prayson, R, and Hart, W: Pathologic considerations of uterine smooth muscle tumors. Obstet Gynecol Clin North Am 22(4): 637, 1995.

Strohbehn, K, Jakary, J, and Delancey, J: Pelvic organ prolapse in young women. Obstet Gynecol, 90(1): 33, 1997.

Vavilis, D, et al: Adenomyosis at hysterectomy. Clin Exp Obstet Gynecol 24(1):36, 1997.

CHAPTER 9

MENOPAUSE

Menopause is not a disease of the endocrine system marked by estrogen deficiency. Rather, it is a transition, and an indicator of continuing maturity. The term menopause refers to the cessation of menses, usually defined retrospectively after 12 months of amenorrhea. Menopause marks the end of reproductive years for women.

More than 30 million U.S. women are now at or beyond menopause. At least 6 million women will reach this stage of life in the next decade. A woman at the age of 50, the average age for menopause in the United States, has a life expectancy of approximately 30 more years. Menopause is, therefore, a transition to approximately 30 postreproductive years. Reproductive capability ceases with menopause, but women's sexuality does not change. Women can remain sexually active throughout their lifetime. Presence of a partner has been shown to be the most important indicator for sexual activity in postmenopausal women.

Perimenopause is a term used to define the period of time surrounding the menopause. Perimenopause begins with changes that indicate a transition is occurring, and ends after the cessation of menses and perimenopausal symptoms.

Midlife is a term used to define the perimenopausal and early menopausal years.

Natural menopause refers to menopause occurring without medical intervention. **Surgical** menopause refers to menopause occurring as a result of surgical removal of ovaries.

The average American woman now lives one-third of her life after menopause. (The median age for menopause in the United States is 50–51 years.) Women do not report depression related to loss of reproductive function. They do report concern about the symptoms related to menopause. Loss of reproductive function is reported to be a "relief" to many women.

A decrease in estradiol and progesterone levels produces perimenopausal symptoms. Most notably those symptoms are hot flashes or flushes, sleep disturbance, genitourinary complaints, skin changes, changes in muscle strength, and changes in memory.

Variability of women's symptoms indicates that pure biology is not the only explanation. Other factors that may influence symptoms are heredity, diet, weight, exercise patterns, and stress levels.

The impact of menopause on women's health and overall well-being is currently being studied. Of note is a lack of research on non-Caucasian women and health and menopause. What is known to date is that any woman with an early natural menopause has a stronger risk for vasomotor symptoms (hot flashes and night sweats), more sexual difficulties, and more trouble sleeping. All types of symptoms are more common in women who have had a hysterectomy or are users of hormone replacement therapy (Kuh, Wadsworth, and Hardy, 1997).

Signs and Symptoms of Perimenopause

IRREGULAR BLEEDING

Menstrual cycles become irregular prior to menopause. Irregularity is usually related to anovulatory cycles. Bleeding may become infrequent, prolonged, heavy, or intermenstrual. Therapies for irregular bleeding include reassurance, hormonal treatment, or endometrial ablation (Fig. 9–1). Pap smear and endometrial sampling should be performed prior to treatment to rule out carcinoma.

HOT FLASHES

The most frequently reported symptom of perimenopause is hot flashes. This symptom brings perimenopausal women to health-care providers most often. Hot flashes are experienced by approximately 75% of women around the time of menopause. This symptom is often the first indicator of the transition.

- Hot flashes can occur for 30 seconds or for several minutes at intervals lasting for months or years. They can occur at any time of the day or night.
- Hot flashes are sudden transient feelings of warmth accompanied by flushing and sweating. Women will feel a need to remove their coats or sweaters or to kick off their blankets. Estrogen withdrawal is related to hot flashes, but exactly how is poorly understood. Estrogen replacement can relieve hot flashes, but low estrogen levels are not sufficient to produce hot flashes. (Prepubertal girls with low estrogen levels do not experience hot flashes. Women with hypothalamic amenorrhea do not experience hot flashes.) However, in perimenopausal women, the lower the estrogen level, the more likely the symptom.
- Episodes usually diminish in frequency and severity over time.
- Hot flashes increase in warm weather; confined spaces; and after consumption of caffeine, alcohol, or spicy foods.
- Women who experience surgical menopause tend to have more hot flashes than women who experience natural menopause.

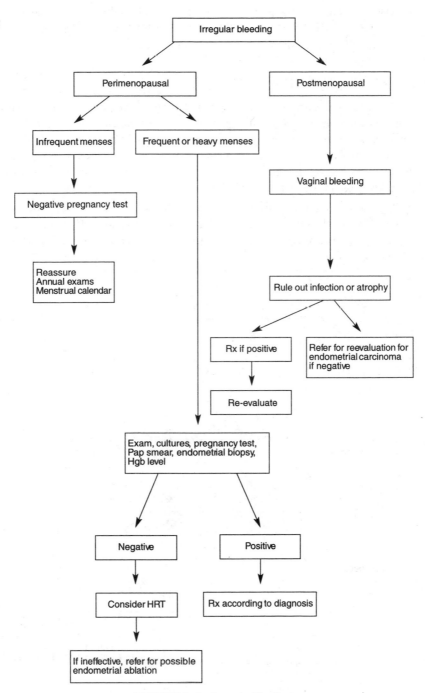

FIGURE 9–1   Irregular bleeding.

- After menopause, the prevalence of hot flashes is highest in the first 2 years.
- Treatment for hot flashes includes reassurance, hormone replacement therapy (HRT), alternative therapies, and weight loss in overweight women.

UROGENITAL CHANGES

Decrease in estrogen causes tissue changes. The tissues of the vagina, urethra, vulva, and trigone of the bladder contain large numbers of estrogen receptors. These tissues atrophy when estrogen is reduced. The vulva loses subcutaneous fat and the epidermis and vaginal epithelium thin. Vaginal glycogen level decreases, leading to a less acidic vagina. (A less acidic environment increases susceptibility to infection.) General lubrication and lubrication accompanying sexual arousal also decreases (Fig. 9–2).

- Topical or systemic estrogen decreases these symptoms. Sexually active women have less vaginal atrophy than women who are not sexually active.
- Regular consumption of cranberry juice (300 mL daily) reduces the risk of bladder infection.

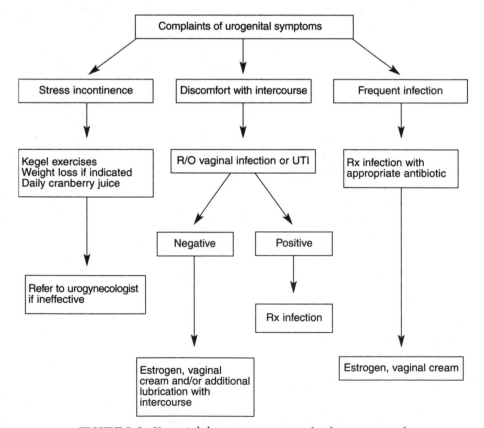

FIGURE 9–2 Urogenital changes, perimenopausal and postmenopausal.

- Stress incontinence may be related to perimenopausal changes. To reduce stress incontinence, the urethral sphincter can be strengthened with Kegel exercises (see Appendix and Chap. 10). Stress incontinence is not affected by estrogen levels.

CHANGE IN PHYSICAL STRENGTH AT MENOPAUSE

Decrease in grip strength has been noted in postmenopausal women. Women report less physical strength following menopause. A regular exercise routine is recommended for all perimenopausal and postmenopausal women to overcome the natural tendency for decreased strength.

MEMORY PROBLEMS AND DIFFICULTY CONCENTRATING

Cerebral perfusion declines with age. Women have higher blood flow values than men until menopause occurs. The connections between menopause and memory are being studied. Estrogen may be related to short-term memory. There is currently conflicting information on whether HRT is helpful. The information on estrogen is conflicting and the information on progesterone is lacking.

Exogenous estrogen may retard the likelihood and severity of Alzheimer's disease. More studies are needed on this important finding.

SLEEP CHANGES

Night "sweats," psychologic distress, and sleep apnea can create sleeping problems in perimenopausal and postmenopausal women.
- Hot flashes, often called night sweats, can disrupt sleep.
- Apnea caused by blockage of the air passage during sleep causes arousal in order to breathe. Apnea is associated with upper-body obesity in women. Symptoms of apnea are daytime sleepiness, persistent tired feelings, and loud snoring at night with gasps.
- Sleep disruption can be reduced by treating hot flashes. Stress management (see Chap. 2) may decrease sleep disruption. Any indicator of sleep apnea requires referral for evaluation and treatment.

VISUAL CHANGES

Less ability to accommodate to close items is common in women over 40 years. **Presbyopia,** difficulty seeing things close up, is a common diagnosis. For women who have never worn glasses, drugstore nonprescription glasses may be all that is necessary. If these are not effective, prescriptive lenses are necessary.

Cataracts are protein deposits in the lenses of the eyes. Early cataract signs are blurred vision and night vision problems. Cataracts require diagnosis and surgical treatment. Decreased exposure to the sun decreases the likelihood of cataract formation. Daily consumption of vitamin C also decreases the likelihood of cataract formation.

Glaucoma is an increase in pressure within the eye. This pressure can damage the optic nerve. Glaucoma can be controlled if diagnosed early. The pressure within each eye should be checked at all eye examinations.

Risk Assessment

The leading causes of death for women aged 45–54 in order of incidence are malignancy, heart disease, cerebrovascular disease, accidents, liver disease, suicide, chronic obstructive pulmonary disease (COPD), diabetes, pneumonia, and homicide. For women aged 55–64, the causes of death in order of incidence are malignancy, heart disease, COPD, pneumonia, diabetes, liver disease, accidents, suicide, and homicide. Women with a natural menopause at age 40–44 years experience an increased risk for cancer-related mortality. No age-related increased mortality rate is seen among women who experience surgical menopause.

Refer to Chapter 2 for discussion of screening for malignancy in these age groups. Secondary prevention strategies for malignancy include breast examination and mammography (see Chap. 2). Regular Pap smears and pelvic examination are part of the screening process for malignancy.

Screening for cancer includes accurate taking of both personal and family history. Tamoxifen has been found to be a useful drug for women who are a significant risk for breast cancer (see Chap. 2). Referral for tamoxifen treatment should be considered for all high-risk perimenopausal women.

Perimenopausal and postmenopausal women should be encouraged to have regular screening for breast cancer, but should also be warned concerning the risk of false positives. A recent research article in the *New England Journal of Medicine* (Elmore et al, 1998) revealed that in each woman the cumulative risk of a false-positive breast cancer screening after 10 screenings was 49.1% for mammograms and 22.3% for breast examination.

Cardiovascular disease in women is related to obesity, plasma lipid levels, hypertension, diabetes, cigarette smoking, sedentary lifestyle, and lack of estrogen. Improvement in any of these factors improves cardiovascular status. Blood pressure screening should be performed at every health-care encounter. The following is a discussion about health promotion related to reducing the risk of cardiovascular disease in women.

Health Promotion

CARDIOVASCULAR

A significant health risk facing perimenopausal and menopausal women is cardiovascular disease. The risk for heart disease begins to rise at age 45. The Framingham Study reported that the risk for cardiovascular disease for women triples after menopause and premature menopause increases the risk. Modifiable risk factors for cardiovascular disease are exercise, diet, smoking, and estrogen levels.

EXERCISE

More active and physically fit women experience less cardiovascular disease. When active people do develop cardiovascular disease, it occurs later in life and is less severe. Fitness can also prevent bone mineral loss. Exercise helps prevent depression and anxiety. Perimenopausal and menopausal women who exercise have fewer hot flashes and less difficulty sleeping. They also have fewer digestive complaints. The Centers for Disease Control tell us that American women are sedentary and that activity level decreases at midlife. Thus, increasing physical activity for women is an objective for all women's health nurse practitioners.

Women's leisure time is often filled with the priorities of others, making time for exercise difficult to find. Finding a mode of activity suitable for each woman is a challenge for practitioners. Women in midlife who are successful in exercising regularly often choose activities that can be done in and around their homes, using time as it becomes free. Examples of these activities are walking, exercising with videos, and riding a stationary bicycle. Exercising for 20–30 minutes three to four times per week is the current recommendation (see Chap. 2). Suggest to women that they explore exercise activities that are reasonable for them to pursue within their current lifestyle, and suggest that the exercise activity be something that they enjoy.

NUTRITION

- Limiting fat intake, particularly after the effective protection of estrogen is removed at menopause, is an important dietary goal. The nutritional goal for menopausal women is 15% protein, 55% carbohydrates, and 30% or less fat.
- Daily calorie requirements for maintenance decrease at menopause. Weight will increase after menopause unless there is increased activity or decreased intake of calories. The recommended daily allowance (RDA) for women over 50 is 80%–85% of the 2200 calories recommended for young adults.
- Calcium intake of 800 mg/day is sufficient for active women under 50. After 50, calcium intake should be increased to 1200–1500 mg/day. Postmenopausal women not on HRT should consider 1500 mg/day of calcium intake.
- The need for iron decreases to 10 mg/day from 15 mg after menopause.
- A diet high in complex carbohydrates (high fiber) may reduce the incidence of colon cancer and may avoid constipation that is common in women in midlife.
- Eight to ten 8-oz glasses of water daily is recommended.
- Weight reduction should be encouraged in overweight perimenopausal and menopausal women. Obesity is associated with cardiovascular disease.

SMOKING CESSATION

Smoking is associated with lung cancer, coronary artery disease, cerebrovascular disease, cervical cancer, hypertension, and respiratory disease. Women in midlife who smoke are more likely to be heavy smokers and less likely to quit than younger women. Quitting smoking for 10 years reduces the risk of lung cancer by 30%–50% according to the Centers for Disease Control. Women who quit smoking reduce their risk for cardiovascular disease by 24% within 2 years of stopping.

Women report that they smoke to reduce their weight and to reduce stress. Advise midlife women to stop smoking and address these two concerns. Other avenues for stress reduction and maintenance of weight should be explored. Address a woman's concerns and barriers to stopping. Help her decide on a quit date. Provide her with reassurance. Nicotine gum and patches may be helpful both with stopping smoking and with preventing weight gain.

HORMONE REPLACEMENT THERAPY

Clearly inform each woman of the risks and benefits of HRT. HRT is reported to alleviate vasomotor symptoms and vaginal symptoms, prevent coronary heart disease, and prevent bone loss. Questions remain concerning the association between HRT and breast cancer and the effectiveness of estrogen replacement with progestin added.

The rationale for HRT is that hormone shifts cause menopausal symptoms and increase the risk for osteoporosis and heart disease. HRT may also be beneficial in preventing tooth loss and need for dentures in postmenopausal women. Women with perimenopausal symptoms interfering with their daily lives and women at risk for heart disease and/or osteoporosis should consider HRT.

Contraindications for HRT are stroke, breast cancer, liver disease, pancreatic disease, history of thrombophlebitis, recent myocardial infarction, endometrial adenocarcinoma, estrogen-dependent tumors, and undiagnosed vaginal bleeding (Table 9–1).

HRT can be supplied in oral form, patches applied to the skin, and in cream form.

- Oral administration is usually estrogen 0.625 mg daily with 2.5 mg progesterone daily. Progesterone is necessary to protect the uterus. It is not necessary to prescribe progesterone following hysterectomy.
- Skin patches are applied once or twice per week on a dry, hairless area of the body, but not on the breast. Patches are a lower dose of estrogen than oral administration, 0.05 mg most commonly, and the estrogen is absorbed directly. Estrogen skin patches are given with oral progesterone when the uterus is present.
- Cream containing estrogen 0.3 mg is used for vaginal effect only; 2 g daily for 1–2 weeks intravaginally followed by 2 g once or twice weekly for maintenance is the recommendation.

TABLE 9–1 CONTRAINDICATIONS TO ESTROGEN THERAPY

Absolute	Relative
Unexplained vaginal bleeding	Seizure disorders
Acute liver damage	High levels of triglycerides
Recent vascular thrombosis	High levels of lipids
Carcinoma of the breast	Migraine headaches
Carcinoma of the endometrium	Atraumatic thrombophlebitis
	Current gallbladder disease

Prolonged estrogen therapy unopposed by progestin causes hyperplasia of the endometrium and a four- to sixfold increase in endometrial cancer. Regular addition of a progestin negates the risk and provides protection.

Women report reasons for stopping HRT (high dropout rates of approximately 30% are reported) as fear of developing cancer and displeasure with side effects, including bleeding, tender breasts, bloating, irritability, mood swings, and indigestion. Therefore, careful education and counseling is necessary prior to beginning HRT and throughout the course of therapy (see Appendix).

Considerations for HRT Therapy

The woman's history of coronary heart disease, osteoporotic fractures, and cancer must be carefully considered in counseling regarding HRT. Her perimenopausal or postmenopausal symptoms must also be considered (Fig. 9–3).

- HRT alleviates vasomotor and urogenital discomfort. This finding is well established.
- HRT has been shown to be the mode of choice to reduce bone loss. Raloxifene, a new drug designed to prevent osteoporosis, appears in the latest studies to be effective and *not* increase the risk of cancer. It may have a role in the prevention of heart disease. It is a selective estrogen receptor modulator that acts as an estrogen in some respects and not in others. The Food and Drug Administration (FDA) has approved this drug for osteoporosis, but at this time HRT or alendronate (Fosamax) are utilized to treat the disease and decrease the fracture risk. It is too early to tell if raloxifene is as effective for treatment of osteoporosis. Raloxifene, according to early studies, may be effective in preventing breast cancer. The risk of breast cancer has been shown to be reduced in early studies. This may be the drug of choice for women at risk for breast cancer and osteoporosis. Raloxifene does not reduce hot flashes and may increase them.
- Estrogen therapy reduces the risk of heart disease. HRT, in some research studies, reduces the risk of coronary heart disease by 50%. Estrogen increases the bioavailability of endothelium-derived nitric oxide, an agent that

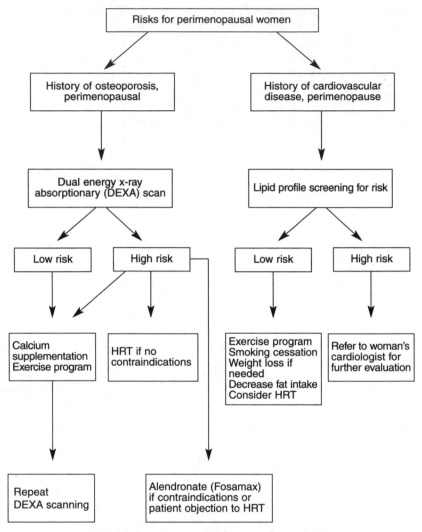

FIGURE 9–3   Hormone replacement therapy (HRT).

slows atherogenesis, inhibits platelet aggregation, and reduces vascular smooth muscle cell proliferation. Early studies reveal that it has little or no effect on women who already have heart disease; thus, it is currently not recommended for that purpose (Hulley, 1998).

- Estrogen therapy can reduce cardiovascular death in postmenopausal women. A report from the Nurses' Health Study suggests that progesterone added to the estrogen therapy does not negate the benefit. Confirming studies are yet to be performed (Hulley, 1998).
- HRT is starting to show positive effect on psychologic function and risk for osteoarthritis.

- HRT is starting to show a connection with a decrease in colon cancer.
- HRT may reduce the incidence of Alzheimer's disease.
- Cancer and HRT connections are under investigation.

The right medication for the correct period of time is the issue for women who choose HRT. History and symptoms will dictate what drug or combination of drugs and in what form. The most commonly prescribed regimes provide a baseline from which to begin therapy. Side effects and decrease in symptoms guide the modification of dose and route of administration (see Appendix).

OSTEOPOROSIS

Loss of bone mineral density begins in women around the age of 30. The rate increases past age 40, and escalates further after menopause. Bone loss is influenced by age, menopausal status, heredity, race, and weight. African-American women have denser bones than Caucasian women; 20 million women currently have osteoporosis.

Modifiable risk factors for both cardiovascular disease and bone mineral density are physical activity, diet, calcium intake, alcohol consumption, and smoking. According to the National Osteoporosis Foundation, the overall cost of acute and long-term care associated with osteoporosis exceeds $10 billion annually. (Health-care costs are primarily related to the morbidity and mortality associated with fractures [Hulley, 1998].)

Dual-energy x-ray absorptiometry, also know as a bone density test (see Chap. 2) should be done for all women with risk factors for osteoporosis (see Appendix).

The treatment of osteoporosis includes calcium, exercise, alendronate (nontoxic, nonhormone therapy capable of stabilizing osteoporotic bone), and HRT.

- Calcitonin, a naturally occurring polypeptide, acts to suppress osteoclast activity and subsequent bone resorption. For many years, calcitonin in injection form was used to treat osteoporosis. Recently, the FDA has approved calcitonin in an intranasal form. The medication is administered in doses of 200 IU daily in the form of one puff in one nostril daily (alternating nostrils). Calcitonin should be used with calcium and vitamin D.
- Oral sodium fluoride works to stimulate bone formation by increasing the number of osteoblasts and has been used in Europe for many years. This should also be used with calcium and vitamin D.
- Alendronate, a bisphosphate, acts to decrease bone resorption and prevent bone loss. The recommended dose for alendronate is 10 mg/day one-half hour before breakfast with a full glass of water. This should be taken with calcium and vitamin D.

CONTRACEPTIVE CONCERNS FOR
PERIMENOPAUSAL WOMEN

Pregnancy is possible when women are ovulating irregularly. During the perimenopausal period, contraception should be discussed.

- The diaphragm may cause irritation because of vaginal dryness during midlife.
- Condoms may be uncomfortable related to lack of lubrication. (Condoms may be necessary, however, if the woman is at risk for human immunodefiency virus [HIV].)
- The intrauterine device (IUD) may be an acceptable contraceptive method, but it must be removed before uterine atrophy occurs.
- Oral contraceptives can be used by many perimenopausal women. If a woman is healthy and nonsmoking, low-dose oral contraceptives can be considered.
- Progestin-only contraceptives can be used. They can produce amenorrhea, which may be helpful in women with irregular bleeding.

ALTERNATIVES TO HYSTERECTOMY

Hysterectomy is the second most frequently performed operation in the United States. Hysterectomy involves the removal of the entire uterus, a total hysterectomy, through an abdominal incision. Hysterectomy can also be performed via laparoscope. (The uterus is removed in pieces via the vagina.)

Hysterectomy is performed most commonly for fibroids, dysfunctional uterine bleeding, prolapse, and endometriosis. For discussion of treatment options for these conditions, see Chapter 8.

Experts agree that hysterectomy is necessary for invasive cancer of the uterus, cervix, or ovaries. Cancer accounts for approximately 15% of hysterectomies performed. Other reasons for hysterectomy require discussion of other therapies.

Options Concerning Hysterectomy

- If the ovaries are removed, which happens in one-half of hysterectomies, the loss of estrogen creates menopausal symptoms. Careful consideration of removal of healthy ovaries should be discussed if hysterectomy is chosen as the treatment method.
- Leaving the cervix behind following hysterectomy reduces the risk of infection. It also reduces the chance of decreased sexual response after hysterectomy.
- Myomectomy is an option for women with fibroids. The fibroid is removed, and the uterus remains intact. The operation has a higher risk of complications than a hysterectomy. The surgeon must be familiar with methodology for the surgery. Fibroids can grow back after myomectomy. Of women who have myomectomy, 25% need further surgery. Myomectomy preserves fertility in women who desire future pregnancies.
- Endometrial ablation can be used to treat excessive uterine bleeding. The endometrium is destroyed in this procedure, along with fibroids within the endometrium and polyps. Ablation can be performed in one of three ways. *Cryotherapy* destroys the uterine lining with freezing. In *thermal* ablation, a balloon is inserted into the uterus and filled with hot water that burns and

destroys the endometrium. The endometrium can also be destroyed with *electricity*. About 50% of women who undergo ablation will never menstruate again; 25% will have a reduction in flow.

ALTERNATIVES TO MEDICAL THERAPY

Of respondents to a 1998 survey conducted by the American Medical Association, 40% reported using alternative therapies to improve their health (Astin, 1998). The most common use was chiropractic, followed by diet, exercise, and relaxation therapies. Only 4% of the respondents used alternative therapy alone. Most combined alternatives with traditional medicine. More educated people than poorly educated people used alternatives. Clearly alternative therapies are not alternatives at all. They are adjuncts. Providers of health care should be informed and open-minded about nonmedical therapies for perimenopause and postmenopause. The National Menopause Society tells us that one of three women with menopausal symptoms tries alternatives for symptom relief (Wilbur et al, 1998).

The following is a discussion of a few of the more common alternative therapies employed by perimenopausal and postmenopausal women.

- Black cohosh is an herb that can be used to relieve hot flashes and vaginal dryness. Black cohosh is a source of natural plant estrogen. The recommended dose is 40 mg daily. Long-term effects have not been determined.
- Soy is also a source of plant estrogen. The daily dose of soy to reduce menopausal symptoms has not been established. There are some indications that soy reduces hot flashes and prevents heart disease and osteoporosis as well as reduces the risk of breast cancer.
- Flaxseeds are a source of a substance similar to plant estrogen. Flaxseeds can help treat hot flashes and vaginal dryness. Taking two tablespoons a day reduces these symptoms.
- Progesterone can be found in wild yams. Natural progesterone can be placed in a cream form and applied topically for relief of perimenopausal symptoms.
- Vitamin E can be utilized for hot flashes and breast tenderness. It may also treat vaginal dryness. Recommended dose is 400 IU twice daily.

Natural or alternative medicines were perceived by perimenopausal and menopausal women to be safer and "somewhat effective" in surveys. Personal control of menopausal symptoms was a major issue for surveyed women. Menopausal women expressed a desire to feel in control of their health. A need for informed choice of treatments was clearly demonstrated in a survey published in the *Canadian Family Physician* in 1998 (Seidl and Stewart).

Conclusion

Perimenopausal and postmenopausal women require comprehensive care including a complete history, thorough physical examination, risk factor assessment, age-appropriate screening, and education.

Women may not be well informed about menopause. A recent Harris survey indicated that only one-half of working women of menopausal age were able to name any long-term health concerns related to the postmenopausal years. Of those who could, 27% mentioned osteoporosis and only 6% mentioned heart disease. A study published by the American College of Obstetricians and Gynecologists showed only 1 in 40 women interviewed knew about an increased risk of heart disease after menopause (American College of Obstetricians and Gynecologists, 1996).

There is need to explain "changes" that occur in a woman during the perimenopausal and postmenopausal years. Reassurance and education may be the only therapy required in many cases.

A one-size-fits-all therapeutic regime clearly will not work for women in midlife. There is a great variety in symptomatology and risk factors. Plans of care must be individualized that include health promotion strategies, screening, and therapies such as HRT and/or herbal remedies.

The final decision for health maintenance and promotion rests with the woman. Guidance is provided based upon current symptoms and personal and family history. Fewer than 20% of postmenopausal women have had hormone therapy prescribed. Of those, 40% continue the therapy for more than 1 year; 30% of women never fill the prescriptions for HRT. A better job of education and explanation is clearly needed, as is creating a long-term partnering in the health-care relationship with midlife women. Women wish to make informed choices about the health management of midlife. HRT or not? Surgery or not? Alternatives or not? Forming a health-promotion strategy is needed for all midlife women. The practitioner and the woman working together and exploring all options for increasing the quality and longevity of life is ideal.

BIBLIOGRAPHY

Allen, K, and Phillips, J: Women's Health Across the Lifespan. Lippincott, Philadelphia, 1997.

American College of Obstetricians and Gynecologists: Guideline for Women's Health Care. ACOG, Washington, DC, 1996.

Astin, J: Why patients use alternative medicine. JAMA 279(19):1548, 1998.

Baker, A, Simpson, S, and Dawson, D: Sleep distribution and mood changes associated with menopause. J Psychosom Res 3(44):359, 1997.

Barile, L: Theories of menopause. J Psychosoc Nursing Mental Health Serv 35(2):36.

Calaf, I, and Alsina, J: Benefits of hormone replacement therapy. Int J Fertil Women's Med 42(Suppl 2):329, 1997.

Clark, A, Flowers, J, Boots, L, and Shettar, S: Sleep disturbances in mid-life women. J Adv Nursing 22(3):562, 1995.

Cooper, G, and Sandler, D: Age at natural menopause and mortality. Ann Epidemiol 8(4):229, 1998.

Cornell University Medical College, The Center for Women's Healthcare: Women's Health Advisory September, 1998.

Damewood, M: Hormonal strategies of the menopause. Maryland Med J 46(8):415, 1997.

Elmore, J, et al: Ten year risk of false positive screening mammograms and clinical breast examination. N Engl J Med 338(16):1089, 1998.

Hammond, C: Management of menopause. Am Fam Physician. 55(5):1667, 1997.

Hulley, S, et al: Randomized trial of estrogen plus progestin for secondary prevention of coronary heart disease in postmenopausal women. JAMA 280:605, 1998.

Kessenich, C: Update on pharmacologic therapies for osteoporosis. Nurse Pract 21(8):19, 1996.

Kuh, DL, Wadsworth, M, and Hardy, R: Women's health in midlife: The influence of the menopause, social factors and health in earlier life. Br J Obstet Gynecol 104(8):923, 1997.

Lewis, J, and Bernstein, J: Women's Health. Jones and Bartlett, Sudbury, MA, 1996.

Pelisser, A: Menopause, hormone replacement therapy (HRT), stomatologic pathologies. Contraception Fertil Sexual 26(6):439, 1998.

Rodgers, M, and Miller, J: Adequacy of hormone replacement therapy for osteoporosis prevention. Br J Gen Pract 47(416):161, 1997.

Seidl, M, and Stewart, D: Alternative treatments for menopausal symptoms. Can Fam Physician 44:1271, 1998.

Waldman, T: Menopause: When hormone replacement therapy is not an option. J Women's Health 7(5):559, 1998.

Wilbur, J, et al: Sociodemographic characteristics, biological factors, and symptom reporting in mid-life women. Menopause 5(1):43, 1998.

CHAPTER 10

HEPATIC AND RENAL

Hepatic Assessment

The liver serves a variety of important functions related to synthesis, energy generation and storage, catabolism, and disposal of toxic substances and waste products. Acute or chronic liver dysfunction leads to biochemical abnormalities. Some liver functions are more sensitive to injury and infection than others. Because the liver performs many functions, a carefully elicited history and thorough physical examination are important screening tools for liver dysfunction. History obtained from every woman should include the following:

- Family history of jaundice or anemia
- Occupation reviewed in detail (contact with animals and exposure to toxins in particular)
- Travel habits
- Alcohol intake
- Contact with jaundiced persons
- History of injections
- Intravenous (IV) drug use
- Onset of illness (if appropriate)

Physical examination should note:

- Pallor.
- Jaundice.
- Spider angioma—a few in women is normal; many can indicate liver dysfunction.
- Mental status.

- Abdominal examination to rule out ascites, enlarged liver, and tenderness (the liver edge is tender in hepatitis, congestive heart failure [CHF], alcoholism, and malignancy). The abdomen should be auscultated for bruits and friction rubs.

Women's health nurse practitioners play a key role in referring women with liver disease or increased risk of liver disease. Prevention and early diagnosis of hepatitis in particular is a component of assessment for every woman at every health-related visit. Testing women for hepatitis during pregnancy and recommending vaccination of newborns have become important functions in the delivery of health care to women and their families.

Renal Assessment

Urinary tract infections are among the most common reasons women seek care. Assessment of the urinary tract includes history, physical examination, and urine testing. History must include the following:

- Dysuria, frequency, urgency
- Suprapubic pain
- Fever
- Hematuria
- Previous urinary tract infection(s)
- Unusual vaginal discharge
- Last menstrual period

Physical examination should include the following:

- Pelvic examination to rule out vaginitis or pelvic inflammatory disease
- Abdominal examination, noting any areas of tenderness
- Examination of the back to rule out costovertebral angle tenderness
- Examination of the urine

Examination of urine has a long-standing tradition in health-care screening. Dipsticks have made assessment of bacteria in urine quick and inexpensive. Since urinary tract infections are known to be a significant source of morbidity for diabetic, pregnant, and older women, most authorities recommend screening of these populations.

Treatment of urinary infection in diabetic women may decrease long-term morbidity. Treating asymptomatic bacteriuria in pregnant women has proved beneficial; therefore, pregnant women should be routinely screened with both dipstick and culture (see Chapter 17). Treatment of asymptomatic bacteria in the urine in the institutionalized elderly woman has not demonstrated a decrease in morbidity. Dipstick tests for bacteria can be inaccurate if the organism does not produce nitrate, the specimen is not first morning, or the urine is dilute. Sensitivity for dipstick urinalysis is 72%–97%; specificity is 64%–82%. Dipstick screening can indicate the need for urine culture in asymptomatic women.

Screening is also advocated to detect hematuria, an indication of urinary tract malignancy. These malignancies, which increase in occurrence after age 40, are more common in men than in women. The sensitivity of dipstick testing for hematuria is good (91%–100%).

Urine screening should be done on an early morning specimen and collected via "clean catch." First, cleanse the vulvar region, followed by a cleansing of the urinary meatus with moistened cotton balls. Avoid the use of soap. Use a clean container and collect the specimen "midstream." Perform the urinalysis as soon as possible after collecting the specimen.

Microscopic examination of urine from women with urinary tract infection may reveal the presence of leukocytes (>10 white blood cells [WBCs] per high-power field), erythrocytes, and bacteria. The specimen may or may not be Gram's-stained. The presence of any or all of these factors assists in the diagnosis of urinary tract infection.

Urine culture confirms urinary tract infection. The presence of an organism in amounts greater than 10^2 or 10^5 (the higher value is used in some laboratories) indicates infection with high sensitivity, specificity, and predictive value.

Acute Pyelonephritis

Acute pyelonephritis is an infectious disease involving the collecting system and the renal parenchyma of the kidney.

Etiology: Bacterial infection, usually with a gram-negative organism. *Escherichia coli* is the most common causative agent.

Occurrence: Surveys of office practices and hospital admissions demonstrate 250,000 episodes of acute pyelonephritis annually in the United States.

Age: Between the ages of 15 and 24, the prevalence of bacteriuria is about 2%–3%, increasing to about 10% by age 60, 20% after the age of 65, and 25%–50% after age 80.

Ethnicity: Not significant.

Gender: Infection of the urinary tract is more common in women than in men by a ratio of 8:1.

Contributing Factors: Advanced age, inefficient bladder emptying, decreased functional ability (dementia, incontinence, neurologic deficits), nosocomial infections, pregnancy, diabetes, sickle cell trait, cystic renal disease.

Signs and Symptoms: Chills, fever, unilateral or bilateral costovertebral angle tenderness, dysuria, frequency of urination, urgency of urination, cloudy malodorous urine. At times, women experience nausea and vomiting.

Diagnostic Tests: Urinalysis, urine culture.

Differential Diagnosis: Cystitis, other causes of flank pain.

Treatment: For mild symptoms, use oral fluoroquinolone for 10–14 days. For severe symptoms, women may require hospitalization for treatment with parenteral antibiotics.

Follow-up: No follow-up is necessary for a mild infection that resolves prior to completion of the course of antibiotics. Severe infections require a repeat urine culture at 5–7 days after initiation of therapy, and at 4–6 weeks after discontinuation of therapy. Recurrence of symptoms requires a renal ultrasound or CT scan.

Sequelae: In 30% of patients with acute pyelonephritis, bacteria invade through the mucosa into the bloodstream, causing bacteremia.

Prevention/Prophylaxis: Prompt treatment of lower urinary tract infection.

Referral: All cases of acute pyelonephritis require consultation for management.

Education: Between 10% and 30% of all patients relapse after a 14-day course of therapy. Individuals who relapse are usually cured with a second course of antibiotics.

Asymptomatic Bacteriuria

Asymptomatic bacteriuria, the persistent colonization of the urinary tract without urinary symptoms, poses a significant health risk for pregnant women. If untreated, 20%–40% of pregnant women develop acute pyelonephritis.

Etiology: In most pregnancies, dilation of the upper collecting system occurs and extends down to the level of the pelvic brim. The dilated ureters may contain over 200 mL of urine and contribute to persistence of bacteriuria in pregnancy.

Occurrence: Occurs in 5%–10% of pregnant women.

Age: The incidence in young women is 1%–2%. The incidence in women more than 60 years of age is 6%–10%. The incidence in institutionalized elderly women is 25%–50%.

Ethnicity: Not significant.

Contributing Factors: Diabetes, hypertension, obstruction of the urinary tract, disseminated infection, pregnancy.

Signs and Symptoms: None.

Diagnostic Tests: Voided urine is easily contaminated by urethral and perineal flora. Cultures must be obtained on clean voided urine and quantified (Fig. 10–1).

Differential Diagnosis: Contaminated urinary specimen for culture.

Treatment: See "Symptomatic Lower Urinary Tract Infection."

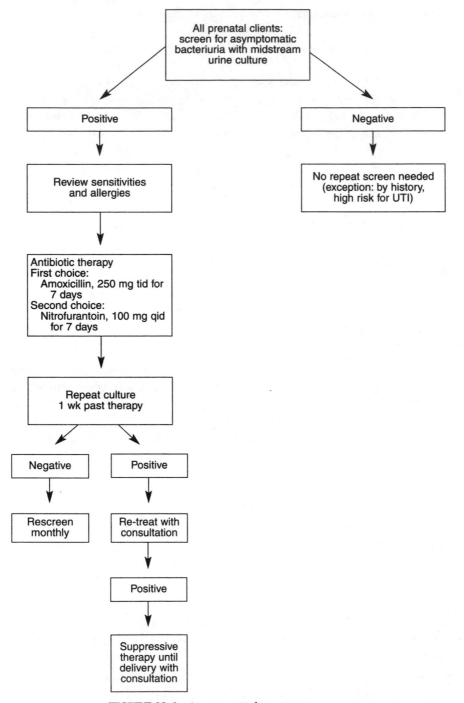

FIGURE 10–1   Asymptomatic bacteriuria in pregnancy.

Follow-up: Repeat urine culture after therapy.

Sequelae: Among women with bacteriuria identified early in pregnancy, up to 40% develop pyelonephritis if not treated. Women with bacteriuria are nearly twice as likely to deliver a low-birth-weight infant. No short-term or long-term adverse outcomes exist that are attributable to asymptomatic bacteriuria in nonpregnant women.

Prevention/Prophylaxis: Screening for asymptomatic bacteriuria is recommended for pregnant women, all women who have been recently catheterized, and women with known renal calculi or other structural abnormalities of the urinary tract.

Referral: All women with asymptomatic bacteriuria require consultation for management.

Education: Pregnant women should be aware of the importance of early prenatal care.

Cystitis

Acute cystitis is a superficial mucosal infection of the bladder.

Etiology: Bacteria reach the bladder by ascending through the urethra.

Contributing Factors: Bacteria that commonly cause cystitis are found at the introitus in 20% of cases. Entry of bacteria into the relatively short female urethra can happen spontaneously. Infection depends on the virulence of the organism, the number of organisms, and the state of the host's defensive system. The most important host defense mechanism is the ability of the bladder's mucosal surface to phagocytize bacteria coming in contact with it. Sexual intercourse and diaphragm and spermicide use have been correlated with cystitis.

Occurrence: Surveys of office practices estimate 7 million episodes of acute cystitis occur annually in the United States.

Age: Between 20% and 30% of women have cystitis in their lifetime.

Ethnicity: Not significant.

Signs and Symptoms: Dysuria, frequency, urgency, and suprapubic discomfort. Of women with cystitis, 40% have hematuria.

Diagnostic Tests: Urinalysis, urine culture and sensitivity on a clean voided specimen, microscopic examination of urine sediment (Fig. 10–2).

Differential Diagnosis: Urethritis diagnosed by negative urinary culture, vaginitis diagnosed by pelvic examination, and local trauma or irritation.

Treatment: A 3-day course of antibiotics achieves a higher rate of cure than single-dose therapy. Short courses of antibiotics improve compliance, lower cost, and lower the frequency of adverse reactions. Table 10–1 describes treatment.

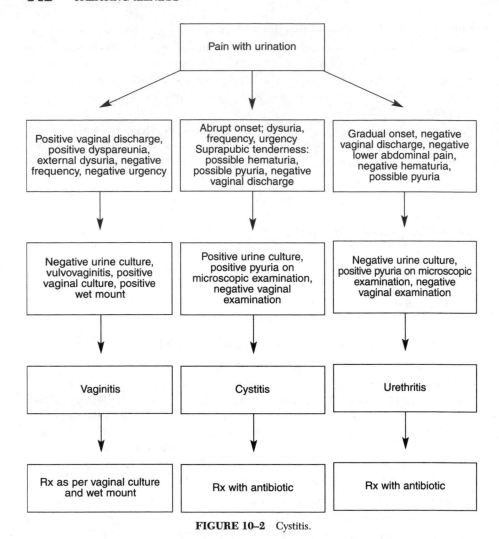

FIGURE 10–2   Cystitis.

TABLE 10–1   MEDICATIONS FOR URINARY TRACT INFECTION

Three-Day Therapy for Nonpregnant Women	
Drug	**Dosage**
Nitrofurantoin	100 mg bid
Ciprofloxecin	250 mg bid
Ofloxacin	200 mg bid
Norfloxacin	200–400 mg bid
Sulfamethoxazole-trimethoprim	160–800 mg bid

Follow-up: No follow-up is necessary if resolution of symptoms occurs following therapy. Recurrence of symptoms requires a repeat urine culture and sensitivity.

Sequelae: Of women who experience cystitis, 40% have a recurrence.

Prevention/Prophylaxis: Contraceptive method that does not include the use of a diaphragm and spermicide.

Referral: Recurrent infections require referral.

Education: Increase fluid intake, void after intercourse, complete antibiotic regime.

Interstitial Cystitis

Interstitial cystitis is a symptom complex characterized by pelvic pain, urinary urgency, urinary frequency, and nocturia. There is an absence of any definable cause for these symptoms. Onset is gradual.

Etiology: Unknown.

Occurrence: Between 44,000 and 450,000 diagnosed cases in the United States. Female-to-male ratio is 9:1.

Age: Average age is 40–46 years.

Ethnicity: Predominately Caucasians. There is a 400% increased incidence in Jewish people.

Contributing Factors: Unknown.

Signs and Symptoms: Urinary frequency, bladder pain, and nocturia.

Diagnostic Tests: Interstitial cystitis is a diagnosis of exclusion. Evaluation includes ruling out other disorders that produce similar symptoms. Diagnosis is assisted by cystoscopy.

Differential Diagnosis: Urinary infection, carcinoma, radiation- and medication-induced cystitis.

Treatment: Until etiology and pathogenesis of interstitial cystitis are identified, specific therapy is not possible. However, symptomatic treatment is helpful and includes dimethyl sulfoxide, antihistamines, anti-inflammatories, intravesical silver nitrate, heparin, and surgery. Bladder training can be helpful to some women.

Follow-up: Unknown.

Sequelae: Unknown.

Prevention/Prophylaxis: Unknown.

Referral: Interstitial cystitis requires referral.

Education: Symptoms increase with sexual intercourse and with menses. Bladder training to prolong voiding intervals should be attempted.

Symptomatic Lower Urinary Tract Infection

Symptomatic lower urinary tract infection (UTI), also called cystitis or bladder infection, occurs when microorganisms infiltrate the bladder and the urethra. Women commonly seek health care for these infections.

Bladder infections occur frequently, even though the lining of the bladder has antiadherent capacities that prevent the colonization of bacteria if they do enter the bladder, and the washing effect of the urine cleanses the bladder. The establishment of a bladder infection depends on the virulence of the organism, the number of organisms introduced, and the woman's defense mechanisms.

Etiology: Current evidence suggests that most episodes of lower UTI in adult women are secondary to ascending infection. Bacteria that reach the bladder through the urethra may ascend into the bladder and possibly the kidneys through the ureters. About 80% of lower UTIs are caused by *E. coli*, about 15% by *Staphylococcus saprophyticus,* and the rest by organisms such as *Klebsiella pneumoniae* and *Proteus mirabilis.* All of these organisms reside in the GI tract.

Occurrence: Between 20% and 30% of women have a lower UTI in their lifetime, and 40% of women with one episode of lower UTI will have a recurrence.

Age: Adult women.

Ethnicity: Not significant.

Contributing factors: Colonization of bacteria in the vagina has been shown to be an essential first step in the production of bacteriuria. The normal vaginal pH is 4, which decreases the ability of bacteria to colonize. However, several factors known to elevate the vaginal pH increase the likelihood of bacterial colonization and also increase the risk of lower UTI. These factors include a decrease in estrogen, spermicides, vaginal infection, and sexual activity. Milking of the urethra by the penis during intercourse can help transport bacteria from the urethra to the bladder.

Some women are more prone to infection from *E. coli,* an organism that normally resides in the healthy large intestine. *E. coli* has the ability to adhere to uroepithelial cells, attaching to host receptor sites. Susceptible women possess an increased density of these receptors, thus facilitating adherence. These women are not "less clean" than other women; they simply are more prone to this organism ascending and infecting the urinary tract. This tendency could be genetic.

The most consistent behavior associated with lower UTI is sexual intercourse. Coital frequency directly relates to occurrence and recurrence of lower UTIs. Symptoms often develop within 24 hours of coitus. Use of a diaphragm may be related to a decreased urge to void or to residual urine, possibly increasing the risk of developing a lower UTI.

Signs and Symptoms: Women present with pelvic pressure, dysuria, urgency, frequency, and sometimes incontinence and hematuria. A low-grade fever (less than 101°F) may be present. Explore the symptoms by determining their onset, frequency, and duration and the presence of internal or external burning on urination. Most lower UTIs have an abrupt onset of symptoms of frequency and urgency of urination, internal burning, and, perhaps, cramping with urination. They are usually of short duration. Nocturia, suprapubic pain, and mild backache may also be present. Fever, malaise, and back pain probably indicate that the infection has extended beyond the lower urinary tract. Dysuria can indicate acute bacterial cystitis or acute urethritis or both. It can also be associated with gonorrhea, chlamydia, herpes, or vaginitis. Pain with urination can also be related to an allergic reaction to an irritating substance.

Bladder tenderness indicates a lower UTI. The bladder should, therefore, be palpated on all women who present with possible lower UTI. Pelvic examination is essential, noting urethral discharge; vaginal erythema, discharge, or atrophy; and presence of vesicles, cervical discharge, or cervical tenderness with motion.

Urethral infection presents with similar symptoms to lower UTI; however, urinalysis reveals a lower-than-expected colony count and only a few WBCs present in the urine. These women are presenting before true bladder infection has occurred and should be treated as if a lower UTI were present.

Determine the patient's history of previous lower UTIs and recent urinary catheterizations. A UTI that recurs after less than 2 weeks is probably a relapsing infection or a persistent infection. History should reveal if a woman is pregnant, menopausal, or perimenopausal. She should also be asked about diabetes, immunocompromising diseases, and sickle cell trait or disease because these women are at higher risk for renal necrosis (Fig. 10–3).

Diagnostic Tests

Urine Culture and Sensitivity: This test shows greater than 5 WBCs per high-power field and the presence of bacteria without many squamous epithelial cells. The traditional criterion for infection is a colony count of more than 10^5 organisms per milliliter. However, as few as 10,000 colonies have been known to produce symptoms in women. Test results will reveal the causative organism.

Enzymatic (Dipstick) Testing: This is a less reliable but effective method of screening. Dipstick testing with reagent strips indicates hematuria, nitrites indicate presence of bacteria, and leukocyte esterase indicates presence of WBCs. After examination, urine should be sent for culture and sensitivity.

Differential Diagnosis: Sexually transmitted diseases, vaginitis, and lack of estrogen can cause irritation of the perineum with symptoms suggesting UTI. In these cases, pain with urination is pain created by urine touching irritated external genitalia. Other disorders causing similar symptoms include fungal infection

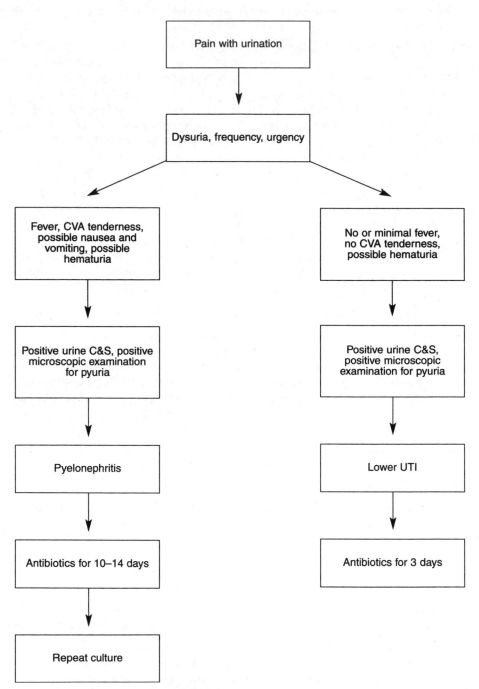

FIGURE 10–3 Urinary tract infection.

of the urethra and bladder, tuberculosis of the bladder, malignancy, interstitial cystitis, and side effects of chemotherapy or radiation therapy. High fever, restlessness, and marked costovertebral angle (CVA) tenderness suggest urinary obstruction or upper UTI.

Treatment: Treatment should be initiated when clinical evidence suggests lower UTI even before results of urine culture are available. Studies show that a 3-day treatment regimen for uncomplicated lower UTI is effective. A single-dose regimen is less effective. See Table 10–1 for recommended antibiotics for therapy. Treatment is chosen based upon cost, safety, side effects, effect on bowel and vaginal flora, and patient allergy. Treatment should also include the recommendation to increase intake of fluids. Intravaginal estrogen may be a recommendation for perimenopausal or postmenopausal women.

Follow-up: Repeat urinalysis after completion of treatment if you suspect persistent lower UTI.

Sequelae: In approximately 30% of cases of sustained bladder infection, further extension of the infection through the ureters to the kidneys can occur.

Prevention/Prophylaxis: Voiding after intercourse and decreased use of spermicide and diaphragm may be helpful in some women. Intravaginal estrogen in perimenopausal and postmenopausal women markedly reduces the incidence of UTIs.

Referral: Refer patients who experience relapse (a recurrence of symptoms of infection after a completed course of antibiotics); pregnant women; women who have a history of pyelonephritis or a chronic disease such as diabetes, suspected renal calculi, or interstitial cystitis; and women who frequently use catheters.

For patients who experience reinfection (infection that occurs weeks or months after treatment of previous lower UTI), referral is recommended only if infections are more frequent than three per year.

Education: Normal voiding eliminates some organisms; not voiding after intercourse may contribute to an increase in lower UTI in some women.

| Urinary Incontinence

Urinary incontinence (UI) is the involuntary loss of urine that results in a social or hygienic problem.

Etiology: Neurologic and/or musculofascial damage.

Occurrence: Approximately 20% of women between 25 and 64 years experience UI.

Age: Of perimenopausal women, 31% report incontinent episodes at least once per month; 46% of women in the age group of 35–44 years; and 60% of women in the age group 45–54. Severity of stress incontinence increases with age.

Ethnicity: Not significant.

Contributing Factors: Women who have delivered vaginally are 2.5 times more likely to report incontinence than women who have never been pregnant. The rate of reported incontinence increases with the number of vaginal deliveries; 38% of mothers report UI after one delivery, 57% after two vaginal births, and 73% after three vaginal births (Sampselle et al., 1997).

Signs and Symptoms: There are three types of urinary incontinence:

Stress UI: Loss of urine during coughing, sneezing, laughing, or physical exercise.

Urge UI: A strong desire to void that is sometimes associated with involuntary detrusor contraction.

Mixed UI: A combination of stress and urge UI (Fig. 10–4).

Diagnostic Tests: Urinalysis, urine culture and sensitivity, pelvic examination.

Differential Diagnosis: UTI diagnosed by urine culture and sensitivity; atrophic vaginitis diagnosed by pelvic examination; urethritis determined by urinalysis, urine culture and sensitivity, and pelvic examination.

Treatment: The treatment of choice for UI includes bladder training and pelvic muscle exercise. Bladder training consists of providing the woman with information about normal bladder function and use of a voiding schedule. The woman is asked to keep a 24-hour voiding schedule and from this a desired initial voiding schedule is established. The initial voiding schedule should match the average frequency (or leakage) of urine demonstrated in the diary. For example, if the average urinary frequency is every 60 minutes, the initial voiding schedule should be every 60 minutes. Systematic delay in voiding is accomplished through distraction and relaxation techniques. The interval between urination is gradually increased until voiding, ideally, occurs every 3–4 hours.

Pelvic muscle exercise, also called Kegel exercise, in recognition of the physician who recommended its use, is a technique that strengthens the supportive pelvic floor muscles. Thirty contractions per day are recommended.

PELVIC MUSCLE CONTRACTIONS OR KEGEL EXERCISE: IDEAL PELVIC MUSCLE CONTRACTIONS HAVE THE FOLLOWING:

- Pelvic floor contracts upward and inward.
- Anus pulls inward and lifts upward.
- Contraction is of moderate to nearly maximum level of intensity.
- Bearing-down or straining-down effort is absent.
- Thigh muscle contraction is absent.
- Gluteal muscle contraction is absent.
- Contraction is held for at least 3 seconds, building to a hold of 10 seconds.
- At least 10 seconds of relaxation is allowed between contractions.

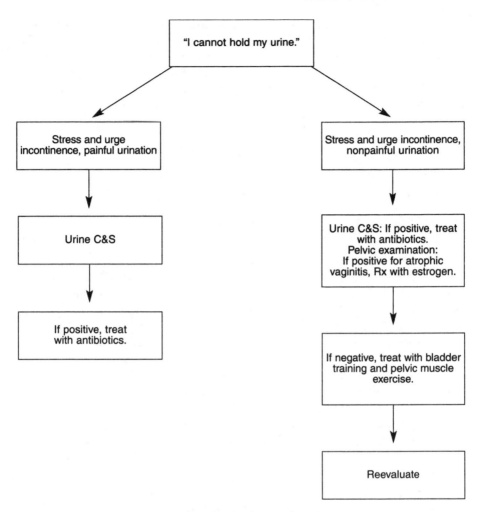

FIGURE 10–4   Urinary incontinence.

Bladder training and pelvic muscle exercises are effective in reducing stress incontinence in women with mild to moderate symptoms. The combination of these two therapies in no way jeopardizes future therapy if referral is necessary.

Follow-up: Several weeks are required before improvement can be expected. Follow-up visits can be scheduled at monthly intervals for 4 months to monitor progress.

Sequelae: Of women who complete a 3-month pelvic exercise program, 56% had a greater than 50% improvement in the number of incontinent episodes.

Prevention/Prophylaxis: Diuretics and caffeine can cause urgency, frequency, and incontinence. Anticholingerics can impair detrusor contractility, resulting in overflow incontinence. Alpha-adrenergic blockers can cause incontinence through lowering urethral tone.

Referral: Minimal or no improvement in symptoms following 16 weeks of therapy is an indication for referral. Refer any women with a positive history of any neurologic deficit, including multiple sclerosis, stroke, or spinal cord injury. Some women are unable to execute even a weak pelvic muscle contraction or cannot implement bladder training and will require referral.

Referral should be made to a health-care provider with specialized knowledge of incontinence. These providers are skilled in the use of supplemental equipment such as vaginal weights, biofeedback, and electrical stimulation. To find such health-care providers, call the National Association for Continence (800-252-3337).

Education: For further information on UI, see the list of agencies in the Appendix.

Viral Hepatitis

Viral hepatitis is a contagious disease estimated to affect more than 500,000 people in the United States each year according to the Centers for Disease Control (CDC). The majority of women infected are either asymptomatic or minimally symptomatic, but a number of women develop serious clinical illness and several thousand die from the disease each year.

Five distinct types of viral hepatitis have been identified: A, B, C, D, and E. Among urban adults with diagnosed hepatitis, 50% have hepatitis B, 15%–30% have hepatitis C, and the remainder have hepatitis A. Prevention of hepatitis requires an understanding of the modes of transmission, periods of communicability, and the use of globulins and vaccines (Table 10–2).

Etiology: Hepatitis is a viral disease. Types A and E are transmitted by fecal-oral route. Type B results from parenteral exposure and/or intimate contact. Type C is the predominant type occurring after transfusion. Type D requires coinfection with hepatitis B.

Occurrence: Hepatitis affects more than 500,000 people in the United States each year. The number of chronic carriers of hepatitis is unknown.

Age: In a study of 6253 pregnant women infected with hepatitis B or C, the incidence of hepatitis B infection was significantly higher in women older than 30 years of age (Alvarez-Munoz et al., 1997).

Ethnicity: Not significant.

Contributing Factors: Handling of infected blood or body fluids, risk of transmission by sexual contact, IV drug use, fecal-oral contamination.

Signs and Symptoms: Acute viral hepatitis is usually a self-limiting illness; 85% of hospital patients and 95% of outpatients with the disease recover completely and uneventfully within 3 months. The majority of women with acute viral infection never become jaundiced. Symptoms include malaise, anorexia, nausea, vomiting, changes in taste and smell, low-grade fever, right upper quadrant discomfort, and fatigue. In 5%–10% of patients with acute hepatitis B, urticaria,

TABLE 10-2 HEPATITIS

Type	Transmission	Chronicity	Susceptibility	Incubation	Facts for Women	Immunity
A	Fecal-Oral	No	Children and adolescents are most susceptible to infection.	30 days	More than 80% of women over age 60 test positive for the antibody to Hep A.	Exposure to Hep A creates an antibody that confers life-long immunity. Initially, the anti-Hep A antibody is IgM, during convalescence it is IgG.
B	Parental, perinatal, and sexual contact. The virus has been found in women's saliva, vaginal secretions, and breast milk.	Yes; approx. 1%–2% of women with clinical disease develop chronic infections.	Spouses of people with Hep B, women with multiple sexual partners, health-care personnel, infants by vertical transmission from from their mothers	12 wks	A large number of infected women never experience apparent illness, making the actual number of chronic cares unknown. Many women are asymptomatic carriers.	Hep B vaccine available
C	Parental, perinatal, vertical transmission rate 18%	Yes	IV drug abusers, intimate contact with infected persons, infants by vertical transmission from their mothers, infants via breast feeding, recipients of transfusions not screened for Hep C	Similar to Hep B		Assays for antibodies turn positive during infection and remain so.
D	Coexists with Hep B	Yes	IV drug abusers, intimate contact with infected persons, infants by vertical transmission from their mothers	Similar to Hep B		Vaccination for Hep B eliminates Hep D.
E	Fecal-oral (found primarily in India and Asia)	?	Younger adults rather than children are affected.	40 days	Pregnant women with Hep E have a high mortality rate.	Unknown

arthralgia, fever, and polyarticular arthritis occur. Hepatitis A and E are the viruses most likely to produce cholestatic disease with jaundice and pruritus.

Diagnostic Tests: The antibody for hepatitis A can be detected in serum. Sensitive screening tests exist for the hepatitis B antibody. Testing can determine chronic versus acute disease. Direct testing for hepatitis C antibody exists. Presence of an antibody to hepatitis D can be detected (Fig. 10–5).

Differential Diagnosis: Nonspecific viral syndrome, drug-induced hepatitis, nonviral hepatitis (an autoimmune mechanism seen in women ages 20–40.)

Treatment: Hepatitis is usually treated on an outpatient basis with diet and decreased activity levels. The diet consists of small, frequent meals; adequate calorie intake; and no alcohol. Activity is as tolerated, with increased rest. Hepatitis

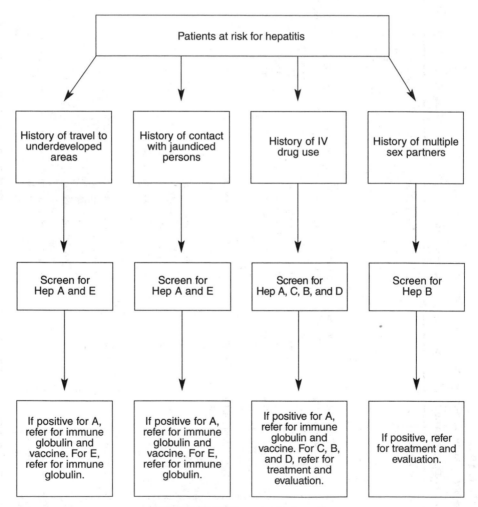

FIGURE 10–5 Screening for hepatitis.

often affects previously active people. Prolonged malaise can lead to depression (see Table 10–2).

Follow-up: After early diagnosis, office visits at 1- to 2-week intervals for evaluation of symptoms and laboratory work.

Sequelae: Acute disease can develop into overwhelming liver cell necrosis and liver failure. This result is most often seen in hepatitis B, but the incidence is also high in pregnant women with hepatitis E.

Chronic hepatitis (not with A or E) occurs with hepatitis infection. The likelihood is higher when acute infection occurs in an immunocompromised host or when the infection occurs at birth. Clinical manifestations of chronic disease usually are the persistence of mild symptoms. Chronic disease can lead to cirrhosis.

Pregnant women infected with hepatitis B or C pose a risk of infecting their newborns. Ever year an estimated 20,000 infants are born to women in the United States with positive hepatitis B antigen. These infants are at risk for hepatitis B infection and chronic liver disease as adults.

Prevention/Prophylaxis: Principles of prevention include minimizing exposure and the use of globulins and vaccines.

Administering immune globulin within 1–2 hours of exposure prevents hepatitis A infection. Immune globulin is 80% effective in preventing clinical disease in nonimmunized individuals. For household contacts and small groups experiencing a common source of outbreak, begin immune globulin prophylaxis and hepatitis A vaccine. Restrict intimate contact and encourage careful hand washing. Routine immunoprophylaxis is not necessary for casual contacts. The CDC recommends administering hepatitis A vaccine to users of illegal injected and noninjected drugs.

To prevent hepatitis B, provide a susceptible person with a protective antibody. Immune globulins containing anti–hepatitis B are given along with the hepatitis vaccine. Hepatitis B vaccine is recommended routinely prior to exposure. Screen for hepatitis B in all pregnant women. Administer the vaccine to all newborns.

Immune globulin and hepatitis B vaccine have not proved to be effective in preventing hepatitis C infection.

Prevention of hepatitis B infection also prevents hepatitis D infection.

Hepatitis E has no immunoprophylaxis available.

Referral: A diagnosis of viral hepatitis requires referral to a medical provider.

Education: Teach the patient the following guidelines:

Hepatitis A and E

- Practice hand washing after the use of the toilet.
- Avoid intimate contact with infected people.
- Infected women should not handle or serve food to others.
- Give immune globulin and/or vaccine to household contacts and people traveling to areas known to have an increased incidence of the disease.

Hepatitis B

- Screen blood donors.
- Follow universal precautions for handling materials that may be infected with hepatitis B.
- Use proper hand washing after direct contact with infected people.
- Avoid intimate contact with infected people.
- All three doses of the vaccine should be received—initial dose, followed by second dose at 1 month, and third dose at 6 months.
- Universal vaccination of all newborns.
- Globulin injection given to nonimmune individuals after exposure.

Hepatitis C precautions are the same as for hepatitis B, and vaccination against hepatitis B prevents hepatitis D.

BIBLIOGRAPHY

General

Goroll, A, May, L, and Mulley, A: Primary Care Medicine. Lippincott, Philadelphia, 1995.
Havens, C, Sullivan, N, and Tilton, P: Manual of Outpatient Gynecology. Little, Brown, Boston, 1988.
Ostergard, D, and Bent, A: Urogynecology and Urodynamics, Theory and Practice. Williams & Wilkins, Baltimore, 1996.

Acute Pyelonephritis

Miller, L, and Cox, S: Urinary tract infections complicating pregnancy. Infect Dis Clin North Am 11(3):13–26, 1997.

Asymptomatic Bacteriuria

Devereaux Melillo, K: Asymptomatic bacteriuria in older adults: When is it necessary to treat? Nurse Pract 20(8):50–68, 1995.
Patterson, T, and Andriole, V: Detection, significance, and therapy of bacteriuria in pregnancy. Infect Dis Clin North Am 11(3):593–599, 1997.

Cystitis

Freeman, S: Common genitourinary infections. JOGNN, 24(8):735–741, 1995.
Hooton, T: Association of acute cystitis with the stage of the menstrual cycle in young women. Clin Infect Dis 23:635, 1996.
Pollen, J: Short term curse for uncomplicated cystitis. Contemp Nurse Pract 1(4):21–30, 1995.

Interstitial Cystitis

Nigro, D, Wein, A, et al: Associations among cystoscopic and urodynamic findings for women enrolled in the Interstitial Cystitis Data Base Study. Urology 49(5A suppl):86–92, 1997.

Symptomatic Lower Urinary Tract Infection

Barger, M, and Woolner, B: Primary care for women: Assessment and management of genitourinary tract disorders. J Nurse Midwif 40(2):231–238, 1995.
Hooton, T, and Stamm, W: Diagnosis and treatment of uncomplicated urinary tract infection. Infect Dis Clin North Am 11(3):551–561, 1997.
Leiner, S: Recurrent urinary tract infection in otherwise healthy women. Nurse Pract 20(2):48–55, 1995.

Urinary Incontinence

Sampselle, C, et al: Continence for women: Evidence based practice. JOGNN 26(4):375–388, 1997.

Viral Hepatitis

Alvarez-Munoz, MT, et al: Infection of pregnant women with hepatitis B and C viruses and risks of vertical transmission. Arch Med Res 28(3):415, 1997.

Balayan, MS: Epidemiology of hepatitis E virus infection. J Viral Hepatitis 4(3):155–165, 1997.

Freitag-Koontz, MJ: Prevention of hepatitis B and C transmission during pregnancy and the first year of life. J Perinat Neonat Nursing 10(2):40–55, 1996.

Hunt, CM: Hepatitis C in pregnancy. Obstet Gynecol 89:883, 1997.

Muller, R: The natural history of hepatitis C: Clinical experiences. J Hepatol, 24(2):52–54, 1996.

Centers for Disease Control and Prevention: 1998 Guidelines for Treatment of Sexually Transmitted Disease. Centers for Disease Control and Prevention, Atlanta, 1998.

CHAPTER 11

MUSCULOSKELETAL

Many autoimmune and connective tissue diseases affect young and middle-aged women. The role of the women's health nurse practitioner (NP) is to detect and refer for diagnosis and therapy disorders of the musculoskeletal system that affect women. This chapter discusses screening and evaluation for diseases that frequently occur in women—fibromyalgia, osteoporosis, rheumatoid arthritis, and systemic lupus erythematosus.

Assessment

- Musculoskeletal assessment requires careful attention to the distribution of joints involved. Musculoskeletal disorders vary in the joints in which they typically present.
- Inflammation of the joints must be noted (Fig. 11–1).
- Duration of symptoms is an important part of assessment. Some disorders have prolonged symptoms, and some are episodic with acute attacks that resolve in time.
- Range of motion must be evaluated.
- Radiographs are helpful in revealing characteristic changes. Laboratory results are often supportive of a diagnosis, but not diagnostic. Diagnoses of musculoskeletal disorders are made primarily based on history and physical examination.

Women's health NPs must be aware of the musculoskeletal disorders that commonly affect women. Appropriate referral for evaluation and treatment flows from such knowledge. Providers of care for women must be aware of osteoporosis, since the prevention of fractures resulting from osteoporosis is a goal for every woman's health NP.

156

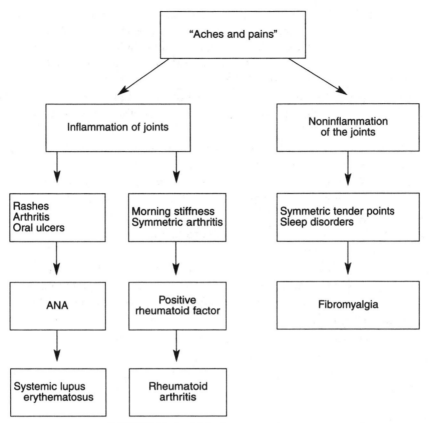

FIGURE 11–1 Multiple joint pain in women.

Fibromyalgia

Fibromyalgia, a common soft tissue pain syndrome seen in women, is a chronic, but not a progressive, disease.

Etiology: Unknown.

Occurrence: Of people with fibromyalgia, 80%–90% are women. It occurs in 2%–5% of the female population.

Age: Fibromyalgia usually affects young and middle-aged women.

Ethnicity: Not significant.

Contributing Factors: Change in weather exacerbates symptoms of fibromyalgia.

Signs and Symptoms: Diffuse aches and pains. Typically, the woman has difficulty localizing her chief complaint. There is an underlying sleep disorder in this disease. The woman complains of overwhelming daytime fatigue. Women have difficulty falling asleep and difficulty staying asleep. Women may also have symptoms of irritable bowel syndrome and cystitis in the absence of infection. Dysmenorrhea can accompany fibromyalgia. Examination reveals paired tender points. The points will be symmetric. Other than the tender points, the musculoskeletal examination will be normal.

Diagnostic Tests: No single test or combination of tests makes the diagnosis. The diagnosis is made clinically, based on history and physical examination and exclusion of other disorders.

Differential Diagnosis: Rheumatoid arthritis, Lyme disease, overuse syndrome, chronic fatigue syndrome, hypothyroidism, and depression.

Treatment: Improve the underlying sleep disorder with medication. Cardiovascular fitness training, which raises the pain threshold, is an important part of the treatment program.

Follow-up: Fibromyalgia is a chronic disease that requires a lifetime of close follow-up evaluation and care.

Sequelae: Fibromyalgia is a chronic disease. Symptoms increase and decrease based upon changes in the weather, degree of stress, and amount of rest. The number and location of tender points appear to be stable throughout time.

Prevention/Prophylaxis: None.

Referral: Diagnosis and treatment should be under the direction of a physician.

Education: A program to improve physical fitness is important to the therapy. Such a program must be designed specific to the woman's life-style.

| Osteoporosis

Osteoporosis is a systemic skeletal disorder characterized by low bone mass and structural deterioration of bone, resulting in bone fragility and an increased risk for fracture.

Etiology: Multifactorial, related to osteoclastic resorption of bone. When bone formation does not keep pace with bone resorption, osteopenia and osteoporosis result. Bone strength is directly proportional to its density.

Occurrence: Approximately 1 in 10 people in the United States has osteoporosis; 80% are women; 150,000–250,000 hip fractures occur annually in women over 65. More than 1 million fractures in women occur per year because of this disease.

Ethnicity: White or Asian women are at increased risk for osteoporosis.

Age: Women at age 50 have a 40% lifetime fracture risk. Risk increases with age. Skeletal mass begins to decline in women past age 40. The rate of decline is most rapid within 2 years after menopause.

Contributing Factors
- Family history
- Thin body mass

- Smoking
- Low calcium intake
- Anorexia or bulimia
- Physical inactivity
- Alcoholism
- Use of corticosteroids
- Early menopause
- Excessive exercise inducing amenorrhea

Signs and Symptoms: Osteoporosis is asymptomatic until fracture occurs. Fracture occurs with minor trauma. Spinal osteoporosis creates multiple compression fractures over time, thus creating the classic "dowager's hump" of osteoporosis.

Diagnostic Tests: Bone mineral density can be tested for at several skeletal sites. Women at risk should be tested. Tests to measure bone density are safe and acceptable to most women. Fracture risk can be predicted from bone density testing; 30% of bone mass loss is required before a standard radiograph can diagnose osteopenia (reduced amount of bone). Testing for bone loss should be done, therefore, with x-ray absorptiometry or computed tomography (CT) scan (see Appendix).

Treatment: The best treatment is prevention. The goal is to reduce the risk of fracture by reducing loss of bone mass. If fracture has occurred, symptomatic relief and aggressive therapy to prevent further bone loss are indicated.

Follow-up: Osteoporosis is a chronic disease that requires close follow-up throughout the woman's life.

Sequelae: Fractures necessitate prolonged hospitalization and surgery with the resulting risks. Of women with hip fractures, 15%–25% require long-term nursing home placement.

Prevention/Prophylaxis
- Calcium supplementation, in doses of 1.5–2 g daily, reduces bone loss. Calcium can be found in many food sources or can be supplemented with over-the-counter preparations. Calcium supplements should be consumed with meals to increase their absorption.
- Hormone replacement therapy is the treatment of choice for postmenopausal osteoporosis. Estrogen reduces bone loss and decreases fractures. The dose required to reduce bone loss is 0.625 mg daily. (Estrogen must be given with progesterone if the woman's uterus is present. Progesterone does not alter the therapeutic effect of estrogen.) There is an unclear risk of breast cancer related to the use of postmenopausal estrogen. Adverse effects of estrogen include migraine headaches, cholelithiasis, and thrombosis. It is unknown whether adding calcium to the estrogen regimen reduces the amount of estrogen needed for the desired result.
- Exercise plays an important role in preventive therapy. Exercise and physical activity increase skeletal mass. Regular weight-bearing exercise can reduce bone loss.

- Antiresorptive drugs bind to bone mineral and inhibit resorption. In this way, the drug acts to increase density and reduce fracture.
- Refer to Figure 11–2.

Referral: Fractures must be referred to a physician.

Education: There is no universal agreement regarding which women should consider estrogen replacement therapy for osteoporosis. Cardiovascular benefits

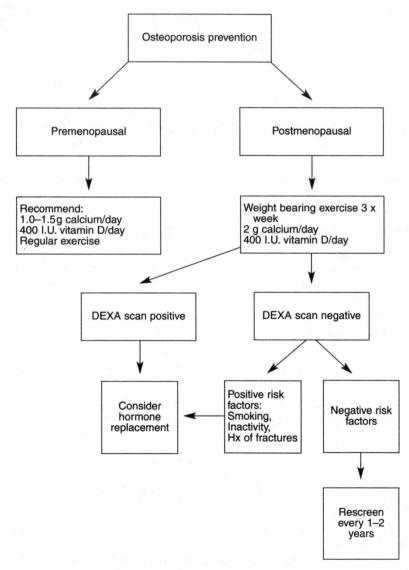

FIGURE 11–2   Osteoporosis prevention.

and cancer risks must be weighed by the NP and the woman at risk. Women who are at risk for osteoporosis must weigh all factors before deciding on estrogen therapy. Postmenopausal women should be taught how to reduce the risk of falling. The home environment should be evaluated for risk of falls.

Rheumatoid Arthritis

Rheumatoid arthritis (RA) is a systemic, immunologically mediated, chronic, and potentially disabling disease.

Etiology: Unknown.

Occurrence: RA is probably the most common cause of chronic inflammatory arthritis, affecting 1%–2% of the general population. Approximately 75% of those affected are women.

Age: Prevalence increases with age. Incidence peaks in the fourth decade.

Ethnicity: Not significant.

Contributing Factors: There is a genetic predisposition to RA.

Signs and Symptoms: Joint stiffness after inactivity is the hallmark of the chronic inflammation associated with this disease. Stiffness occurs in the morning upon awakening and after sitting for long periods. The small joints of the feet and hands are involved. Eventually nearly every joint in the body becomes involved. On physical examination, the joints are "boggy" because of underlying synovitis. RA is a systemic disease and may involve multiple organ systems. The woman may experience low-grade fever, fatigue, and mild weight loss.

SYMPTOMS OF RA

- Morning stiffness
- Pain involving at least three joints
- Symptoms lasting more than 6 weeks
- Serum rheumatoid factor elevated
- Radiologic changes consistent with RA

Diagnostic Tests: Of women with this disease, 80%–85% have detectable rheumatoid factor in their blood. Radiographs of the hands, wrists, and feet are helpful in establishing the diagnosis.

Differential Diagnoses: Osteoarthritis, spondyloarthropathies, gout, Lyme disease, fibromyalgia, tendinitis, and bursitis.

Treatment: RA is treated with corticosteroids and nonsteroidal anti-inflammatory drugs (NSAIDs). At times, surgery is required for treatment.

INSTRUCTIONS FOR THE WOMAN TAKING NSAIDs
- Always take with food.
- Notify provider of abdominal pain or change in bowel movement.
- Avoid aspirin.
- Have blood tested regularly as advised by a doctor.

Follow-up: RA is a chronic disease that requires close follow-up throughout the woman's life. Several issues exist for women with RA who require surgery of any type. Pregnancy with RA requires close follow-up.

Sequelae: The clinical course is one of remissions and exacerbations. Approximately 40% of women diagnosed experience disability within 10 years. Some women experience a self-limiting disease and others suffer a chronic progressive illness.

Prevention/Prophylaxis: None.

Referral: RA is a chronic systemic disease. Therapy must be designed and provided by a physician. A team of care providers that involves an NP, physical therapist, and occupational therapist is a preferable referral source.

Education: Patient education deals primarily with dismissing misconceptions while emphasizing minimizing discomfort and preserving function.

Systemic Lupus Erythematosus

Systemic lupus erythematosus (SLE) is a multisystem disease associated with the production of multiple autoantibodies.

Etiology: Unknown.

Occurrence: More common in women than in men, with a 9:1 ratio.

Ethnicity: More common in African-American and Asian women than in white or Hispanic women.

Age: SLE is most common in women of childbearing age.

Contributing Factors: Genetic, environmental, and hormonal.

Signs and Symptoms
- Arthritis occurs in 76%–88% of the cases (joint involvement similar to that of RA). Arthritis is systemic and inflammatory, involving multiple joints.
- Rashes, including the classic butterfly rash occurring across the nose and on the cheeks. Rashes come and go without scarring.
- Painless oral ulcerations.
- Alopecia.
- Fever, fatigue, weight loss.

Diagnostic Tests: ANA is a useful screening test (greater than 95% sensitive for SLE).

Differential Diagnosis: ANA is positive in RA, thyroiditis, chronic infection, and malignancy.

Treatment: NSAIDs for arthritis, corticosteroids.

Follow-up: SLE is a chronic disease that requires close follow-up after diagnosis.

Sequelae: Ovarian failure related to steroids, renal disease, neuropsychiatric lupus, hypertension, leukopenia, hemolytic anemia, and thrombocytopenia.

Prevention/Prophylaxis: None.

Referral: Refer for diagnosis and treatment. Pregnancy, use of oral contraceptives, or estrogen replacement therapy combined with SLE requires referral.

Education: Avoidance of the sun and use of sunscreen should be advised.

BIBLIOGRAPHY

Barth, W: Office evaluation of the patient with musculoskeletal complaints. Am J Med 102(1A):3S–10S, 1997.

Belilios, E, and Carsons, S: Rheumatologic disorders in women. Med Clin North Am 81(1):77–101, 1998.

Callahan, L, Rao, J, and Boutaugh, M: Arthritis and women's health prevalence, impact and prevention. Am J Prev Med 12(5):401–409, 1996.

Morbidity and Mortality Weekly Report: Prevalence and impact of arthritis among women—United States 1989–1991. Mortality Weekly Report 44(27):517, 1995.

Schaefer, K: Health patterns of women with fibromyalgia. J Adv Nursing 26(3):565, 1997.

CHAPTER 12

PERIPHERAL

VASCULAR

Assessment of the peripheral vascular system is an important component in providing care for women because it can reveal underlying disorders that require referral and treatment. Prevention and treatment of thrombus and prevention of cardiovascular disease are two goals in women's health care. This chapter discusses screening for hyperlipidemia and thrombophlebitis.

Assessment

- All pulses should be palpated at every woman's health examination. (Include the radial, brachial, femoral, popliteal, dorsalis pedis, and posterior tibial arteries.)
- Note the temperature of the feet and legs.
- An important ominous clinical sign is edema of the legs. Compare one leg to the other, noting presence of edema (Fig. 12–1).
- Note the color of the extremities and the presence of ulcers or varicose veins.

Hyperlipidemia

Evidence has accumulated demonstrating that treating hyperlipidemia can reduce atherosclerosis and its resultant cardiovascular complications. The presence of hyperlipidemia does not guarantee the formation of plaques, nor does the absence of

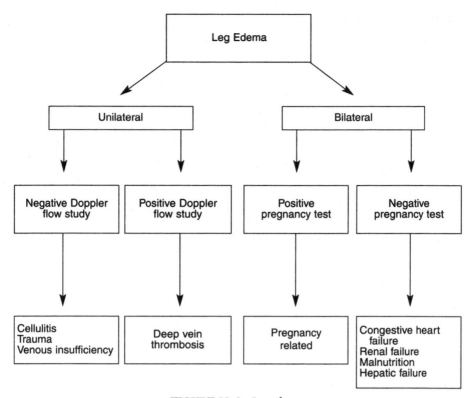

FIGURE 12-1 Leg edema.

excessive lipids reassure against them. Multiple factors create an atherosclerotic condition. The presence of hyperlipidemia requires further evaluation for total cardiovascular risk assessment.

Etiology: Lipoproteins are a combination of lipids such as cholesterol and triglycerides combined with proteins that enable circulation. Lipoprotein can have either low or high density. Low-density lipoproteins (LDLs), the major carriers of cholesterol, are clearly present in atherosclerosis. High-density lipoproteins (HDLs) are believed to function in peripheral tissue as acceptors of cholesterol, which is then diffused out of cell membranes. The proportion of HDL to LDL is an important factor in evaluation of risk for atherosclerosis. Women with high HDL and low LDL have a reduced risk for developing cardiovascular disease.

Occurrence: Elevated or borderline cholesterol levels are present in 20%–30% of women.

Age: Cholesterol levels increase with age. Women carry a higher portion of HDL until menopause, after which the risk for cardiovascular disease rises to the same level as men.

Ethnicity: Not significant.

Contributing Factors

- Genetic variations in lipoprotein structure, metabolic enzymes, and inter-action between lipids and the cell wall.
- Dietary fat and cholesterol intake have a substantial influence on serum cholesterol and LDL levels. Saturated fat in the diet is most noted to affect cholesterol and LDL levels.
- Postmenopausal estrogen replacement therapy increases HDL and lowers LDL level.

Diagnostic Tests: A single measurement should never be used for diagnosis of hy-perlipidemia. Total cholesterol measurement that is borderline or elevated re-quires a lipid profile (Table 12–1 gives the National Cholesterol Program guide-lines). Lipid profile includes total cholesterol, triglyceride, HDL, and LDL levels.

Signs and Symptoms: Hyperlipidemia causes no symptoms. Diagnosis is made through blood screening.

Differential Diagnosis: Hypothyroidism, nephrotic syndrome, and diabetes sec-ondarily lead to hyperlipidemia. Certain drugs can affect lipid levels as well. Beta blockers are an example (Fig. 12–2).

Treatment: Lipid abnormality is a component of total cardiovascular disease risk. Hyperlipidemia can be treated with dietary modifications, exercise, and weight reduction. Pharmacologic therapy is reserved for women in the highest overall risk category.

Follow-up: A diagnosis of hyperlipidemia requires at least annual follow-up. The total cardiovascular risk assessment may necessitate closer follow-up.

Prevention/Prophylaxis: The goal is to reduce coronary morbidity and mortality by reducing the risk for the first coronary event.

Referral: Risk is evaluated based on hyperlipidemia plus blood pressure, smoking, diabetes, family history, age, and presence or absence of cardiovascular disease. Women with hyperlipidemia should be referred for evaluation of risk for car-diovascular disease.

TABLE 12–1 NATIONAL CHOLESTEROL PROGRAM GUIDELINES

	Cholesterol (mg/dL)	LDL (mg/dL)	Recommendations
Desirable	<200	<130	Repeat within 5 years.
Borderline	200–239	130–159	Dietary information and lipid profile, with referral based on results.
Elevated	≥ 240	≥ 160	Refer.

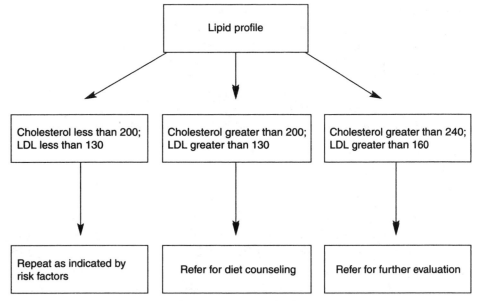

FIGURE 12–2 Hyperlipidemia.

Education: Treatment for hyperlipidemia requires a change in eating and exercise habits. Careful education and monitoring of behavior are required for successful intervention.

Thrombophlebitis

Superficial thrombophlebitis occurs almost always in a varicose vein because of static blood flow. Deep venous thrombosis is an acute thrombus formation. It varies in clinical presentation and is potentially life-threatening.

Etiology: The cause of acute thrombus formation in the venous system is unclear. In most instances thrombus formation is related to damage, stasis, and hypercoagulability.

Occurrence: Venous thrombophlebitis can occur following gynecologic surgery. Studies report that 40% of deaths following pelvic surgery are attributable to venous thrombosis and pulmonary embolus.

Age: The frequency of venous thrombosis increases with age. Venous thrombosis is reported most often in women over 50 years of age.

Ethnicity: Not significant.

Contributing Factors: Varicose veins, sedentary lifestyle, obesity, hypertension, diabetes, pelvic surgery, duration of pelvic surgery, prolonged immobilization, malignancy, hypercoagulable states, and estrogen therapy.

Signs and Symptoms
- Localized warmth, redness, tenderness, and swelling of the extremity.
- Pain in the limb that increases with movement.
- Positive Homan's sign (pain with dorsiflexion of the foot).
- Clinical findings for thrombus are not specific. When thrombosis is suspected, noninvasive testing should be performed. Diagnosis based on history and physical examination alone is reported to be correct only 50% of the time.

Diagnostic Tests: Doppler ultrasound studies enhanced with color flow technology.

Differential Diagnosis: Varicose veins, venous insufficiency.

Treatment: Prophylaxis is preferable to treatment. Thrombosis in a deep vein is treated with anticoagulants. Superficial thrombosis is treated with analgesics, anti-inflammatory medication, elevation, and rest.

Follow-up: Thrombus formation requires close follow-up for evaluation of underlying disorders. Prevention of further episodes is imperative.

Sequelae: Calf vein thrombosis is generally associated with a good prognosis. Thrombosis above the knee is associated with pulmonary embolism.

Prevention/Prophylaxis: Thromboembolitic deterrent stockings (TEDS), heparin therapy prior to pelvic surgery.

Referral: Thrombus formation above the knee requires immediate referral and subsequent hospitalization. Deep vein thrombosis below the knee requires referral for evaluation, treatment, and close follow-up.

Education: The clinical symptom that most closely correlates with diagnosis of thrombosis is unilateral leg swelling. All women should be informed of the significance of this finding. Pain may or may not be present with the swelling.

BIBLIOGRAPHY

Brochier, M, and Arwidson, PA: Coronary heart disease risk factors in women. Eur Heart J 19(Suppl A):45–52, 1998.

Goroll, A, May, L, and Mulley, A: Primary Care Medicine. Lippincott, Philadelphia, 1995.

Martins, I, et al: Smoking, consumption of alcohol and sedentary life style in population grouping and their relationships with lipidemic disorders. Rev Saude Publica 29(1):38–45, 1995.

Seltzer, V, and Pearse, W: Women's Primary Health Care. McGraw-Hill, New York, 1995.

Walsh, J, and Grady, D: Treatment of hyperlipidemia in women. JAMA 274(14):1152, 1995.

CHAPTER **13**

ENDOCRINE,

METABOLIC, AND

NUTRITIONAL

This chapter discusses the assessment and referral of women who have a disorder related to the endocrine system or a metabolic disorder, including those related to nutrition. The discussion includes thyroid disorders, diabetes, primary amenorrhea, hirsutism, premenstrual syndrome, obesity, anorexia nervosa, and bulimia.

Endocrine disorders affect menstrual function. A woman presenting with menstrual dysfunction may, therefore, have an underlying endocrine disorder. The presentation of endocrine disease often differs between women and men. This chapter focuses on clinical presentations in which endocrine disorders must be considered. The physiology of menstruation, infertility, and menopause are discussed in other sections of the book, as are menstrual disorders.

Assessment

Recognition of a possible endocrine or metabolic disorder is an important nurse practitioner (NP) function. Height and weight, an important part of every examination, are simple screening tools for endocrine disorders as well as for obesity, anorexia, and bulimia.

The presence of age-appropriate secondary sex characteristics should be ver-

169

ified at the first visit to an NP. Breast development indicates active estrogen. Pubic and axillary hair indicate active androgens (see Table 5–1). The lack of secondary sex characteristics after age 13 requires referral to a reproductive endocrinologist. Development of secondary sex characteristics prior to age 8, called precocious development, also requires referral to a reproductive endocrinologist. Lack of menses in women more than 16 years old with normal secondary sex characteristics requires referral. After 16 years of age, lack of menses may indicate a difficulty with the genital tract or a failure of the hypothalamic-pituitary-ovarian axis to interact appropriately. Abnormal distribution of body hair may also indicate endocrine dysfunction. Hirsutism indicates increased androgen production.

Primary Amenorrhea

The mean age for appearance of menses, known as **menarche**, is 12 years. Girls who do not experience menses by age 16 or 17, referred to as **primary amenorrhea**, require evaluation.

Etiology: The causes of primary amenorrhea are divided into two categories: those with the absence of secondary sex characteristics, and those with the presence of secondary sex characteristics. If secondary sex characteristics are absent, etiology includes absence of ovarian estrogen, hypothalamic disease, or pituitary disease. In the presence of secondary sex characteristics, amenorrhea is related to anatomic defects, androgen insensitivity syndrome, nutritional amenorrhea, systemic disease, or hyperprolactinemia. The most common reason for primary amenorrhea is polycystic ovarian syndrome, in which a self-perpetuating state of chronic anovulation occurs. This ovulatory dysfunction involves the hypothalamus, pituitary, ovaries, adrenals, and peripheral adipose tissue.

Occurrence: Unknown.

Age: Lack of onset of menses by age 16 or 17 years.

Ethnicity: Not significant.

Contributing Factors: Amenorrhea can be exercise-induced. Body weight low enough to influence hypothalamic function is seen in middle- and long-distance runners, gymnasts, ballet dancers, and swimmers. It is also seen in women with anorexia.

Signs and Symptoms: Lack of menses, hirsutism, lack of development of secondary sex characteristics, infertility, elevated follicle-stimulating hormone (FSH) and luteinizing hormone (LH) levels (Table 13–1).

Diagnostic Tests: Careful physical examination, karyotype, FSH levels, LH levels, and serum prolactin levels. Ovarian ultrasound can assist in diagnosis.

Differential Diagnoses: Delayed physiologic menarche, Sheehan syndrome (postpartum pituitary necrosis), posttraumatic hypopituitarism, radiation-induced hy-

TABLE 13–1 PRIMARY AMENORRHEA

Diagnosis	Secondary Sex Characteristics	Serum FSH Level
Delayed menarche	Yes	Normal
Anatomic defects	Yes	Normal
Gonadal dysgenesis	No	Elevated
Ovarian-hypothalamic-pituitary disease	No	Low
Nutritional amenorrhea	Yes	?

popituitarism, Cushing's syndrome, thyroid disease, central nervous system (CNS) lesions, epilepsy, ovarian tumor.

Treatment: Estrogen replacement therapy is the most common treatment modality.

Follow-up: A reproductive endocrinologist should follow girls with primary amenorrhea.

Sequelae: Loss of bone density can occur with primary amenorrhea.

Prevention/Prophylaxis: None.

Referral: Girls should be referred to a reproductive endocrinologist if they have not experienced menses by age 16 or 17.

Education: All women should be educated concerning puberty and menarche. Teach mothers when to refer their daughters for evaluation.

Anorexia and Bulimia

Anorexia and bulimia are psychosomatic illnesses than involve extreme weight loss.

Etiology: Anorexia is related to a body image distortion and a great fear of becoming obese. Bulimia is characterized by consuming large quantities of food over a short interval (binging) followed by vomiting and/or use of laxatives or diuretics and/or restricted eating.

Occurrence: One to two percent of women meet the *DSM-IV* criteria for anorexia or bulimia. One woman per 100,000 is anorectic, while 4.5%–18% of high school and college women are bulimic.

Age: The most common age group for anorexia is 12–30 years. The most common age group for bulimia is 17–25 years.

Ethnicity: Anorexia and bulimia occur 90%–95% of the time in Caucasian females.

Contributing Factors: Emotional distress, depression, anxiety, conflictual relationships, and social isolation. Current or past substance abuse has been associated with anorexia and bulimia. A history of sexual abuse has also been associated with anorexia and bulimia.

Signs and Symptoms: The anorectic woman usually denies that she is ill, but her thinness attracts the NP's attention. The woman usually does not complain of hunger, but may complain of difficulty sleeping, bloating after eating, constipation, or cold intolerance. Amenorrhea is common in anorectics. Most women with anorexia are restless, physically active, and some exercise to excess.

History will reveal an inability to maintain a recommended weight, secretive eating, frequent weighing, persistent feelings of dissatisfaction with weight, and mood changes associated with food (Table 13–2, also see Appendix).

Diagnostic Tests: History, physical examination, laboratory studies to detect complications, such as electrolyte levels; electrocardiogram (ECG); complete blood count (CBC); and thyroid-stimulating hormone (TSH), glucose, alkaline phosphatase, and serum estrogen levels.

Differential Diagnoses: Malignancy, chronic infection, intestinal disorders, endocrinopathies, tumors of the CNS, psychiatric illness.

Treatment: Medical management, pharmacotherapy, nutrition therapy, behavioral therapy, cognitive therapy, and family therapy. Hospitalization is necessary if weight loss is severe and rapidly progressing or signs of complications such as cardiac arrhythmia or hypokalemia occur.

Follow-up: Treatment is a multidisciplinary team effort. Follow-up with the team will be necessary for long-term resolution.

Sequelae: Of women with anorexia, 9% do not survive. Amenorrhea of hypotha-

TABLE 13–2 EATING DISORDERS

	Anorexia Nervosa	Bulimia	Obesity
Characteristics	Refusal to maintain normal weight, fear of gaining weight, amenorrhea	Binge eating, self-induced vomiting, use of laxatives or diuretics, fasting	Compulsive overeating not related to hunger
History	Cannot maintain weight, resists giving diet history, excessive exercise, amenorrhea	Binge/purging patterns, weight fluctuations	History of unsuccessful diets, restricted social activities because of weight
Physical findings	Low weight, pale and emaciated, lanugo, atrophied or poorly developed breasts, arrhythmias, overuse muscular injuries, amenorrhea	Normal weight or slightly overweight, "chipmunk" appearance, conjunctival hemorrhage, dental enamel eroded, overuse muscular injuries, menstrual irregularities	Excessive body fat, hypertension, hirutism, varicosities, abdomen protuberant, arthritis, depression
Treatment	Medications, diet, exercise, psychotherapy	Medications, diet, counseling and therapy	Medications, diet, exercise, group therapy

lamic origin occurs with severe weight loss. Loss of bone density occurs with extreme weight loss. Outcome studies show that 60% of anorectics achieve normal weight and menstruation, 49% achieve normalized eating patterns, and 20% endure chronic symptoms. Bulimia can produce dental erosion, swollen salivary glands, gastrointestinal irritation, and electrolyte imbalance. Of all bulimics, 20% endure chronic symptoms.

Prevention/Prophylaxis: Overall advice to prevent an eating disorder includes the following guidelines:

- Eat a variety of nutritious meals and snacks throughout the day.
- Eat favorite foods in moderation.
- Avoid skipping meals.
- Keep healthy foods on hand.
- Find alternatives for managing uncomfortable feelings.
- Avoid dieting.

Referral: The shortest time between onset of symptoms and the beginning of treatment is associated with a more favorable outcome. Refer to a multidisciplinary team that involves mental health professionals and nutrition specialists as soon as you suspect an eating disorder.

Education: NPs can educate all women about the importance of proper nutrition and the hazards of dieting.

Screening for Diabetes

Diabetes mellitus is a metabolic disorder characterized by abnormal metabolism of carbohydrates, fats, and proteins. Type I is insulin-dependent diabetes mellitus. Type II is non–insulin-dependent diabetes mellitus (NIDDM). Type I is generally diagnosed in childhood or early adulthood. Type II is generally diagnosed in adulthood.

Etiology: Type II is related to the destruction of the beta cells in the islets of Langerhans. Type II is related to a defect in insulin receptors or an altered state of response to insulin in the beta cells.

Occurrence: Diabetes occurs in 3%–7% of the U.S. population. Type II is 10 times more common than type I. Similar rates of diabetes occur in men and women.

Age: The incidence of NIDDM, which increases with age, is usually diagnosed after age 40.

Ethnicity: NIDDM is ethnic group–related. The prevalence of the disease in Puma Indians is 35%, Native Americans 17%, Hispanics 12%, and African-Americans 5%. Mexican-Americans have a 1.6–1.9 times greater incidence of diabetes than Caucasians.

Contributing Factors: Risk factors for NIDDM are overnutrition with resulting obesity. Of diabetics, 80% are obese or have a history of obesity. Steroids reduce the receptor affinity for insulin. Other risk factors for NIDDM include family history of NIDDM, gestational diabetes, history of impaired glucose tolerance, history of coronary heart disease.

Signs and Symptoms: The appearance of symptoms may be acute or subacute in type I diabetes. The deficiency of insulin leads to a breakdown of protein (an increase in amino acids), a breakdown in fats (increase in free fatty acids), and a breakdown in glycogen to glucose metabolism. These changes create hyperglycemia and metabolic ketoacidosis, which, if not treated, can lead to coma and death.

In type II diabetes, the disease may be insidious at the start. The classic symptoms of diabetes include polyuria, polydipsia, and polyphagia. Weight loss is another symptom of diabetes (Table 13–3).

Diagnostic Tests: Fasting blood glucose, random blood glucose, and oral glucose tolerance tests. Screening is recommended for those women at risk for the disease (see Contributing Factors).

DIAGNOSTIC CRITERIA FOR DIABETES MELLITUS IN THE NONPREGNANT ADULT

- Random plasma glucose level ≥ 200 mg/dL plus classic diabetes symptoms—polydipsia, polyuria, polyphagia, and weight loss.
- Fasting plasma glucose level of ≥ 140 mg/dL on two occasions.
- Fasting plasma glucose level of < 140 mg/dL, but sustained elevated plasma glucose levels as determined by glucose tolerance testing.

TABLE 13–3 CHARACTERISTICS OF TYPE I AND II DIABETES

	Type I	Type II
Age at onset	<20	>40
Incidence in patients diagnosed with diabetes	1 in 10	9 in 10
Symptoms	Acute or subacute	Slow onset
Obesity at onset	Uncommon	Common
Family history	Uncommon	Common
Ketoacidosis	Frequent	Rare
Insulin	Decreased	Variable
Treatment	Diet, insulin	Diet, oral hypoglycemic medication, insulin

Differential Diagnoses: Hypoglycemia.

Treatment: The goals of therapy for a diabetic include normalizing metabolism and preventing complications. Methods of therapy include education, meal planning, exercise, and the use of hypoglycemic agents or insulin.

Follow-up: Diabetes requires management throughout the woman's life.

Sequelae: Complications of untreated or undertreated diabetes include retinopathy, nephropathy, neuropathy, coronary heart disease (increased four times in women over men), cerebral vascular accident, and peripheral vascular disease.

Referral: Abnormal blood glucose levels require referral to an endocrinologist for evaluation.

Education: Management of diabetes requires in-depth education about the disease, diet management, risk factors, exercise management, and methods used to evaluate the disease process. Experts should provide education about diabetes.

Hirsutism

Hirsutism is excessive hair growth in women. Excessive hair is facial, pubic, axillary, abdominal, and chest.

Etiology: Increased androgenic activity causes the increased hair growth. The increase in androgen may indicate an underlying endocrine disease. The source of androgen may be the ovary, the adrenal gland, or both. Anabolic steroids can produce hirsutism, as can danazol, a drug used to treat endometriosis.

Occurrence: Excessive androgen action is the most common endocrinopathy of women, affecting 10%–20% of U.S. women.

Age: Hirsutism usually begins after age 25.

Ethnicity: Hirsutism has familial, racial, and ethnic patterns. Eastern European women are more hirsute than Scandinavian women are; white women are more hirsute than black women.

Contributing Factors
- Insulin resistance can trigger excessive ovarian androgen production. A link between obesity and hirsutism exists.
- Hirsutism in conjunction with oligomenorrhea or amenorrhea may represent polycystic ovarian syndrome.
- Cushing's syndrome can produce hirsutism, as can congenital adrenal hyperplasia.

Signs and Symptoms: Increased hair growth. Acne and androgenic alopecia can occur with hirsutism. The ovaries may be normal sized or enlarged and contain multiple cysts.

Diagnostic Tests: Physical examination, free serum testosterone, LH:FSH ratio.

Differential Diagnoses: Virilization defined as temporary hair recession, acne, deepening voice, increased muscle mass, and clitoromegaly.

Treatment: Mild hirsutism not related to endocrine disease can be treated with hair bleaching, waxing, or electrolysis. Medical therapy is required for hirsutism related to endocrine disease. Appropriate oral contraceptives or antagonizing androgen levels with several medications are used for therapy.

Follow-up: Hirsutism related to endocrine disease requires lifetime follow-up.

Sequelae: There is an increased incidence of type II diabetes in women with hirsutism as well as unfavorable lipid patterns.

Prevention/Prophylaxis: Obesity is a modifiable risk factor.

Referral: Any woman with significant hirsutism should be referred to a reproductive endocrinologist for evaluation.

Education: Hirsutism can indicate a loss of femininity to women. After endocrine pathology has been ruled out or treated, referral for hair reduction, particularly in the facial area, is recommended.

Female Obesity

Obesity is an excessive accumulation of body fat. Obesity is a multifactorial disease that involves genetics and biochemistry as well as environmental and cultural factors.

Etiology: Obesity is increasingly becoming a major public health problem in the United States. It can create a number of health-related problems for women. Obesity is rarely the result of an endocrine disorder; rather, obesity is usually a disease of appetite regulation and metabolism.

Occurrence: Obesity is the most prevalent nutritional disorder of affluent nations, including the United States. Obesity affects over one-third of adult women in the United States.

Age: Obesity can occur at any age.

Ethnicity: Obesity is more common in African-American and Mexican-American women than in Caucasian women. Of African-American and Mexican-American women, 50% are obese.

Contributing Factors: Familial tendency, emotional problems.

Signs and Symptoms: Mild obesity is defined as 20%–40% above the average weight for women of the same height and build. Moderate obesity is defined as 41%–100% above the average. Severe obesity is defined as more than 100% above the average. (See Table 13–2 and Appendix.)

Diagnostic Tests: Height and weight, measurement of skinfold thickness, diet history, physical examination, thyroid screening.

Differential Diagnosis: Cushing's syndrome, hypothyroidism, polycystic ovarian syndrome, hypothalamic injury, congestive heart failure, and renal failure.

Treatment: Competently designed treatment programs tailored to individual needs have the greatest success rate. Therapy includes dietary approaches, behavior modification, and exercise. Therapy may include pharmacologic treatment. A multidisciplinary approach is recommended.

Follow-up: Motivation is a key factor to weight reduction. Long-term follow-up with a multidisciplinary team is needed for weight reduction and maintenance.

Sequelae: Obesity is associated with oligo-ovulation, polycystic ovarian syndrome, endometrial cancer, and after menopause breast cancer. (Obesity increases the production of estrogen, increases the free testosterone levels, and increases the androgen levels.) Obesity is associated with infertility.

Obesity increases the risk for morbidity and mortality in women. Pregnancy in obese women is handled as high risk. Coronary artery disease in middle-aged women, sleep apnea, surgical risk, osteoarthritis, and gallbladder disease have an increased incidence in obese women.

Referral: Refer obese women to a multidisciplinary team for weight loss.

Education: Realistic goals and expectations are critical. The woman must be willing to alter eating and exercise patterns permanently.

Premenstrual Syndrome

Premenstrual syndrome (PMS) is a cyclic recurrence in the luteal phase of the menstrual cycle of distressing symptoms (physical, psychologic, and/or behavioral) that interfere with normal activities.

Etiology: Unknown.

Occurrence: Most women (80%–90%) have some distressing symptoms prior to menses. Of these, 30% report severe temporary distress, with 3%–5% reporting disabling temporary symptoms.

Age: PMS can occur at any age, but it is most common in later reproductive years.

Ethnicity: Not significant.

Contributing factors: Deficient diet, lack of exercise, chronic illness, stress.

Signs and Symptoms: Symptoms can include any combination of the following: Breast swelling and tenderness, lower abdominal bloating and constipation, loose stool or diarrhea 24 hours prior to menses; and for the first 1 to 2 days of menstrual bleeding, increase in appetite and cravings, fatigue, emotional lability and depression, irritability, insomnia, menopausal-like hot flashes, night sweats, and migraine-like head-aches. Dysmenorrhea does not usually occur with PMS, although it may in adolescence (Fig. 13–1).

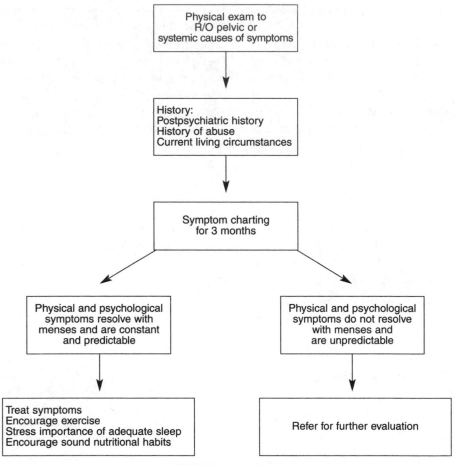

Physical exam to
R/O pelvic or
systemic causes of symptoms

History:
Postpsychiatric history
History of abuse
Current living circumstances

Symptom charting
for 3 months

Physical and psychological
symptoms resolve with
menses and are constant
and predictable

Physical and psychological
symptoms do not resolve
with menses and
are unpredictable

Treat symptoms
Encourage exercise
Stress importance of adequate sleep
Encourage sound nutritional habits

Refer for further evaluation

FIGURE 13–1   PMS.

Diagnostic Tests: Reviewing a symptom calendar makes the diagnosis. Diagnosis is made by the nature, severity, and timing of the symptoms. Symptoms occur at the onset of or after ovulation and resolve 6–7 days following the onset of menses. There is at least 1 week without symptoms. Symptoms do not occur suddenly; they gradually increase over the years. The symptoms are consistent and predictable. The symptoms do not resolve without intervention.

There are no laboratory tests that help diagnose PMS. A CBC and thyroid screen can be used to rule out anemia and thyroid disease.

Differential Diagnosis: Depression, chronic pelvic pain, post–tubal ligation syndrome, and perimenopausal symptoms.

Treatment: Treatment of PMS includes counseling and reassurance. A decrease in salt and sugar intake can be helpful in relief of symptoms. Eliminating caffeine and increasing exercise can reduce symptoms.

Medications can be utilized. Vitamin B$_6$, pyridoxine, 100–200 mg daily, may help relieve symptoms. Headache can be treated with medication. Oral contraceptives are not helpful for relief of this syndrome. Luteinizing hormone–releasing hormone (LHRH) agonists and continuous oral progesterone have been utilized to reduce PMS. Antidepressants can be utilized for severe PMS.

Follow-up: After initiation of therapy, monthly visits for 3 months are recommended for evaluation.

Sequelae: None.

Prevention/Prophylaxis: Normal physiologic changes in the menstrual cycle precipitate the symptoms. No prevention can be recommended.

Referral: Referral to a physician is appropriate if there is no relief of symptoms after 3 months. A mental health referral may be appropriate. A referral to a nutritionist may be helpful. Support groups for PMS have been helpful to some women.

Education: An understanding of the normal menstrual cycle may enhance understanding of PMS.

Thyroid Disease

Disease of the thyroid can create hypothyroidism or hyperthyroidism. The thyroid gland is a possible site for malignant growth.

Etiology: The most common cause of hypothyroidism is an autoimmune disease, which results in gradual destruction of the thyroid gland. The most common cause of hyperthyroidism is Graves' disease, an autoimmune disease. Cancer of the thyroid is a relatively rare disease with a low mortality rate.

Occurrence: All thyroid disorders, benign and malignant, are more common in women than in men. Hyperthyroidism is 5 times more common in women and hypothyroidism is 10 times more common. Thyroid tumors occur twice as frequently in women.

Age: The incidence of thyroid cancer has a bimodal and age-specific index with a peak in the 30s, increasing with age after the third decade.

Ethnicity: African-Americans are at a lower risk for thyroid cancer.

Contributing Factors: Radiation to the head and neck increases the probability of thyroid cancer.

Signs and Symptoms: Signs of hypothyroidism are fatigue, lethargy, weakness, cold intolerance, weight gain, and menorrhagia. The woman may also have bradycardia and/or loss of axillary, pubic, and scalp hair. The thyroid gland may or may not be enlarged. TSH level will be elevated and T_4 level low.

Signs of hyperthyroidism include nervousness, increased sweating, heat intolerance, palpitations, fatigue, and weight loss. The woman may also have a goiter, tremors, or tachycardia. Exophthalmos may be present. T_4 level will be high and TSH level low.

Singular or multiple thyroid nodules may indicate thyroid cancer (Table 13–4).

TABLE 13–4 THYROID DISEASE

	Hypothyroid	Hyperthyroid
Symptoms	Nonspecific presentation; one-third present with cold intolerance, weight gain, dry skin, fatigue, menstrual irregularity	Tremulousness, palpitations, heat intolerance, weight loss, amenorrhea
Laboratory results	High TSH, low T_4 level	Low TSH, elevated T_4 level
Treatment	Thyroid hormone replacement	Antithyroid drugs, beta blockers, radioactive iodine

Diagnostic Tests
- Total serum T_4 measures levels of free and bound T_4
- Total serum T_3
- TSH
- Thyroid scan
- Ultrasound

See Appendix.

Differential Diagnoses: Euthyroid goiter, mild transient enlargement of the thyroid gland postpartum, benign adenoma.

Treatment: Hypothyroidism treatment involves thyroid replacement, usually for life. Hyperthyroidism is treated with medications that interfere with thyroid hormone synthesis, radioactive iodine, or surgery. Thyroid cancer requires surgery.

Follow-up: Thyroid disease requires lifelong medical management. Thyroid testing and medication adjustment occurs at regular intervals throughout the woman's life.

Sequelae: Extremes of thyroid dysfunction are associated with ovulatory and menstrual disturbances. Hypothyroid can delay puberty and create a state of chronic anovulation. Hyperthyroid can delay puberty and create amenorrhea and chronic anovulation.

Prevention/Prophylaxis: None.

Referral: Endocrine disorders require medical management. Refer any suspected cases of thyroid disease to a medical physician.

Education: Emphasize the importance of long-term follow-up after diagnosis and referral.

BIBLIOGRAPHY

General

Carr, B, and Blackwell, R: Textbook of Reproductive Medicine. Appleton & Lange, Stamford, CT, 1998.
Goroll, A, May, L, and Mulley, A: Primary Care Medicine. Lippincott, Philadelphia, 1995.

Primary Amenorrhea

Marantides, D: Management of polycystic ovary syndrome. Nurse Pract 22(12):34, 1997.
Redmond, G. Androgens and women's health. Int J Fertil Women's Med 43(2):91, 1998.

Anorexia, Bulimia, and Obesity

Allen, K, and Phillips, J: Women's Health across the Lifespan. Lippincott, Philadelphia, 1997.
Bongain, A, Isnard, V, and Gillet, J: Obesity in obstetrics and gynecology. Eur J Obstet Gynecol Reprod Biol 77(2):217, 1998.
McGilley, B, and Pryor, T: Assessment and treatment of bulimia nervosa. Am Fam Physician 57(11):2743, 1998.
Ricchini, W: For your patients: Recognizing eating disorders. Adv Nurse Pract 6(4):25, 1998.

Diabetes

Harris, M, et al: Prevalence of diabetes, impaired fasting glucose, and impaired glucose tolerance in U.S. adults. Diabetes Care 21(4):518, 1998.

Hirsutism

Young, R, and Sinclair, R: Hirsutes I: Diagnosis. Aust J Dermatol 39(1):24, 1998.
Foreyt, J, and Poston, W: Obesity: A never-ending cycle. Int J Fertil Women's Med 43(2):111, 1998.

Thyroid

Seltzer, V, and Pearse, W: Women's Primary Health Care. McGraw-Hill, New York, 1995.

CHAPTER **14**

PSYCHOSOCIAL

DISORDERS

This chapter discusses psychologic and social issues that directly impact on women's health. Addressing women's health concerns involves recognizing and responding to mental as well as physical health needs. (Health is generally defined as both mental and physical well-being.) Gender-based research guides the women's health nurse practitioner (NP) in identifying mental health issues for women. This chapter discusses mood disorders, substance abuse, and the physical and emotional results of violence against women. Screening each woman for mental health concerns is an important component of women's health care.

History

At every therapeutic encounter with every woman, evaluate her mood. What do you note about its intensity, lability, and appropriateness? If you suspect depression, administer a series of questions to evaluate the level of depression and guide referral. Ask every depressed woman about suicide. Asking about suicide does not plant the idea. It is a myth that discussing suicide gives ideas that were not previously present. It is also a myth that women who talk about depression do not commit suicide.

Assess the logic of thought in all women. Is she relevant, organized, and coherent at each encounter?

At each encounter, question each woman about previous psychiatric illnesses and about psychosocial stressors such as domestic violence, substance abuse, sexual assault, and recent significant losses.

RISK FACTORS FOR SUICIDE IN WOMEN

Age 55–65
History of prior attempts
Living alone
Depression
Unemployment
History of chronic pain, chronic illness
History of recent surgery or terminal illness
Substance abuse
Psychotic history
Positive family history of suicide
Specific plan for suicide formulated

From: Phillip Long, MD, www.mentalhealth.com

Physical Examination

Careful physical examination follows a detailed history, including mental status examination.

Anxiety

Second only to depression in women seeking mental health services, anxiety is two to three times more likely to occur in women than in men. Mild anxiety motivates people to perform well and serves a protective function. Severe anxiety can incapacitate and disable.

Etiology: Anxiety can be situational or general. Anxiety can occur in the form of panic attacks, phobias, or obsessions.

Occurrence: Anxiety is reported by 5%–15% of the population.

Age: Anxiety can occur at any age.

Ethnicity: Not significant.

Contributing Factors: Traumatic events, including domestic violence and sexual assault; psychosocial stressors.

Signs and Symptoms: Apprehension, agitation, and heightened arousal are the classic symptoms of anxiety.

Somatic complaints occur with anxiety, including fatigue, insomnia, weakness, dizziness, tremulousness, restlessness, palpitations, chest pain, tachycardia, hyperventilation, dry mouth, diarrhea, nausea, and urinary frequency.

SYMPTOMS OF ANXIETY

Tachycardia
Dyspnea
Diaphoresis
Sweating palms
Urinary urgency
Diarrhea
Decreased appetite
Dizziness
Tremulousness
Fatigue
Apprehension
Restlessness
Tension
Difficulty concentrating
Lack of interest
Insomnia

Situational anxiety is a normal reaction to an anxiety-provoking situation.

General anxiety is anxiety lasting more than 6 months. The woman does not report being worried about one specific thing. She is fearful and panicked with an impulse to flee. She has a feeling of impending doom.

Panic attacks are often associated with a positive family history. Of people experiencing panic attacks, 80% are women. Panic attacks affect 3% or 4% of women. During a panic attack, the woman experiences palpitations, diaphoresis, shakiness, chest pain, and dizziness. (The hypervigilance associated with panic attacks may mimic cardiac or neurologic disease.)

Phobia is an irrational fear of a specific stimulus. Women will seek to avoid the stimulus.

Obsessive-compulsive disorder (OCD) affects 3% of the population. Obsessions and compulsions impair the ability to function. Obsessions are unwanted thoughts. Compulsions are ritualized repetitive behaviors.

Posttraumatic stress disorder (PTSD) occurs after a traumatic event (outside the range of the normal human experience). PTSD occurs in 17%–30% of women who are exposed to trauma. The woman re-experiences the event through thoughts or dreams; she also has intrusive memories and flashbacks. She avoids behavior related to the event, and experiences states of hyperarousal (hypervigilance). She may experience panic attacks, and she may have difficulty sleeping.

PTSD in women is most closely associated with loss of a loved one and assaultive violence. Women are at higher risk for PTSD than men.

Diagnostic Tests: Psychosocial history should be a part of all history taking, but it

ANXIETY DISORDERS

Generalized Anxiety

Lasting > 6 months
Concern over many issues

Panic Attacks

Extreme anxiety episodically
Avoidance behavior

Phobia

Irrational fear of a specific stimulus

Obsessive-Compulsive Disorder

Obsession, intrusive thoughts
Compulsion, repetitive ritualistic behaviors
Symptoms that impair functioning

Posttraumatic Stress Disorder

History of trauma
Re-experiencing of trauma
Avoidance
Increased arousal

should be emphasized in women with somatic complaints that may be related to anxiety.

Differential Diagnosis: Depression, psychosis, drug effect, diet related (caffeine, monosodium glutamate [MSG]), hyperthyroidism.

Treatment: A combination of psychotherapy, behavioral therapy, and education are indicated for anxiety disorders. Women seek treatment for anxiety more often than men. Women are most frequently treated with a combination of medication and psychotherapy.

Follow-up: Anxiety disorders require multiple visits for treatment.

Prevention/Prophylaxis: Prevention of violence against women.

Sequelae: Substance abuse is a common sequelae to anxiety in women. Women who abuse substances show high rates of PTSD (30%–59%).

Referral: Women experiencing anxiety that interferes with functioning should be referred to a source that deals with anxiety disorders.

Education: The use of illicit drugs, prescription drugs, and alcohol to reduce anxiety should be decreased. The source of the anxiety should be discovered in order to reach resolution of the symptoms.

Depression

Depression, the most common severe mental disorder in women, occurs in women twice as often as in men.

Etiology: Depression can be related to genetic, cognitive, social, or economic factors. The genetic factors include neurotransmitter and neuroendocrine functions. Cognitive factors include powerlessness, learned helplessness, and decreased self-concept. Social factors include trauma, abuse, and multiple roles.

Occurrence: Depression affects more than 1 million women in the United States. Approximately 2 million visits to a psychiatrist per year are made by depressed women. Approximately 1 woman in 10 is severely depressed.

Age: Mean onset of depression in women is 40 years. One-half of women initially diagnosed with depression are between the ages of 20 and 50 years of age. Depression in elderly women is an underdiagnosed and undertreated problem. Depression in the elderly population affects nutrition, activity, and medical treatment. Two-thirds of depressed and hospitalized elderly persons are female. Every elderly woman, particularly those living alone, should be screened for signs of depression.

Ethnicity: Depression is higher in black women ages 18–24.

Contributing Factors
Learned helplessness is related to decreased education, decreased socioeconomic level, unemployment, and young age.

Lack of intimacy has been identified as an important provoking agent that increases the risk for depression in women.

High levels of recent stress are also predictive of depressive symptoms. Life stress plays a larger role in the provocation of recurrent episodes of depression for women than men.

Depression in girls ages 14–18 relates to lack of parental support, low self-esteem, and low levels of attachment.

Depression in women can be related to violence and childhood sexual abuse.

Depression in elderly women relates to loss of a spouse and lack of physical health.

Depression can accompany borderline personality, dissociative disorders, eating disorders, substance abuse, and anxiety disorders.

Depression may be related to infertility, recent surgery, or the postpartum period.

Signs and Symptoms: Sadness is the number one symptom of depression, followed by irritability and loss of interest. Depressed women may be preoccupied with physical complaints, may have changes in memory or concentration, and may have disturbed sleep, disturbed appetite, or lack of energy.

Depression can be mild, moderate, or severe. (See Appendix.)

According to the *DSM-IV*, a diagnosis of major depression is made based upon the following (at least five of these symptoms must be present):

- Depressed mood
- Loss of interest in pleasure
- Sleep disturbances
- Significant weight loss
- Psychomotor retardation and agitation
- Decreased energy
- Feelings of worthlessness
- Impaired concentration
- Recurrent thoughts of dying

Diagnostic Tests: Careful physical examination including a mental status exam.

SYMPTOMS DIAGNOSTIC OF DEPRESSION

Depressed mood most of the day, nearly every day

Diminished interest in all or almost all activities most of the day nearly every day

Significant weight loss when not dieting or significant weight gain

Insomnia or hypersomnia nearly every day

Psychomotor agitation or retardation

Fatigue or loss of energy nearly every day

Feelings of worthlessness or excessive guilt

Diminished ability to think or concentrate nearly every day

Recurrent thoughts of death

Adapted from *The Diagnostic and Statistical Manual of Mental Disorders, Fourth Edition.* Copyright 1994 American Psychiatric Association.

Differential Diagnosis

Chronic fatigue, Lyme disease, fibromyalgia, rheumatoid disease, endocrinopathies.

Adjustment disorder in which mood is depressed following a significant life stressor. In adjustment disorder, coping mechanisms will develop and the woman will have a depressed mood for less than 6 months.

Bereavement creates severe depression that persists for less than 6 months.

Treatment: Medications and psychotherapy.

Follow-up: Depression must be closely followed during treatment.

Sequelae: Suicide can be a consequence of depression. Every depressed woman must be asked directly about suicide. Does she have suicidal thoughts? Does she intend to commit suicide? Does she have any plans for suicide? A history of prior attempts and living alone increase the risk for suicide. (See "Risk Factors for Suicide in Women" earlier in this chapter; also see Appendix.)

Prevention/Prophylaxis: Early diagnosis and treatment may prevent suicide.

Referral: Women who express intent and a plan for suicide require immediate referral. Any women expressing feelings of complete failure, immobilization, or feeling trapped or paralyzed require immediate referral. All women with severe depression require referral for evaluation and treatment.

Education: Relief from the stigma of depression is an important goal for women suffering from depression. Women's health providers should encourage compliance with treatment.

Insomnia

Insomnia is defined as difficulty falling or staying asleep that interferes with daytime functioning.

Etiology: Psychiatric disorders such as depression, anxiety, and character disorders account for one-half of insomnia complaints. The remaining cases of insomnia, in the general population, are related to chronic pain, drug reactions, sleep apnea, and physical symptoms such as urinary frequency. The National Sleep Foundation reports that, in women, insomnia is largely a result of biological events such as menstruation, pregnancy, and menopause.

Occurrence: Women are 50% more likely to experience insomnia than men.

Age: Insomnia can occur at any age.

Ethnicity: Not significant.

Signs and Symptoms
Seventy-one percent (71%) of women report sleep disturbance in the first few and last few days of the menstrual cycle. Just prior to menses and at the beginning of menses, women report difficulty falling asleep, waking up in the middle of the night, and having trouble getting out of bed.

Seventy-nine percent (79%) of pregnant women report disturbed sleep related to heartburn, fetal kicks, and anxiety.

Fifty-six percent (56%) of menopausal women report disrupted sleep with hot flashes as the primary reason for sleep loss followed by the need to urinate. Menopausal and postmenopausal women report trouble falling asleep and waking in the middle of the night.

Diagnostic Tests: A positive history is the most important diagnostic test for insomnia. Asking the woman to keep a sleep log may help make the diagnosis. Any history of pain, urinary frequency, and drug use should be explored in relationship to sleep loss.

Differential Diagnosis: Endocrine disorders, psychiatric disorders.

Treatment

Use medication to reduce insomnia only in severe sleep disorders. Avoid sedatives and hypnotics, especially in the elderly population.

Hormone replacement therapy may assist menopausal women with insomnia.

Special pregnancy pillows may assist pregnant women with interrupted sleep.

If anxiety or depression is the reason for insomnia, treatment of these underlying conditions will reduce sleep loss.

Follow-up: Follow-up visits for improvement of insomnia are important. Treatment of underlying conditions should improve insomnia. Pregnancy requires planned napping to "catch up" on lost sleep.

Sequelae: Interference with functioning in the daytime.

Referral: Women who report symptoms of sleep apnea—waking with air hunger—should be referred to a sleep specialist for evaluation.

Education: Of women with insomnia, 20% use over-the-counter sleep aids, 13% use prescription drugs, and 8% use alcohol to induce sleep. Reduction of the use of alcohol and medications is preferable. Treatment of underlying conditions and counseling regarding good sleep habits is preferable to use of medication whenever possible.

Sexual Dysfunction

Interruption or absence of any stage in the sexual response cycle (desire, arousal, orgasm, resolution) can result in sexual dysfunction. Dissatisfaction with a sexual relationship is a common complaint of women. Discomfort with intercourse may have a physical or a psychologic origin. (See Chap. 5.)

Etiology: Prior negative sexual experiences, fear of sexual failure, interpersonal issues, situational stress, and anxiety.

Occurrence: Unknown.

Age: Sexual dysfunction can occur in any sexually active female.

Ethnicity: Not significant.

Signs and Symptoms

Lack of desire related to negative experiences, fear of failure, or interpersonal reasons.

Lack of arousal related to insufficient foreplay, distraction, or undesirable forms of stimulation.

Lack of orgasm related to lack of arousal or inability to achieve an orgasm may be symptomatic of an underlying problem.

Vaginismus may occur following a major trauma such as rape or sexual abuse.

Lack of vaginal lubrication related to menopause can make intercourse uncomfortable.

Diagnostic Tests
History of the sexual dysfunction is needed for diagnosis.
A detailed account of discomfort with intercourse, lack of desire, or lack of orgasm must be obtained. History of sexual abuse must be obtained.
Current and recent stressors may be related to sexual dysfunction. (See Chap. 5 for further discussion of sexual history.)
Complete pelvic examination must be performed.

Differential Diagnosis: Vaginal infection, atrophic vaginitis, urinary tract infection.

Treatment: Education about sexual functioning and the human sexual response cycle. Treatment of any underlying condition such as anxiety may be required.

Follow-up: Follow-up visits following education, treatment, or referral are necessary. In most cases, sexual dysfunction can be resolved.

Prevention/Prophylaxis: Primary prevention of sexual abuse.

Sequelae: None.

Referral: Women with complex sexual problems of a psychologic nature require referral to a sex therapist. Sexual dysfunction that involves both partners requires referral.

Education: Teaching about normal sexual responses and taking the opportunity to answer questions and address concerns often resolves sexual dysfunction.

Substance Abuse and Dependence

Substance abuse is the use of a psychoactive substance not consistent with medical guidelines or nonmedical use of prescription medications. Dependence is the need for repeated doses to avoid feeling "bad" both physically and psychologically.

Etiology: Genetic, biologic, biochemical, sociocultural, psychologic, and learned behavior are all components of substance abuse.

Occurrence: Three to five percent of women have problems with alcohol. A National Health Interview Survey found that 4.3% of women interviewed were alcohol-dependent. A Gallup poll found that among 26,000 women interviewed, 50% were nondrinkers, 45% were light drinkers, 3% were moderate drinkers, and 2% were heavy drinkers. Of the women who drank, 21% were "binge" drinkers and 4% drank during pregnancy.

In women, alcohol is still the most widely abused drug. Tobacco is the second most frequently used drug. In women, marijuana is the most commonly utilized illicit drug, followed by cocaine. Use of a prescription drug for nonmedical reasons frequently occurs in women. Up to 70% of all prescription drugs in the United States are used without a prescription.

Age: Alcoholism can affect women at any age. Little is known about alcohol abuse in women older than 65. Drugs are disproportionately prescribed for older women. Drugs are prescribed for elderly women 2.5 times more often than they are for older men. Elderly women are approximately 7% of the population, but 17% of psychoactive drug prescriptions are given to them, as are 20% of all prescribed sedatives and hypnotics.

Ethnicity: American Indian women are more susceptible to alcohol-related health problems. Alcohol mortality rates are significantly higher for women who are Native American.

Contributing Factors: Alcohol abuse is seen 10% less in women than in men. Smoking rates appear to be about the same in women as in men. There is a minimal difference between men and women in the use of illicit drugs. Men drink more beer in a negative emotional state, particularly loneliness. Women drink more beer and wine when experiencing positive emotions. Women most frequently begin using cocaine in a social situation. Women often begin illicit drug use with their partners.

Signs and Symptoms: Withdrawal creates agitation, anxiety, restlessness, tremors, anorexia, and insomnia. Symptoms of alcohol abuse may include excessive use of mouthwash or perfume, frequent complaints of not feeling well, elimination of or change in social interactions, protection of places in the home where alcohol may be hidden, changes in physical appearance, and a positive response to the CAGE questionnaire for screening.

THE CAGE QUESTIONNAIRE

Have you ever felt the need to **C**ut down on drinking?

Have you ever felt **A**nnoyed by criticism of drinking?

Have you ever had **G**uilty feelings about drinking?

Have you ever taken a morning **E**ye opener?

Women are twice as likely as men to receive prescriptions for tranquilizers, analgesics, barbiturates, and amphetamines. Direct questions related to drug use are required to evaluate drug misuse appropriately.

Diagnostic Tests: Careful history of drugs used and amount, frequency, and duration of use. Direct questions such as: "In the past three months, have you consumed more than five drinks containing alcohol on a single occasion?" and "Do you use drugs for recreation?" should be asked.

Alcoholics Anonymous interviews tell us that the disease process of alcoholism progresses in 2.8 years for men, but only 1.1 for women. The number of years from onset to problem drinking is 11 for men and only 3.6 for women. Early diagnosis and referral reduce complications. There appears to be less time to formulate early diagnosis in women.

Screen each woman who abuses substances for anemia, hypertension, diabetes, cancer, liver disease, eating disorders, and dental problems. All women should be screened for smoking. At every opportunity, ask women about their smoking habits.

Differential Diagnosis: Use of cocaine, marijuana, or opiates must be considered in women with amenorrhea, anovulation, or spontaneous abortion. Cocaine and opiates can be related to hyperprolactinemia. Alcohol can affect estrogen and progesterone levels, but the relationship is not well understood.

Treatment: Offering brief but specific advice can motivate women to reduce their alcohol intake or reduce their use of drugs. One-third of Alcoholics Anonymous participants are women.

Follow-up: Family planning must be discussed with every woman who abuses substances. Carefully follow women who identify themselves as having the ability to quit smoking or drinking or drug use "on their own." Carefully monitor their progress.

Prevention/Prophylaxis: Identification of women with drug and alcohol problems leads to intervention. Complications can be prevented with early intervention.

Women reporting alcohol dependency also report receiving prescriptions for hypnotics and sedatives. Use of alcohol should be questioned prior to prescribing medication. Prescription drugs can be abused and should therefore be prescribed with caution.

Advise all smokers to stop. Supply self-help quitting materials to every woman smoker.

Sequelae

Alcohol abuse takes a great physical toll on women. Female alcoholics have death rates 50% higher than those of men. Causes of death for female alcoholics are suicide, alcohol-related accidents, cardiovascular disease, and cirrhosis of the liver.

Alcohol abuse is associated with hepatitis B infection, gastrointestinal bleeding, malnutrition, and pancreatitis.

Fetal alcohol syndrome is caused by alcohol abuse during pregnancy.

Alcohol impairs judgment and increases risky behavior that can lead to unwanted outcomes.

Cocaine causes abruption, preterm labor, fetal distress, and stillbirth. Babies are born in withdrawal. Cocaine causes hypertension, respiratory distress and arrhythmias, seizures, psychiatric problems, hyperprolactinemia, menstrual irregularities, and infertility.

Heroin is associated with human immunodeficiency virus (HIV), hepatitis, subacute bacterial endocarditis (SBE), tuberculosis (TB), accidents, suicide, and homicide. Heroin causes central nervous system (CNS) damage, respiratory depression, constipation, and anorexia. Heroin creates the risk of death from overdose. Withdrawal of heroin creates, in 9–15 hours, sweating, increased respiratory rate, increased blood pressure, insomnia, nausea and diarrhea, pain, and drug craving.

Of women with AIDS, 27% are intravenous (IV) drug users.

Cigarettes are the leading cause of preventable death in the United States. Cigarettes kill more women than alcohol, drugs, auto accidents, homicides, suicides, and HIV combined. Cigarettes kill through cancer, coronary heart disease (CHD), peripheral vascular disease (PVD), chronic obstructive pulmonary disease (COPD), and intrauterine growth retardation (IUGR). Lung cancer is the most fatal cancer in women. (The lung cancer mortality rate exceeds that of breast cancer.) Cigarettes are related to infertility, peptic ulcers, and skin wrinkling.

Referral

If the patient is pregnant and is abusing a substance, treat the pregnancy as high-risk, requiring case management and social services.

Alcohol and drug dependency can be treated on an inpatient or outpatient basis.

If women cannot stop smoking without assistance, refer to a smoking cessation program. Women who are pregnant and/or raising children require referral to stop smoking.

Education: Women who abuse substances should be educated about HIV, sexually transmitted diseases (STDs), prenatal care, childhood safety and injury prevention, nutrition, and general health.

The following is a list of classes of over-the-counter drugs in order of most frequent sales:

- Vitamins
- Analgesics
- Antacids
- Laxatives
- Agents used to promote sleep

Women use a high proportion of these medications. Careful drug history should reveal inappropriate use of these substances. Education about nonpharmacologic approaches to common discomforts may reduce the intake of these medications.

Violence against Women

Violence against women encompasses physical, emotional, and sexual abuse. Perpetrators of these acts may be known to the woman or they may be strangers. Violence against women occurs in all ages, races, socioeconomic groups, educational levels, and occupations.

Etiology: Theories about violence against women arise from sociology, psychology, and feminism. Sociology describes violence as learned behavior. The perpetrator learns to be violent in the family of origin. Psychology discusses pathology related to the abuser. Feminism believes that violence arises in a culture that tolerates such behavior.

Occurrence: Crimes of rape, sexual assault, and physical assault by a perpetrator known to the victim are infrequently reported. Crime surveys conducted by the Justice Department tell us that violent crimes against women are experienced by 2.5 million women annually. The number of women who report these crimes is lower than 2.5 million, whereas the number of women who seek care for their injuries is even lower. For example, according to the Justice Department, reporting of rape to the police followed by emergency room examination takes place just 17% of the time.

Women are more frequently victimized by offenders they know than by strangers. Two out of three women who respond to Justice Department surveys report knowing the offender.

Age: Younger women are at greater risk for sexual assault and domestic violence. Although sexual assault can and does occur against children and elderly persons, it is most likely to occur in women aged 14–24 years.

Ethnicity: Not significant.

Contributing Factors: See "Etiology."

Signs and Symptoms: Women who have been raped or sexually assaulted may report to the police and may then be escorted to an emergency facility that houses a sexual assault response team.

Victims of domestic violence may or may not report their physical abuse to health-care providers. Domestic violence always includes emotional abuse with physical abuse. Sexual abuse occurs with physical and emotional abuse 50% of the time. The woman may be fearful of reporting. She may be fearful of how the abuser will respond to reporting, and she may be fearful of what action the abuser will take when she reports. Every woman should be screened for domestic violence. Direct questions are appropriate.

DOMESTIC VIOLENCE SCREENING QUESTIONS

Do you feel safe in your home?

Do arguments in your home sometimes get physical?

Are you presently in a relationship with a person who threatens you or physically hurts you?

Did someone cause these injuries?

*Screening must take place in the absence of the person accompanying the woman.

The woman who has been victimized may display:

- Expressions of helplessness and powerlessness
- Symptoms of depression
- Inappropriate affect
- Unclear history of injury
- Multiple injury sites
- Incongruent explanation and examination

Diagnostic Tests: Careful history and physical examination.

Differential Diagnosis: Depression, PTSD, psychiatric disease.

Treatment: Physical injuries are treated as appropriate. Individual and/or group counseling is necessary after victimization.

Follow-up: Keep careful records and photographs of all women when abuse is suspected or reported. Counseling or therapy after victimization requires multiple visits and long-term follow-up.

Prevention/Prophylaxis: Primary prevention is accomplished through education. For example, teaching about dating violence and sexual assault to college and high school populations increases awareness in these groups. Secondary prevention reduces the incidence of violence in at-risk populations, such as people unable to give consent for sexual activity. Tertiary prevention reduces the consequences of adverse effects after violence. Examples include domestic violence shelters and sexual assault response teams.

Sequelae: One-third of all women killed are killed by their spouses, former spouses, or boyfriends. Injuries in both domestic violence and sexual assault are primarily in the form of contusions, abrasions, and lacerations. More severe episodes can result in fractures, head injuries, and death. Long-term somatic complaints that arise from violence against women include chronic pelvic pain, gastrointestinal symptoms, back pain, and headache.

Psychologic sequelae of violent victimization are PTSD, major depression, alcohol or drug abuse, anxiety disorders, and eating disorders. Sexual abuse among women is associated with depression, anxiety, suicidal ideation, suicide attempts, and PTSD. Physical abuse is associated with depression, anxiety, suicidal ideation, and PTSD (see Appendix).

Referral: In cases of domestic violence, carefully evaluate the woman's strengths, support systems, and safety in her home. Refer all victims of domestic violence to resource centers specializing in domestic violence. All victims of sexual assault or rape should be referred to a sexual assault response team. This team will take a history of the event, treat and detect injuries, collect forensic evidence, prevent sexually transmitted diseases, and pregnancy and provide referral resources for follow-up.

Education: See "Prevention/Prophylaxis."

BIBLIOGRAPHY

General

Allen, K, and Phillips, J: Women's Health across the Life Span. Lippincott, Philadelphia, 1997.

Frank, J, et al: Women's mental health in primary care. Depression, anxiety, somatization, eating disorders and substance abuse. Med Clin North Am 82(2):359, 1997.

Goroll, A, May, L, and Mullery, A: Primary Care Medicine. Lippincott, Philadelphia, 1995.

Horton, J: The Women's Health Data Book. The Jacob's Institute of Women's Health, Washington, DC, 1995.

Kroenke, K, and Spitzer, R: Gender differences in the reporting of physical and somatoform symptoms. Psychosom Med 60(2):150, 1998.

Wyshak, G, and Modest, G: Violence, mental health, and substance abuse in patients who are seen in primary care settings. Arch Fam Med 5(8):441, 1996.

Anxiety

Breslau, N, et al: Sex differences in posttraumatic stress disorder. Arch Gen Psychiatry 54(110):1104, 1997.

Foa, E: Trauma and women: Course, predictors and treatment. J Clin Psychiatry 58 Suppl (9):25, 1997.

Hutchings, P, and Dutton, S: Symptom severity and diagnoses related to sexual assault history. J Anxiety Disorders 11(6):607, 1997.

Najavitis, L, Weiss, R, and Shaw, S: The link between substance abuse, posttraumatic stress disorder in women. Am J Addict 6(4):273, 1997.

Yonkers, K, et al: Is the course of panic disorder the same in women and men? Am J Psychiatry 155(5):596, 1998.

Depression

Gil-Rivas, V, et al: Sexual and physical abuse: Do they compromise drug treatment outcomes? J Substance Abuse Treatment 14(4):351, 1997.

Koenig, H, and Kuchibhatla, M: Use of health services by hospitalized medically ill and depressed patients. Am J Psychiatry 155:871, 1998.

Kornstein, S: Gender differences in depression. J Clin Psychiatry. 58 Suppl (15):12, 1997.

Little, J, et al: How common is resistance to treatment in recurrent, nonpsychotic geriatric depression? Am J Psychiatry Aug:1035, 1998.

West, M., et al: Anxious attachment and self reported depressive symptomatology in women. Can J Psychiatry 43(3):294, 1998.

Insomnia

Baker, A, Simpson, S, and Dawson, D: Sleep disruption and mood changes associated with menopause. J Psychosom Res 43(4):359, 1997.

Hall, M, et al: Intrusive thoughts and avoidance behaviors are associated with sleep disturbances in bereavement-related depression. Depression Anxiety 6(3):106, 1997.

National Sleep Foundation: Sleep Tips for Women. National Sleep Foundation, Washington, DC, 1998.

Sexual Dysfunction

American College of Obstetricians and Gynecologists: Guidelines for Women's Health Care. The American College of Obstetricians and Gynecologists, Washington, DC, 1996.

American College of Obstetricians and Gynecologists: Sexual Dysfunction. ACOG Technical Bulletin. ACOG, Washington, DC, 1995.

Substance Abuse and Dependency

Stein, M, and Cyr, M: Women and substance abuse. Med Clin North Am 81(4):979, 1997.

Taj, N, Devera-Sales, A, and Vinson, D: Screening for problem drinking: Does a single question work? J Fam Pract 46(4):328, 1998.

Violence against Women

Browne, A: Violence against women by male partners. Am Psychologist 48(10):1077, 1993.

Campbell, J, and Lewandowski, L: Mental and physical effects of intimate partner violence on women and children. Psychiatric Clin North Am 20(20):353, 1997.

Skinner, C, et al: The coexistence of physical and sexual assault. Am J Obstet Gynecol 172(5):1644, 1995.

Sutherland, C, Bybee, D, and Sullivan, C: The long-term effects of battering on women's health. Women's Health 4(1):4170, 1998.

Williams, L: Failure to pursue indications of spousal abuse could lead to tragedy. Can Med Assoc J 152(9):1488, 1995.

CHAPTER 15

HEMATOLOGIC AND

IMMUNE SYSTEMS

This chapter discusses anemia, the most common hematologic disorder seen in women, and human immunodeficiency virus (HIV), the most serious of immune diseases seen in women. Refer to a general text for discussion of other hematologic disorders.

The nurse practitioner (NP) can work toward prevention of HIV by providing counseling or referring for counseling any women revealing high-risk behaviors related to HIV infection. As treatment methods for HIV improve, early diagnosis and referral are important NP functions.

Assessment

History of any of the following may indicate a hematologic or immunologic disorder:
- Weakness, malaise, fatigue
- Dyspnea on minor exertion
- Bleeding history, including unexplained bruising, excessive bleeding after injury, and excessive menstrual bleeding
- Increased frequency of infection

Physical examination in women with a hematologic disorder may reveal any or all of the following:
- Skin pallor
- Pale conjunctiva
- Petechiae
- Lymphadenopathy
- Enlargement of spleen or liver

198

Anemia

Normal hemoglobin levels in women are 12–14 g/dL. During pregnancy, blood volume increases beginning as early as 6 weeks. Erythropoietin levels increase during pregnancy by 30%. Plasma volume also increases. Normal hemoglobin levels in women who are not pregnant differ from those of pregnant women. A hemoglobin level less than 11.5 g/dL in a woman who is not pregnant and less than 10 g/dL for a pregnant woman is considered low and reflective of anemia.

Etiology: The most common cause of anemia in women is iron deficiency.

Occurrence: Iron-deficiency anemia, an insufficient supply of iron to the cells of the body, is the single most prevalent nutritional disorder in women. Iron-deficiency anemia affects millions of people worldwide. Of nutritional anemia cases, 85% are iron-deficiency anemia; the remaining 15% are iron-deficiency anemia combined with folate and other nutritional deficiencies.

Age: Infants, small children, adolescents, women of childbearing age, and pregnant women are the most vulnerable.

Ethnicity: Iron-deficiency anemia is seen more commonly in women of Caribbean, Latin American, Asian, Mediterranean, and African descent.

Contributing Factors: Low stores of iron in women are related to menses and pregnancy. It takes about 4 months for adult women to display a drop in hemoglobin after iron stores have been depleted.

Signs and Symptoms: Fatigue may be a symptom. Pale skin and pallor of the conjunctiva may be present. Many women with low hemoglobin levels are asymptomatic. Anemia is discovered with screening. The most common time for screening is during pregnancy.

Diagnostic Tests: Hemoglobin and hematocrit, serum iron, total iron-binding capacity (Fig. 15–1).

Differential Diagnosis
- Pernicious anemia
- Chronic anemia related to HIV, diabetes, or chronic infection
- Chronic renal failure (creates serious anemia)
- Sickle cell anemia

Treatment
- Give oral iron therapy at 60–180 mg daily.
- Recheck hemoglobin in 2–3 weeks. If no change, further investigation is required.
- Treat pernicious anemia with daily injections of vitamin B_{12}.
- Give folate, needed during pregnancy and periods of rapid growth, at 1–2 mg daily.

Follow-up: After initiating iron therapy, recheck the hemoglobin level in 2–3 weeks.

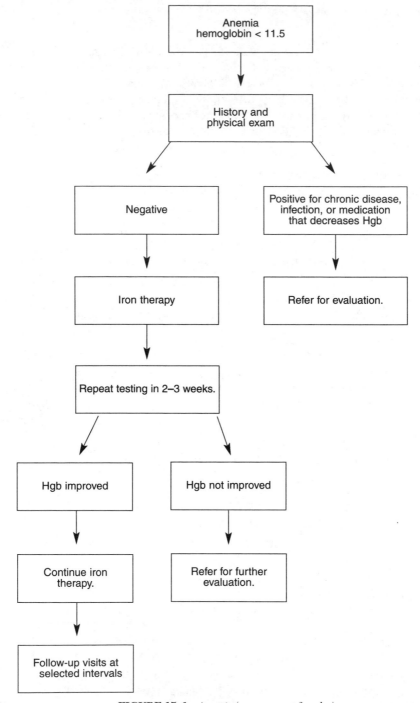

FIGURE 15–1 Anemia (nonpregnant females).

Sequelae: None for iron-deficiency anemia if diagnosed and treated.

Prevention/Prophylaxis: Periodic screening of hemoglobin levels should be performed on all women with a history of excessive menstrual bleeding. Hemoglobin levels are screened on every prenatal client.

Referral: Women unresponsive to iron therapy should be referred for further evaluation.

Education: Folate is needed during pregnancy for the health of both mother and baby. Establishment of early prenatal care allows for early supplementation of iron and folate.

Sickle cell anemia creates severe recurrent bone pain. Pregnancy increases the risks associated with sickle cell anemia (increased urinary tract infections and pulmonary infections).

Genetic counseling for the father of the baby is recommended to help determine the risk of disease for the fetus. Sickle cell anemia and pregnancy create a high-risk situation. Early diagnosis and referral are necessary.

Human Immunodeficiency Virus (HIV-1, HIV-2)

Women represent the fastest-growing group of adults with AIDS (symptomatic HIV). How many women are infected with HIV is unknown. Typically, the woman infected may not progress to the symptomatic stage of the disease for 10 years, although individual variation is wide and the range is 1–20 years.

Etiology: HIV is a viral disease.

Occurrence: In 1995, 71,818 women were diagnosed with AIDS in the United States.

Age: HIV infection can occur at any age.

Ethnicity: AIDS is more prominent in African-American and Latin-American women than in Caucasian women.

Contributing Factors: Poverty, drug abuse (injection with a contaminated needle), victims of violence, sexual contact, contact with infected body secretions, receipt of infected blood.

Signs and Symptoms: Three phases of the disease exist:

- Acute or primary—This phase lasts 2–12 weeks. Viral replication is high in this phase and viral load is high. Of people infected, 20%–70% report non-specific symptoms such as fever, malaise, lymphadenopathy, sore throat, and maculopapular rash on the upper thorax. Plasma is HIV-positive in this phase. Antibody screening is negative.
- Clinical latency—This phase lasts for 1–20 years. Viral load decreases. Antibodies become detectable. Replication of the virus occurs primarily in the

lymphoid tissue. The women are asymptomatic other than painless lymphadenopathy.

- Symptomatic phase—This phase is commonly referred to as AIDS. Symptoms include opportunistic infections, neoplasms, neurologic complications, and severe wasting.

Diagnostic Tests: Enzyme-linked immunosorbent assay (ELISA) is the initial screening test. If this test is positive, the Western blot confirms infection with HIV. Informed consent must be obtained prior to HIV testing (Fig. 15–2).

Differential Diagnosis: Epstein-Barr virus infection, cytomegalovirus (CMV) infection, and mononucleosis.

Treatment: HIV is treated with antiretroviral agents including protease inhibitors and nucleoside reverse transcriptase inhibitors. A combination of agents is utilized because it is difficult for the virus to develop multiple mutations simultaneously. The goal of treatment is to slow the decline of the immune system.

Follow-up: HIV infection is a chronic disease. Women infected with the virus are followed carefully throughout their lives.

Sequelae: Progressive immunosuppression results in opportunistic infections. (Table 15–1). Women with HIV have an increased incidence of genital tract neoplasms. Women with HIV have a higher mortality rate than men with HIV. Access to care may account for the difference.

Prevention/Prophylaxis: Reduction of risk factors. HIV-infected women have an increased susceptibility to sexually transmitted diseases. Sexually transmitted diseases increase susceptibility to HIV. A woman who is diagnosed with any sexually transmitted disease should be counseled about HIV infection and screened for HIV.

Referral: Women diagnosed with HIV require referral into a team centered on the care of HIV-positive women. The team should include medical, nursing, and social services. Women with HIV require special care during pregnancy, during considerations for birth control, and during any infection, including sexually transmitted diseases and pelvic inflammatory disease.

Education: Early diagnosis and facilitation of care are critical in the care of women and children. Of those treated with combination drugs, 60%–90% have prolonged periods of undetectable levels of HIV RNA. Early identification of HIV-infected women can greatly reduce the number of infected infants. Of HIV infection in infants, 60%–70% occurs at delivery; 30% of infections occur earlier in the prenatal course. Prenatal therapy for HIV can reduce transmission by 60%–70%. Pregnancy is a window of opportunity for prevention of vertical transmission. Counseling and referral for testing for all pregnant women is recommended. Breastfeeding, which contributes to the risk of transmission of HIV, accounts for one-third to one-half of vertical transmission worldwide.

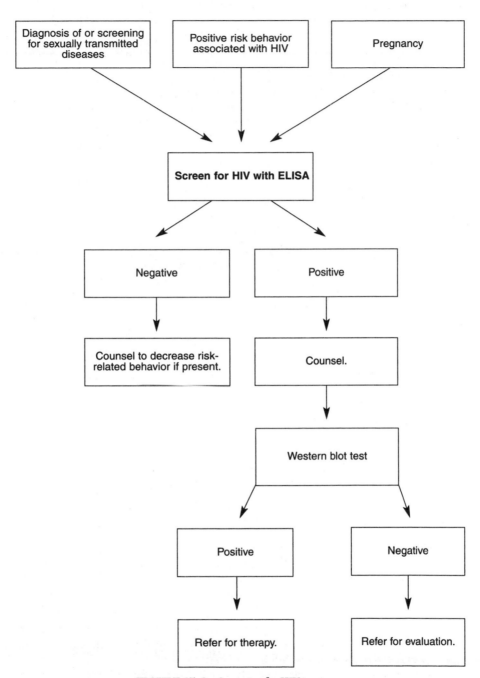

FIGURE 15–2 Screening for HIV in women.

TABLE 15-1 OPPORTUNISTIC DISEASES

CD4 number	Condition
200–500 mm³	Thrush Kaposi's sarcoma Tuberculosis reactivation Herpes zoster Bacterial sinusitis/pneumonia Herpes simplex
100–200 mm³	*Pneumocystis carinii* pneumonia All of the above
50–100 mm³	Systemic fungal infections Primary tuberculosis Cryptosporidiosis Cerebral toxoplasmosis Progressive multifocal leukoencephalopathy Peripheral neuropathy Cervical carcinoma
0–50 mm³	Cytomegalovirus disease Disseminated *Mycobacterium avium* complex Non-Hodgkin's lymphoma Central nervous system lymphoma AIDS dementia complex

BIBLIOGRAPHY

General

Seltzer, V, and Pearse, W: Women's Primary Health Care. McGraw-Hill, New York, 1995.

Anemia

Viteri, F: A new concept in the control of iron deficiency. Biomedical and Environmental Sciences 1(1):46–60, 1998.

HIV/AIDS

Bulterys, M, and Lepage, P: Mother to child transmission of HIV. Curr Opin Pediatr 10(2): 143, 1998.

Cohen, M: Natural history of HIV infection in women. Obstet Gynecol Clin North Am 24(4): 743, 1997.

Hoyt, L: HIV infection in women and children. Postgrad Med 102(4):165, 1997.

Korn, A, and Abercrombie, P: Gynecology and family planning care for women infected with HIV. Obstet Gynecol Clin North Am 24(4):855, 1997.

Kreiss, J: Breast feeding and vertical transmission of HIV-1. Acta Paediatr Suppl 421:113, 1997.

Norse, C, and Butler, K: Perinatal transmission of HIV and diagnosis of HIV infection in infants. Ir J Med Sci 167(1):28, 1998.

Phair, J, and Murphy, R: Contemporary Diagnosis and Management of HIV/AIDS Infections. Handbooks in Health Care, Newtown, PA, 1997.

CHAPTER **16**

SYMPTOM-BASED

PROBLEMS

Nurse practitioners (NPs) are called upon to diagnose and treat or refer women who present with a vague complaint. Pain is a common female presentation with an unspecified qualifier such as headache, "belly" pain, or pain with intercourse. The NP must, through guided interview and examination, qualify the complaint and establish a treatment or referral plan.

The most common symptom-based complaints from women to the women's health NP include abdominal pain, pelvic pain, breast pain, and headache. For each of these complaints, an important NP function is to differentiate between acute and chronic conditions and recognize which women require immediate referral for treatment.

Abdominal Pain

NPs in women's health are frequently challenged when a woman presents with abdominal pain. A woman's definition of abdominal pain, particularly lower abdominal pain, includes both the abdomen and the pelvis. Women do not consider the abdomen and pelvis as separate areas, so they frequently visit the women's health NP with a complaint of "belly" pain. The pain that may be diffuse or localized is frequently associated with nausea and vomiting. The woman's previous experience with pain, her culture, and her educational background influence her interpretation of pain. All of these factors make diagnosis a challenge.

The three categories of abdominal pain include:

Visceral pain. This pain tends to be localized and is perceived as dull, burning, diffuse, and sometimes crampy. It can produce nausea, vomiting, and diaphoresis.

Somatic pain. This pain is described as sharp, knifelike, and well localized.
Referred pain. This is pain located in an area other than the source; for example, pain under the diaphragm can be related to a ruptured ovarian cyst.

Etiology: Cholecystitis, diverticulitis, pancreatitis, perforated ulcer, obstruction, appendicitis, and irritable bowel (Table 16–1).

Occurrence: Depends on etiology.

TABLE 16–1 ETIOLOGY OF ABDOMINAL PAIN

Disease	Age	Symptoms	Diagnostic Aides
Cholecystitis	30–60	Pain commonly starts a few hours after a meal that includes fatty foods. Nausea and vomiting are common. Pain is located in right upper quadrant (RUQ) and may radiate to the scapulae or shoulder. Deep inspiration increases the pain.	Ultrasound
Diverticulitis	50–60	Pain in the left lower quadrant (LLQ). Nausea is common. Elevated WBC count.	CT scan
Pancreatitis	30–50	Commonly associated with chronic alcoholism or biliary tract disease. Pain is epigastric and radiates to the back. Nausea and vomiting are common. Severe tenderness on palpation. Elevated amylase and WBCs.	Abdominal ultrasound and CT scan
Perforated ulcer	Any age	Pain is sharp, epigastric, and radiates out over the entire abdomen. Shoulder pain may be present. Nausea and vomiting are common. Fever. Serum amylase and WBCs are elevated. The abdomen is rigid with rebound tenderness in all four quadrants.	Abdominal x-ray and CT scan
Large bowel obstruction	More than 40 years	Pain has a gradual onset accompanied by constipation, absence of flatulence, and abdominal distention. Abdomen is tympanic.	Abdominal x-ray or CT scan
Appendicitis	Teens to early twenties	Pain begins in the periumbilical area and migrates toward the right lower quadrant (RLQ). Atypical location can and does occur during pregnancy and retrocecal appendix. In these cases, pain is in the RUQ. Mild fever may be present. WBCs may be elevated.	Abdominal ultrasound

Age: See Table 16–1.

Ethnicity: Gallstone formation is more common in Native American women over 30 years of age than in other American women.

Contributing Factors: High-fat diet; gallstones occur more frequently in women who have been pregnant than in nonparous women. Women who use oral contraceptives for at least 4 years have a twofold increased incidence of cholecystitis.

Signs and Symptoms: Fever suggests sepsis, pelvic abscess, pelvic inflammatory disease (PID), appendicitis, or pyelonephritis. The woman will be able to identify where the pain is most intense. Auscultation of the abdomen may reveal increased or decreased bowel sounds. Palpation of the abdomen may reveal direct, rebound, or referred tenderness. Masses may be present. Note any guarding and rigidity. Direct and/or rebound tenderness points to an inflammatory process (Fig. 16–1).

Diagnostic Tests: History is the most important diagnostic test for abdominal pain. Carefully elicit the nature, onset, location, severity, duration, quality, radiation pattern, and effect on activity. The woman should describe her activities prior to onset of the pain, including whether the onset of pain was gradual or sudden. Ask the patient how eating, urination, and defecation affect the pain. Obtain a detailed description of the pain. In addition, obtain the menstrual history.

Complete blood count (CBC) with differential, urinalysis, amylase, liver function tests, pregnancy test, and abdominal or pelvic ultrasound assist with diagnosis. Abdominal x-ray series or computed tomography (CT) scan of the abdomen or pelvis or both may be required.

Differential Diagnosis: PID, ectopic pregnancy, acute gastroenteritis, ruptured ovarian cyst, mittelschmerz.

Treatment: Depends on diagnosis. Hospitalization may be required. Surgical or medical therapy may be indicated.

Follow-up: Surgical therapy requires frequent, but short-term, follow-up visits. Medical therapy requires long-term follow-up for adjustment of diet and medication.

Sequelae: Depends on the severity of the illness.

Prevention/Prophylaxis: Low-fat diet, weight control, stress management.

Referral: Abdominal pain requires referral to either a surgeon or a medical doctor. Any evidence of peritoneal irritation or obstruction is an indication for immediate hospitalization and surgical consultation.

Education: Stress the importance of follow-up after diagnosis and treatment, counseling for low-fat diet if prescribed, methods of weight reduction or maintenance, and strategies for stress reduction.

Right Upper Quadrant
Cholecystitis
Pancreatitis
Perforated ulcer
Appendicitis
Pneumonia
Ischemic bowel
Intraperitoneal bleeding

Left Upper Quadrant
Gastritis
Pancreatitis
Perforated ulcer
Pneumonia
Ischemic bowel
Gastric ulcer disease
Intraperitoneal bleeding

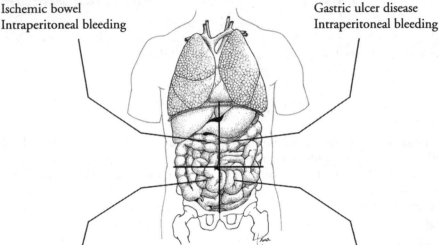

Right Lower Quadrant
Large bowel obstruction
Appendicitis
Irritable bowel
Ectopic pregnancy
PID/Tubo-ovarian abscess
Ruptured ovarian cyst
Mittelschmerz
Ureteral calculi
Ischemic bowel
Intraperitoneal bleeding

Left Lower Quadrant
Large bowel obstruction
Diverticulitis
Irritable bowel
Ectopic pregnancy
PID/Tubo-ovarian abscess
Ruptured ovarian cyst
Mittelschmerz
Ureteral calculi
Ischemic bowel
Intraperitoneal bleeding

FIGURE 16–1   Possible sources of abdominal pain.

Pelvic Pain

Diagnosis and treatment of acute pelvic pain are discussed elsewhere in this book. Common causes of acute pelvic pain include PID (see Chap. 8), ectopic pregnancy (see Chap.17), urinary tract infection (see Chap. 10), and mittelschmerz (painful ovulation). Refer to the box for a more complete listing of the causes of acute pelvic pain.

PELVIC PAIN

Acute	Chronic
PID	Primary dysmenorrhea
Torsion of tube or ovary	Secondary dysmenorrhea
Ovarian cysts	Irritable bowel syndrome
Appendicitis	Pelvic adhesions
Kidney stones	Pelvic relaxation
UTI	Interstitial cystitis
Diverticulitis	Levator spasm
Intestinal abscess	
Mittelschmerz	

This section discusses pelvic pain of a more chronic nature, most specifically, factors related to dysmenorrhea and dyspareunia.

History

When a woman presents with pelvic pain, you must rule out an acute condition. Acute abdominal pain with fever, hypotension, tachycardia, rigid abdomen on palpation, and decreased bowel sounds requires immediate referral. Signs of ectopic pregnancy with positive pregnancy test and acute unilateral pelvic pain also require immediate referral. In addition, torsion of the ovary causing unilateral acute pain with negative elevated white blood cell (WBC) levels and sedimentation rate requires immediate attention. Signs and symptoms of PID also require immediate attention (see Chap. 8).

A history of constipation, nausea and vomiting, or diarrhea indicates that the cause of the pain is abdominal. A history of flank pain and dysuria indicates that the pain originates in the urinary tract.

The date of the last menstrual period (LMP) must be obtained. A relationship between the pain and the menstrual cycle must be established.

Onset of the pain, quality of the pain, as well as whether or not the pain radiates and to where the pain radiates must be established. (Cervical, uterine, and vaginal pathology can be referred to the back or buttock; tubal or ovarian pathology can cause pain to radiate to the medial thigh.)

Questions must be asked concerning exacerbating factors as well as factors that decrease the pain.

Examination

Perform an abdominal examination, emphasizing points of tenderness. (If raising the head increases tenderness, the pain involves the abdominal wall. If raising the head decreases the pain, the pain is visceral.)

TABLE 16–2   CHRONIC PELVIC PAIN

Source	History	Examination
Endometriosis	Increasing dysmenorrhea	Pelvic tenderness
Primary dysmenorrhea	Pain with menses from menarche	Negative
Secondary dysmenorrhea	Pain with menses	Uterine and/or adnexal tenderness
Pelvic adhesions	Starts months after surgery, localized	Thickening on exam, pain with motion

Perform a pelvic examination, emphasizing areas of adnexal thickening, cervical discharge, uterine masses, fixation of any structures, ovarian masses, or focal tenderness. If the woman can point to the pain, ask her to draw a circle around it indicating how far the pain radiates.

Laboratory testing that assists in diagnosis includes serum human chorionic gonadotropin (hCG) level; CBC, sedimentation rate, urinalysis, culture of the cervix and rectum, and ultrasound examination of the pelvis (Table 16–2, Fig. 16–2).

| Dysmenorrhea

Dysmenorrhea is painful menstruation. Dysmenorrhea is divided into two types, primary and secondary. Primary dysmenorrhea occurs with menses from menarche. Secondary dysmenorrhea occurs with menses after menarche. Primary dysmenorrhea does not imply underlying pathology. Secondary dysmenorrhea, especially if it occurs after years of minimal or no discomfort, can indicate an underlying pathology (Fig. 16–3).

Etiology: Dysmenorrhea is caused by an increase in prostaglandin levels. Increased uterine tone and dysrhythmic contractions create a "cramping" sensation with menses.

Occurrence: Dysmenorrhea affects one-half of menstruating women. Of menstruating women, 10% report being incapacitated by dysmenorrhea.

Age: Dysmenorrhea can occur in any menstruating female.

Ethnicity: Not significant.

Contributing Factors: Endometriosis, PID, adenomyosis, ovarian cysts.

Signs and Symptoms: Painful menses "crampy" in nature occurring with the onset of menses and lasting 48–72 hours. The cramping is felt in the suprapubic area, low back, and inner thighs.

Diagnostic Tests: CBC and differential, sedimentation rate, urinalysis, serum hCG, pelvic ultrasound.

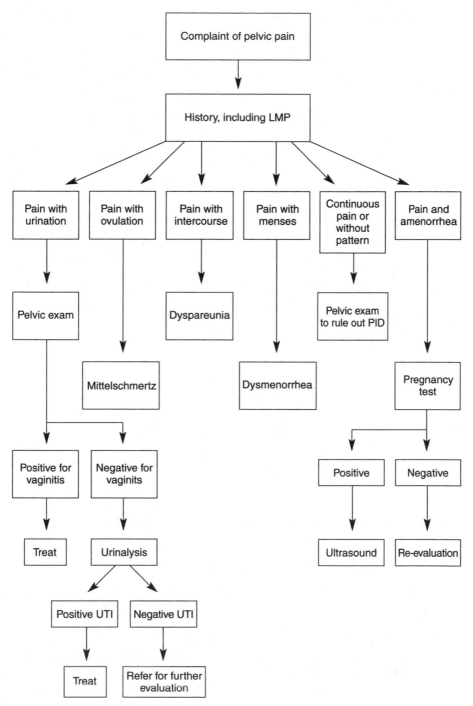

FIGURE 16–2 Pelvic pain.

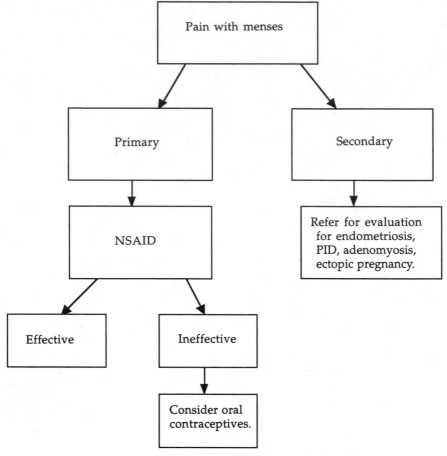

FIGURE 16–3 Dysmenorrhea.

Differential Diagnosis: PID, ectopic pregnancy, torsion of the ovary, ruptured ovarian cyst, acute abdomen, pelvic mass.

Treatment: Nonsteroidal anti-inflammatory agents are effective for relief of dysmenorrhea. Oral contraceptives reduce dysmenorrhea.

Follow-up: Follow-up visits for efficacy of therapy are advised for dysmenorrhea.

Sequelae: None.

Prevention/Prophylaxis: None.

Referral: Secondary dysmenorrhea requires consultation for further diagnosis and treatment.

Education: Dysmenorrhea is a common complaint among menstruating women. Cramping with menses that interferes with usual activity is an indication for evaluation and treatment. Cramping with menses, in women who have no prior episodes, is an indication for evaluation.

Dyspareunia

Dyspareunia is pain with intercourse; it is a pain syndrome, not a sexual dysfunction. Many conditions can create dyspareunia, including infection and allergy.

Etiology: There are two types of dyspareunia. The first type that creates pain on insertion is caused by lack of lubrication, lack of stimulation, or vulvar irritation and inflammation. The second type that creates pain on deep penetration is caused by endometriosis, ovarian cysts, adhesions, or PID (Fig. 16–4).

Occurrence: Of women surveyed, 60% report experiencing dyspareunia at least once in their lives; 30% of women surveyed labeled dyspareunia as a chronic problem.

Age: Dyspareunia can occur in any sexually active female.

Ethnicity: Not significant.

Contributing Factors: Vaginal infections; allergens, such as deodorants, soaps, douching agents, bubble bath, and contraceptive foams and creams; obesity; incontinence; shaving in the pelvic area; history of sexual abuse.

Signs and Symptoms: Infection or allergy (erythematous and edematous vulva; rashes such as macules, papules, scaling, ulcers, lesions; lice; palpable inguinal lymph nodes); evidence of incontinence; vulvar atrophy; pelvic relaxation (see Chap. 8); vulvodynia, that is, chronic vulvar discomfort with burning and stinging producing irritation and "rawness"; Bartholin's cyst and abscess, which presents as a tender, cystic mass in the area of the Bartholin's gland.

Diagnostic Tests: CBC, sedimentation rate, cervical and vaginal culture.

Differential Diagnosis: Infected episiotomy, retained suture material, urethritis or cystitis, vulvar cancer.

Treatment
Treat bacterial infection with topical or systemic antibiotics.
Treat fungal infection with antifungal medication.
Treat atrophy with supplemental lubrication, Kegel exercises, position changes for intercourse, and/or estrogen cream.
Treat Bartholin's cyst or abscess with warm soaks to encourage drainage.

Follow-up: All women with pelvic pain should have a follow-up visit(s). The multiple causes of this condition require follow-up for assurance of correct diagnosis, treatment, and resolution.

Sequelae: Resolution occurs in most cases with appropriate therapy. Vulvodynia occurs in 9% of women with vulvar symptoms. This syndrome has no known etiology and is, therefore, difficult to treat. Vulvodynia is a chronic condition.

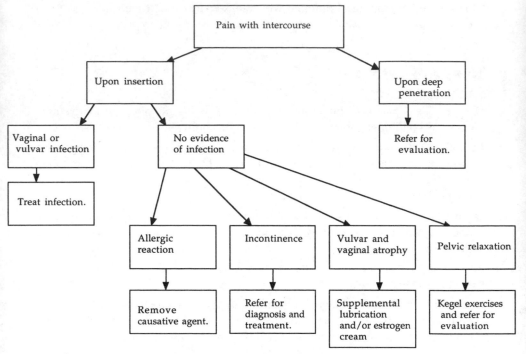

FIGURE 16-4   Dyspareunia.

Prevention/Prophylaxis: Supplemental lubrication in the menopausal period. Prevention of vaginal infection.

Referral

Women with deep dyspareunia require referral for diagnosis of any of the etiologic agents, such as PID, ovarian cysts, adhesions, or endometriosis.

Women with vulvodynia, a diagnosis made by exclusion, should be referred to a provider specializing in this disease.

Pelvic relaxation should be referred to a gynecologist for treatment.

Sexual dysfunction, particularly if the partner also has a dysfunction, should be referred to a specialist.

Women with a history of sexual abuse should be referred to a provider skilled in dealing with this issue.

Bartholin's cysts that do not respond to local therapy or require incision and drainage (I&D) should be referred for therapy. Therapy includes I&D or marsupialization or insertion of a Word catheter.

Education: As a part of their education process, all women should learn about the human sexual response cycle. Pain with intercourse is not a "normal" occurrence and may indicate an underlying disorder.

Other Symptom-Based Problems

Two other symptom-based complaints are common in women. One is breast pain (mastalgia) and the second is headache. Good history-taking skill that will guide decisions about treatment and referral is the key to providing adequate care for women with these complaints.

Refer to Chapter 2 for a discussion of breast examination. Discussion of neurologic examination is beyond the scope of this text. Refer to a text that describes eye examination, examination of the head and neck, and neurologic examination for review prior to evaluating headache.

Cyclic Mastalgia

Cyclic mastalgia is the most common breast-related complaint seen in women's health practice. The breast is a complex organ that is sensitive to hormones. Estradiol and progesterone stimulate breast tissue. Breast pain that positively correlates with menses is called cyclic mastalgia. Cyclic mastalgia and fibrocystic changes are not the same (see Chap. 7). One can exist without the other. Cysts and pain are different entities that may or may not occur together.

Etiology: Premenstrual breast tenderness and swelling in the luteal phase most commonly occurs 1–4 days premenstrually. It may occur anywhere from 5–14 days premenstrually. The severity and intensity can vary.

Occurrence: In a study of more than 1000 women reporting to an Ob/Gyn clinic, 69% described premenstrual breast discomfort; 36% reported seeking help for this condition; 20% reported seeking out more than one health-care provider for advice related to this symptom. Cyclic mastalgia, when defined as a part of premenstrual syndrome, is better established than mood disorders.

Age: Cyclic mastalgia can occur in any menstruating female.

Ethnicity: Not significant.

Contributing Factors: Caffeine consumption, hormone replacement therapy, oral contraceptives.

Signs and Symptoms: Breast pain prior to menses. The pain may decrease normal activities. Women report wearing loose clothing and avoiding touching of the breasts during sexual activity premenstrually. The pain does not usually interfere with work or school or with social activities.

Physical examination does not reveal mass or discharge. The breast is tender upon palpation.

Diagnostic Tests: None are indicated; however, women less than 36 years old with cyclic mastalgia are five times more likely to have a mammogram than asymptomatic women.

Differential Diagnosis: Breast infection, duct obstruction, breast cancer with inflammatory mass, periareolar infection, trauma.

Treatment: Support bra, avoidance of caffeine, vitamin E supplementation up to 400 IU daily. Reassurance is part of the treatment plan for cyclic mastalgia. Medications such as danazol, tamoxifen, and bromocriptine have been utilized for breast tenderness. These medications have many adverse reactions such as hot flashes, hirsutism, and dysfunctional uterine bleeding. They should be utilized only in the most severe cases of cyclic mastalgia.

Follow-up: Follow-up is at the discretion of the woman.

Sequelae: The extent to which cyclic mastalgia influences breast screening, self-medication, and use of alternative medicine is unknown.

Prevention/Prophylaxis: Decrease caffeine consumption.

Referral: Severe cases of cyclic mastalgia require referral.

Education: Types of food and drinks containing caffeine should be reviewed. Hazards of overconsumption of vitamin E, a fat-soluble vitamin, should be reviewed.

Headache

Fewer than 1% of headaches in women indicate serious intracranial disease. Headaches have multiple possible causative factors; the NP is frequently asked to help female clients "sort out" the possible etiology of their particular headache.

Etiology: Headache can be caused by intracranial or extracranial factors. Intracranial factors are derived from cranial nerves, dura, and cranial arteries. Extracranial factors are derived from skin; muscles; eyes; blood vessels; extracranial arteries; mucous membranes of nose, ears, sinuses; or the temporomandibular joint.

Occurrence: Unknown.

Age: Headache can occur at any age.

Ethnicity: Not significant.

Contributing Factors: Stress, menses, food allergies, sinus infection, temporomandibular joint dysfunction, systemic infection, hypertension, eye muscle strain.

Signs and Symptoms: Headache can be mild, moderate, or severe; unilateral or bilateral; generalized or localized; and with sudden or gradual onset.

Diagnostic Tests: History, including a description of the intensity of the headache, presence of aura, character of the pain, precipitants, aggravating and alleviating factors, and a medication history.

Examination should include blood pressure and temperature, eyes, mouth, ears and sinuses, neck, and tests for neurologic signs. Include CT scan of the head to rule out a mass if appropriate.

Differential Diagnosis

Migraine headache: Migraine affects 10% of adults, with more women than men affected. In two-thirds of women with migraines, there is a family history of the disease. Migraine can begin in childhood or in early adulthood. Sixteen % of women with migraine reporting their first migraine in the perimenopausal years. One in seven women with migraines is affected by them only around the time of menses. Many women with migraines report an increase in number and severity of headaches surrounding menses.

Migraines can occur with or without aura. Migraine symptoms include nausea, anorexia, and photophobia. Migraine headache is described as unilateral, pulsing, moderate to severe, and increasing with activity. Migraine is described with the following phases: prodrome, aura, headache, termination, and postdrome. Precipitants include emotional upset, particular foods, and menses.

CHARACTERISTICS OF MIGRAINE HEADACHES

Prodrome	Aura	Headache	Termination	Postdrome
Irritability	Visual symptoms	Unilateral	24–48 hours	Fatigue
Nausea	Vertigo	Throbbing		Irritability
Difficulty concentrating	Aphasia			

Source: Sturm, J, and Donnan, G: Diagnosis and investigation of headache. Aust Fam Physician 27(7): 587, 1998.

Tension headache: A tension headache is described as dull and steady, chronic or recurrent, bilateral pressure about the head that increases as the day progresses. Precipitating factors include anxiety and stress.

Sinus infection: Sinus infection creates headache that is throbbing, acute at onset, worse upon awakening, better after rising, and worse as the day progresses. Sinus headache is accompanied by purulent nasal discharge.

Temporomandibular joint dysfunction: This condition creates headache from tension induced by jaw clenching and nocturnal teeth grinding. Masticator muscles fatigue and spasm, creating a chronic dull aching headache and difficulty opening the mouth in the morning.

Ocular headache: Ocular headache occurs from eye muscle strain or acute glaucoma.

Masses: Masses in the head create headache one-third of the time. When masses create headache, the headache is in one location, progressive, and increases in duration and severity. Eventually changes in mental status occur.

Meningitis: This inflammation creates a severe, generalized, and constant headache.

Systemic fever and infection: Systemic fever and infection create cranial vasodi-latation and a diffuse throbbing headache.

Hypertension: High blood pressure creates an occipital headache that is worse in the morning.

Treatment: The causative factor can be removed, thus eliminating the headache in ocular headache, hypertension headache, and headache related to infection and fever. Medication is available to reduce the frequency and severity of migraine headache. Tension headache is treated with nonsteroidal anti-inflammatory medication or acetaminophen.

Follow-up: Migraine headache requires frequent follow-up for management of medication.

Sequelae: There is an increased probability of stroke during migraine headache.

Prevention/Prophylaxis: Women with a history of migraine headache should carefully consider the use of oral contraceptives and supplemental estrogen. The incidence of migraine may increase with increased estrogen.

Referral: Headache must be quickly referred if it is sudden, severe, or persistent. A new headache of acute onset or a headache that progresses over days or weeks, or any headache with an abnormal neurological examination requires immediate referral. Neck stiffness, altered mental state, ataxia, and severe nausea and vomiting all require immediate referral.

Education: Frequency of analgesic use, whether prescription or over-the-counter, should be assessed in all women who complain of headache.

BIBLIOGRAPHY

Abdominal Pain

Barrenetexa, G, Schneider, J, and Rodriquez-Escudero, F: Abdominal mass in a young woman. Pitfalls and delayed diagnosis. Eur J Gynaecol Oncol 17(6):507, 1996.
Goroll, A, May, L, and Mulley, A: Primary Care Medicine. JB Lippincott, Philadelphia, 1995.
McFadyen, B, et al: Laparoscopic management of the acute abdomen. Surg Clin North Am 72(5): 1169, 1992.
Seltzer, V, and Pearse, W: Women's Primary Health Care. McGraw-Hill, New York, 1995.
Silen, W: Early Diagnosis of the Acute Abdomen. Oxford Press, London, 1991.
Taylor, K, and Kelner, M: The emerging role of the physician in genetic counseling and testing for heritable breast, ovarian, and colon cancer. CMAJ 154(8):115, 1996.

Breast Pain

Adler, D, and Browne, M: Prevalence and impact of cyclic mastalgia in a United States clinic based sample. Am J Obstet Gynecol 177(1):126, 1997.
Tavaf-Motamen, H: Clinical evaluation of mastalgia. Arch Surg 133(2):211, 1998.

Pelvic Pain

Apgar, B: Dysmenorrhea and dysfunctional uterine bleeding. Primary Care Clin Office Pract 24(1):161, 1997.
Baggish, M, and Miklos, J: Vulvar pain syndrome: A review. Obstet Gynecol Surv 50(8):618, 1995.

Fisher, G: The commonest causes of symptomatic vulvar disease: A dermatologist's perspective. Aust J Dermatol 37(1):12, 1996.

Hill, D, and Lense, J: Office management of Bartholin gland cyst and abscesses. Am Fam Physician 57(7):1619, 1998.

Jamieson, D, and Steege, J: The prevalence of dysmenorrhea, dyspareunia, pelvic pain, and irritable bowel syndrome in primary care practices. Obstet Gynecol 87(1):55, 1996.

Jamieson, D, and Steege, J: The association of sexual abuse with pelvic pain complaints in primary care populations. Am J Obstet Gynecol 177(6):1408, 1997.

Lecks, K: Vulvodynia: Diagnosis and management. J A Acad Nurse Pract 10(3):129, 1998.

Steege, J: Office assessment of chronic pelvic pain. Clin Obstet Gynecol 40(3):554, 1997.

Other Symptom-Based Disorders

Marks, D, and Rappoport, A: Practical evaluation and diagnosis of headache. Semin Neurol 17(4):307, 1997.

CHAPTER 17

ANTENATAL CARE

Demographic trends, pressures to reduce medical costs and improve access to care, and women's choices surrounding health care are creating important changes in prenatal care. According to the U.S. Department of Health and Human Services, there has been a general upward trend in the number of births in the last decade. Although three-quarters of the births in the United States are in women between the ages of 20 and 35, there has been a trend toward childbearing in the late 30s and early 40s. Childbearing outside of marriage has increased during the last two decades. In the last 10 years, the teenage birthrate has increased, particularly among girls ages 15–17. These demographic trends are affecting prenatal care both directly through numbers of clients and age of clients, and indirectly through the formation of public policy. If the trends continue, the demand for obstetricians, nurse midwives, and nurse practitioners will remain high and possibly increase. Pressures to reduce cost and increase access are creating a demand for nurse practitioners with creative nurse-centered strategies.

The objective of prenatal care is to ensure that every wanted pregnancy culminates in the delivery of a healthy baby without jeopardizing the health of the mother. Creative strategies are necessary for reaching this objective and simultaneously meeting the requests of the prenatal client. Reaching the objective and creating an experience that the woman perceives as positive is best accomplished with a team approach. A balance between technology and sensitivity is best achieved through a team approach, with the team consisting of the pregnant woman, advanced practice nurses specializing in women's health, obstetricians, perinatologists, nurses, social workers, and dietitians. Each of these team members contributes a unique perspective to the case management of each prenatal client. Each team member will represent a segment of the entire clinical picture. In a well-functioning team, plans for care can be devised that meet the health needs of the prenatal client and her fetus in a manner that is acceptable to the woman.

220

Assessment

Prenatal Assessment

The purpose of prenatal assessment is to evaluate the status of the woman and her fetus during pregnancy, to identify risks, and to plan for early intervention. Initial evaluation of the prenatal patient should include a comprehensive history, a physical assessment, diagnostic testing, and an overall risk assessment. A plan of care is formulated at the first visit, reviewed with the patient, and updated as needed throughout her prenatal course.

HEALTH HISTORY

Health history should be obtained at the first prenatal visit and updated at each prenatal visit. The history should include at least the following information. Additional information should be obtained based on the health-related characteristics of the patient population.

Name
Age
Race
Gravida and Para
Date of last normal menses, frequency of menses
Contraceptive use prior to last menstrual period
Obstetric history, starting with the first pregnancy and including all pregnancies
  up to the current pregnancy (including health of the children)
Past medical illnesses and/or surgeries
History of chronic illness
Gynecologic history, including past or present genital infections and sexually
  transmitted diseases, previous Pap smears, history of fibroids, exposure to di-
  ethylstilbestrol (DES)
Endocrine disorders
Systems review (see Chap. 5)
Exposure to Viruses during This Pregnancy
Medication use during this pregnancy
Symptoms during this pregnancy, including bleeding, nausea and vomiting
Allergies and/or drug sensitivities
Immunization history
Human immunodeficiency virus (HIV) risk assessment
Work history, including exposure to hazardous agents
Substance abuse history, including past or present use of alcohol, caffeine, to-
  bacco, prescription drug use, over-the-counter drug use, and illicit drug use
Dietary habits before and during pregnancy
Weight, current and before pregnancy

Exercise patterns
Elimination patterns
Sleep patterns
Significant stress
Relationship with the father of the baby
Support persons
Domestic violence screening
Socioeconomic status
Cultural background and network
Educational level
Age, occupation, and race of father of the baby
Family history, including allergies, cardiovascular disease, endocrine disorders, genetic or chromosomal disorders, hematologic disorders, mental retardation, multiple gestations, neurologic problems, psychiatric illnesses, renal disease, and child abuse

PHYSICAL EXAMINATION

Physical examination is performed during the first prenatal visit. This complete exam is essential for formulation of an individualized care plan for each prenatal client. The physical examination must include the following:

Height, weight, blood pressure.
Evaluation of nutritional status.
Skin: Note striae, linea nigra, increased pigmentation of aureole, jaundice, scars, lesions.
Head and neck: Note edema, lesions, lymphadenopathy.
Eyes: Determine reading ability; check pupils; perform ophthalmoscopic examination.
Ears: Test for hearing ability; perform otoscopic examination.
Nose: Note edema, ulcerations, perforation of the septum.
Lips: Note pallor, cyanosis, presence of lesions or inflammation.
Gums: Note gingivitis, bleeding.
Oral mucosa: Note erythema, lesions, or ulcerations.
Tongue: Note lesions, thrush, leukoplakia.
Teeth: Note decay, condition of dental repairs, and quality of hygiene.
Posterior pharynx: Note edema, exudate, presence of tonsils.
Thyroid: Note size and position.
Thorax and lungs: Note respiratory rate and listen to breath sounds.
Heart: Note rate and rhythm, presence of murmurs.
Breasts: Note masses, areola pigment changes, striae, nipple inversion.
Back: Note costovertebral angle (CVA) tenderness, scoliosis, or lordosis.
Abdomen: Note bowel sounds, striae; measure uterine height if appropriate; and listen to fetal heart tones if 10 weeks of gestation or more; determine fetal presentation if appropriate.
Musculoskeletal: Note limitation of movement, swollen joints, or abnormal gait.
Extremities: Note edema or varicosities (see Appendix).

Neurologic: Note affect and orientation; perform cranial nerve examination.

Pelvic examination including external genitalia: Note presence of warts, lesions, varicosities, edema, erythema, or presence of discharge; examine vagina, noting discharge, lesions; examine cervix, noting color, surface characteristics, discharge, tenderness, lesions; examine uterus, noting size, position, mobility, tenderness, masses; examine adnexa, noting size, mobility, and tenderness.

Clinical pelvimetry: Note ischial spines, transverse diameter, and diagonal conjugate measurements.

Rectal examination: Note hemorrhoids or masses.

LABORATORY DATA

Laboratory information assists in formulating a plan of care for each prenatal client. The following are recommendations for laboratory screening for low-risk prenatal clients:

Complete blood count to be drawn at 15–16 weeks' gestation and repeated at 26 to 28 weeks of gestation (see Chap. 10).

Urinalysis and urine culture and sensitivity performed at 15–16 weeks' gestation and repeated as necessary throughout the pregnancy to rule out asymptomatic bacteriuria.

Blood group and Rh type drawn at 15–16 weeks' gestation.

Antibody screen to be drawn at 15–16 weeks' gestation.

Rubella titer drawn at 15–16 weeks' gestation.

Syphilis screen drawn at 15–16 weeks' gestation.

Pap smear if last screening more than 6 months prior to first prenatal visit.

Culture for gonorrhea and *Chlamydia* at first visit with repeat at 36 weeks' gestation.

Screen for HIV at 15–16 weeks' gestation.

Hepatitis B screen to be drawn at 15–16 weeks' gestation.

Pregnancy test if indicated at first visit.

One-hour post 50-g Glucola drawn at 26–28 weeks' gestation.

Culture for group B streptococci at 34–36 weeks' gestation.

Additional testing may include screening for rubeola and cytomegalovirus (CMV); urine culture, sickle cell screen, and toxoplasmosis titer can be ordered.

Assessment of the prenatal population at the practice site will determine the laboratory profile. Plans for laboratory testing are altered according to patient's risk assessment.

Genetic screening should be discussed with each woman. Alpha-fetoprotein (AFP) or triple screen should be offered to each patient (Fig. 17–1). Additional testing for genetic disorders may be indicated based upon the woman's age and risk factors. AFP or triple screen should be drawn at 15 weeks' gestation, and thus the recommendation that other testing be coupled with this drawing of blood. If the patient does not desire AFP or triple screen, specimens for complete blood count (CBC), blood type and antibody screen, rubella, syphilis, hepatitis, and HIV can be drawn at

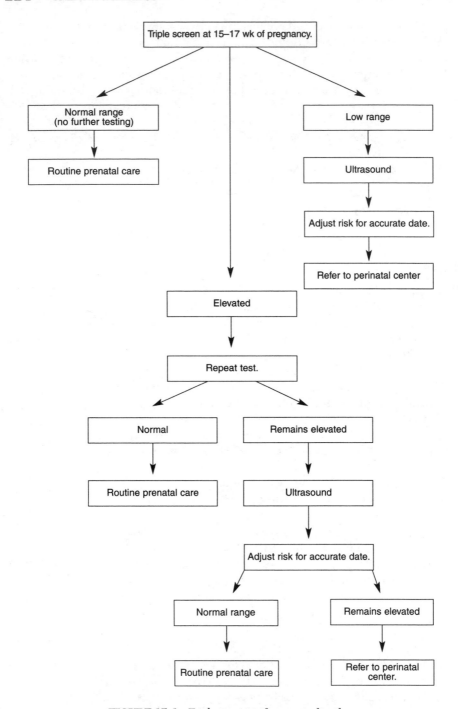

FIGURE 17–1 Triple screening for genetic disorders.

any time. AFP is interpreted by multiple of the mean (MOM), compared to the mean, and is adjusted by gestational age, weight, and presence or absence of diabetes. A low maternal serum AFP level may be an indicator of Down's syndrome. A high serum maternal AFP level may be an indicator for neural tube defects. The sensitivity of the screening requires further testing to determine if Down's syndrome or a neural tube defect is actually present. Triple screen is defined as AFP plus human chorionic gonadotropin (hCG) levels and estriol measurement. Ordering a triple screen enhances the sensitivity and predictive value of the AFP screen. Abnormal triple screen values require ultrasound to confirm gestational age and repetition of the test. A second abnormal screening requires amniocentesis to rule out Down's syndrome, or ultrasound to rule out neural tube defects.

RISK FACTOR ASSESSMENT

The first prenatal visit includes history taking, physical examination, consideration of laboratory testing, and risk assessment. Significant risk factors are determined by history and confirmed by physical examination and/or laboratory or radiologic evidence. Risk factors must be noted on the woman's chart and discussed within a reasonable amount of time with a team of health-care providers that includes an obstetrician. Risk assessment is an important component in the formation of the prenatal care plan for a client. Significant risk factors that can be detected at the first prenatal visit include:

Previous cesarean delivery, including type of uterine incision (Medical records are required to validate type of incision.)
Expected date of confinement (EDC) less than 12 months from previous delivery
Parity of 7 or more
Previous tubal pregnancy
Previous cone biopsy
Previous placental abruption or placenta previa
Severe hypertensive disorder during previous pregnancy
Previous postpartum hemorrhage
Previous abdominal or pelvic surgery
Uterine anomalies
DES exposure
Previous preterm labor, birth, or ruptured membranes
History of prolonged labor
Two or more spontaneous abortions, second-trimester abortions, or multiple first-trimester terminations
A newborn that was small or large for gestational age
Multiple gestation
History including neonatal morbidity or congenital abnormalities
Previous fetal or neonatal death
Previous breast surgery
Nutritional disorders
History of anesthesia complications

History of maternal drug use
History of infertility
Maternal age less than 15 years or more than 40 years
History of sexually transmitted diseases
Psychosocial stress
Chronic disease

CARE PLAN

A prenatal care plan is formulated after the initial visit and consultation with the team. The prenatal care plan includes:

Diagnoses
Anticipated problems
Plan of management including rationale
Predicted outcome for plan of management
Alternative(s) to plan of management including rationale

ONGOING ASSESSMENT

During each prenatal visit following the initial visit, history is updated, a physical exam is performed that includes maternal and fetal assessment, and risk assessment is re-evaluated. Ongoing assessment at each visit will include:

Updating health history
Physical assessment including weight and vital signs
Performing microscopic evaluations of urine at each visit, performing a dipstick urine and examining of vaginal and cervical secretions as indicated
Obtaining and interpreting laboratory tests
Pap smear and follow-up as indicated
Evaluating fetal well-being
Prescribing medications as indicated
Nutritional and diet counseling
Health education
Ongoing risk assessment
Assessing and treating prenatal complication(s)
Counseling as indicated including social work counseling
Implementing emergency procedures if necessary

ONGOING RISK ASSESSMENT

The following risk factors, which can be revealed at any prenatal visit, require consultation with an obstetrician either by telephone or in person. Consultation should be performed during the prenatal visit whenever possible.

Positive antibody titer
Gestation more than 28 weeks at first visit

Clinical evidence of myoma or pelvic or abdominal masses
Suspected polyhydramnios or oligohydramnios
Suspected cardiac murmur
Hematocrit (Hct) less than 28%
Sickle cell (SS) hemoglobin
Abnormal Pap smear
Multiple gestation confirmed by ultrasound
Evidence of fetal chromosomal disorder
Hypertension during pregnancy
Evidence of intrauterine growth retardation confirmed by ultrasound
Gestational diabetes confirmed by glucose tolerance test
Cardiovascular disease including thrombophlebitis, chronic hypertension, heart
    disease, and pulmonary embolus
Urinary tract disorders including renal disease and pyelonephritis
Metabolic or endocrine diseases including diabetes mellitus and/or gestational
    diabetes, thyroid disease, and use of thyroid medications
Chronic pulmonary disease including asthma and chronic bronchitis
Unexplained vaginal bleeding
Abnormal weight gain (less than 12 or greater than 50 lb)
Nonvertex presentation past 37 weeks' gestation
Nondelivery at 41 weeks' gestation
Lack of obstetric follow-up after 28 weeks of gestation
Consistent nonattendance at office visits
Evidence of nutritional disorders such as anorexia or bulimia
Evidence of maternal use of illicit drugs
Neurologic disorders including history of seizures, use of anticonvulsant drugs,
    and severe recurring migraines
Psychiatric disorders including previous psychotic episode, current mental health
    problem judged to be significant by psychiatric evaluation, and drug addiction
Active infection including tuberculosis (TB)
Autoimmune diseases including systemic lupus erythematosus (SLE)

Physiologic Adaptations of Pregnancy

Understanding the physiology of pregnancy is crucial to the development of a care
plan for prenatal clients. The following is a review of the adaptations mandated by
pregnancy presented with a systems approach.

Reproductive Tract

Uterus increases in size from a 10-mL cavity weighing 70 g to a cavity enlarged to
hold 5000 mL and weighing 1100 g. The uterus throughout pregnancy becomes in-

creasingly elastic and fibrous. Growth is in response to estrogen and progesterone and in response to the products of conception. The cervix becomes cyanotic and soft because of increased vascularity and hyperplasia. Pregnancy produces more cervical mucus with more tenacious consistency. Corpus luteum forms in an ovary and must be maintained during the first 6–7 weeks of pregnancy. The vagina produces increased discharge, which is acidic in nature. The vaginal mucosa becomes increasingly thick to allow for distensibility.

Skin

Striae, stretch marks, occur in approximately one-half of all pregnant women. Increased pigmentation occurs in the linea nigra because of melanocyte-stimulating hormone.

Breasts

Nipple enlargement and increased pigmentation occur during pregnancy. Alveolar growth is induced as pregnancy progresses.

Cardiovascular

Blood volume increases up to 32 weeks and then levels off. Blood volume increases 40%–50% during pregnancy. An increase in the plasma component is greater than the increase in the red blood cell (RBC) component, causing a physiologic anemia of pregnancy. A small decrease in systolic blood pressure occurs during pregnancy. A decrease in diastolic blood pressure becomes pronounced in midpregnancy. Blood pressure varies according to position. Blood pressure will be different in sitting position, left lateral position, and supine position because of vena caval compression and decreased venous return. Venous blood pressure increases in the lower extremities because of uterine growth. There is an increased tendency toward stasis, varicosities, and edema during pregnancy. The heart is displaced anteriorly and upward, causing an increased anteroposterior (AP) diameter and cardiothoracic ratio as well as a left axis deviation. Heart sounds change, with the first heart sound becoming louder and more greatly split. Systolic ejection murmurs are not uncommon in pregnancy. The cardiac output in lateral recumbent position increases by 30%–50%, peaking at 20–24 weeks. The uterus receives the largest increase of cardiac output, with increased blood flow from 50–500 mL/min. Renal blood flow increases by 30%. Increased blood flow to the skin during pregnancy may explain heat intolerance.

Hematologic

Red blood cell (RBC) production increases by 33%. Mean corpuscular volume (MCV) increases because of an increased number of reticulocytes. Serum iron level decreases in pregnancy. Iron requirements of 4 mg/day are needed to meet maternal and fetal needs (450 mg to increase RBCs, 350 mg to fetus, and 200 mg lost in delivery). White blood cell (WBC) total count is increased. The WBC value peaks at 30 weeks. Total lymphocyte count decreases, with the vast majority seen in decreased T helper lymphocytes. All coagulation factors increase except factors XI and XIII. Platelets decrease in the third trimester.

Endocrine

Prolactin level increases during pregnancy, up to 150 ng/mL. The pituitary enlarges, as does the thyroid gland, due to increased vascularity and hyperplasia. T_3 uptake decreases and T_4 values increase.

Pulmonary

Increased abdominal pressure causes the transverse diameter of the chest to increase by 2 cm. The costal angles widen and diaphragmatic motion is increased. Total lung capacity is unchanged in the first half of pregnancy but decreased in the second half because of decreased residual volume related to elevation of the diaphragm. Tidal volume is increased, probably mediated by progesterone. Pulmonary capacity is increased by 30%–40%. Respiratory alkalosis is caused by increased ventilation. Diffusion capacity is increased in early pregnancy as a result of increased pulmonary blood flow and subsequently decreases due to increases in HGB concentration.

Renal

During pregnancy the kidneys enlarge approximately 1 cm and weigh approximately 50 g more than in the nonpregnant state because of increased blood and water content. There is dilation of the entire collecting system because of a growing dextrorotated uterus, progesterone influence, and increased volumes of urine.

Renal blood flow and glomerular filtration increase during the first trimester and plateau into the second trimester at 30%–50% increases. Renal blood flow increases to 500 mL/min from 100 mL/min. Glomerular filtration rate (GFR) increases to 150 mL/min from 100 mL/min. Glucose is filtered in the glomerulus and reabsorbed in the tubules. Glucosuria can occur during pregnancy because of GFR overwhelming the capacity for reabsorption. Physiologic proteinuria occurs at rates of up to 300 mg/24 hr because increased GFR overcomes the ability to reabsorb protein in the tubules. HCO_3 has decreased resorption in compensation for respiratory alkalosis. The pregnant woman retains 1000 mEq sodium needed to expand the intravascular and extravascular compartments. She also retains 350 mEq of potassium in competition with the wasting of HCO_3. Serum osmolality decreases to 10 mOsm/kg with increased urine volume of 25%.

Digestive

Gums become edematous and bleed more easily because of increased blood flow and increased mucopolysaccharide levels. The lower esophageal sphincter has increased pressure because of the enlarging uterus and increased progesterone. The stomach has decreased motility and tone because of progesterone. The small and large intestines have decreased motility, allowing for increased absorption. Production of liver proteins is increased, as is the production of alkaline phosphatase. The gallbladder increases to twice its size. Bile becomes more dilute and cholesterol is therefore less soluble, increasing the possibility of stone formation.

Metabolic Changes

Insulin levels are increased 2 to 10 times over the nonpregnant values, but glucose levels stay within 30–40 mg/dL. Fasting states show reduced fasting blood sugar by 5–10 mg/dL compared to the nonpregnant state. Peaks of glucose are delayed from 30–55 minutes as pregnancy progresses. Total caloric cost of pregnancy is 75,000 kcal. A wide range of weight gain is acceptable during pregnancy (20–45 lb). There is no correlation between prepregnant weight and weight gain during pregnancy. Weight gain in the first half of the pregnancy is related primarily to maternal components. During the second half of pregnancy, the largest growth is to the fetal placental unit, with the greatest growth noted between weeks 20 and 30. During the third trimester, maternal fat is stored as a caloric source for breastfeeding.

Medication during Pregnancy

Pregnancy can alter the absorption of oral drugs. Peristalsis is slowed, therefore increasing the amount of exposure and absorption of any drug. Excretion of medication is altered by increased renal plasma flow and increased storage into adipose tissue. Pregnancy can alter the distribution of any drug because of the change in intravascular and extravascular volume. Nausea and vomiting can affect the utilization and absorption of medication. There is no placental barrier to drugs. The fetus relies on the maternal circulation for detoxification and excretion.

FOOD AND DRUG ADMINISTRATION (FDA) CATEGORIES INTENDED TO GUIDE THE PRESCRIBING OF MEDICATION DURING PREGNANCY

Category A represents no risk during pregnancy.

Category B represents no risk identified in animal studies or studies with people, but there are not adequate studies to demonstrate safety.

Category C represents adverse effects in animal studies with no available studies with people, or there are no studies in animals or people.

Category D represents studies demonstrating birth defects in people, but the benefit outweighs the risk.

Category X represents contraindication during pregnancy with risks outweighing benefits.

Anticipatory Guidance during Pregnancy

Danger Signs

The importance of the following symptoms should be explained to each woman upon diagnosis of pregnancy. Written information containing these symptoms should be distributed to each prenatal client.

Pain with urination, frequency of urination, urgency of urination, fever, and backache (symptoms of urinary tract infection or pyelonephritis).

Severe nausea and vomiting, particularly when fluid cannot be retained.

Persistent fever over 100°F.

Lower abdominal pain in the first trimester that may or may not be accompanied by vaginal bleeding (symptoms of ectopic pregnancy).

Vulvar pain or discomfort, change in vaginal discharge, swelling of the vulva, pelvic pain or tenderness (symptoms of vaginal infections and sexually transmitted diseases [STDs]).

Fluid gush from the vagina or leaking of fluid from the vagina. The fluid will not resemble urine (premature rupture of membranes).

Uterine contractions in a regular pattern that are increasing in intensity prior to 36 weeks of pregnancy (premature labor).

Rhythmic backache (premature labor or labor).

Leg pain (thrombophlebitis).

Absence of fetal movement for more than 24 hours.

Swelling of hands, feet, and face; visual disturbance; headache (pregnancy-induced hypertension).

Vaginal bleeding during pregnancy.

Alcohol

Consumption of alcohol during pregnancy can produce fetal alcohol syndrome. Safe advice to give pregnant women is to recommend complete abstention from the consumption of alcohol. Alcoholics Anonymous can be a very valuable resource for women with difficulty abstaining from alcohol.

Smoking

Smoking is related to low birth weight and premature delivery. The adverse effects increase with the number of cigarettes smoked daily. Encourage women to stop smoking during pregnancy. Refer smokers to a support group that will assist them in reducing and eventually stopping smoking.

Drugs

Use of illegal drugs creates risk for prematurity and low birth weight as well as hepatitis B and HIV infection. Refer women using illegal drugs to a drug detoxification center specializing in the needs of pregnant women. Advise pregnant women to consult with a physician or nurse practitioner who specializes in women's health prior to consuming any over-the-counter medication. The use of prescription medication should be reviewed by a woman's health practitioner. Many prescription drugs can be harmful to the embryo or fetus, making review a wise consideration.

Radiation Exposure

There are recognized dangers to the fetus from diagnostic radiation, specifically chromosomal mutations and an increased risk for cancer in later life. Based upon animal experimentation, the only entirely safe dose of radiation is no dose of radiation. Pregnant women should therefore be advised to avoid radiation exposure. If radiation is necessary, shielding of the abdomen is essential. Radiation exposure during pregnancy can occur prior to the woman's knowledge that she is pregnant. The date of the last menstrual period should be elicited from every woman of childbearing age prior to radiation exposure. Special attention should be given to women who work in environments that create exposure to radiation. These women must adjust their work patterns to reduce or eliminate radiation exposure during pregnancy.

Work

As the knowledge base about teratogens increases, pregnant women who work outside of the home should have accurate information. The Reproductive Toxicology Center in Washington, D.C., can be reached at 1-202-293-5137. The Occupational Safety and Health Administration (OSHA) has also compiled information related to work, safety, and pregnancy. They can be reached at 1-800-356-4674.

Women should be encouraged to reduce their exposure to chemicals during pregnancy. They should work in well-ventilated areas and wear protective gloves, clothing, and masks to reduce exposure to possible teratogenic agents. Lead pipes can be a source of lead contamination. Pregnant women, particularly those living or working in buildings constructed prior to 1980, should have their drinking water tested for lead. Neither food nor water should be stored in containers that may have lead contamination. Women should be encouraged to inform their employers of pregnancy as soon as possible. Work modifications should include:

Reduction in hard physical labor, with lifting restricted.

Work days no longer than 8 hours.

Enforcement of at least two 10-minute breaks per day and 1 hour for lunch.

Availability to the pregnant woman of a bathroom and a place to rest and elevate her legs.

Provision of a short period of time every 1 or 2 hours to allow for walking for women who must stand or sit for long periods of time during work hours.

Pregnant women should avoid extremes in temperature, chemical exposure, and any activity that may threaten the pregnancy through trauma.

Several medical diagnoses may inhibit a pregnant woman from working. Obstetrical diagnoses such as multiple pregnancy or cerclage may prohibit working. The type of work that a woman performs and the numbers of hours per day she works must be considered before restriction is implemented. Decisions concerning work safety and a pregnant woman must be made by a team consisting of the pregnant woman, the nurse practitioner (NP), the obstetrician, and the woman's employer.

Exercise

Exercise during pregnancy has multiple physical and psychologic benefits. Exercise patterns established prior to pregnancy can be maintained throughout the pregnancy with the following restrictions:

Heart rate is kept under 140 beats per minute, with elevated heart rate not exceeding 15–20 minutes per exercise session.

The pregnant woman should not exercise in hot, humid conditions.

Hydration must always be considered before, during, and after an exercise session.

The woman should modify the exercise program as the physical demands of the pregnancy increase (as the weeks of pregnancy advance).

The pregnant woman should stop exercising if she has pain, bleeding, prolonged dizziness, prolonged shortness of breath, or palpitations.

Women who have not exercised regularly prior to pregnancy should begin a program that gradually increases in length and intensity. New programs should be followed regularly, not sporadically, and should be supervised by a person familiar with exercise programs designed for pregnant women. Skiing, both snow and water; scuba diving; or any sport performed at elevated altitudes should be prohibited during pregnancy because of risks involved for both mother and fetus.

Saunas and hot tubs should be avoided during pregnancy. Blood being shunted to the skin because of the elevation in body temperature predisposes the woman to syncope.

Complications of pregnancy may inhibit exercise. These include incompetent cervix and premature labor. Medical diseases can also prohibit exercise during pregnancy. Any woman with an obstetric or medical complication of her pregnancy will require evaluation of her exercise program.

Sexual Activity

Sexual activity is not restricted during pregnancy unless a complication such as premature labor or placenta previa develops. Pregnant women should be advised to assume their usual level of sexual activity throughout the pregnancy unless advised not to by a health-care provider. Assure pregnant women that the fetus is not injured by intercourse. Exploration of comfortable positions for intercourse during pregnancy may be suggested.

Prevention of STDs should be discussed with pregnant women. Advise the pregnant woman to use condoms if she has a new sexual partner or multiple partners, or if she is unsure about her partner's drug use or sexual activity.

Travel

Travel is best undertaken in the second trimester when risk for complication is lowest and comfort level during the pregnancy is highest. Advise the pregnant and traveling woman to discuss her travel plans with the nurse practioner (NP). The nurse practitioner should discuss with the woman plans for emergency care if it becomes necessary, and provide her with safety advice dependent upon her destination (drinking water, foods, etc.). Advise her to walk for a few minutes every one or two hours while traveling. She should keep herself well hydrated. Air travel is not restricted during pregnancy.

Seat belts should be used while traveling in a car. The lap portion of the seat belt should be placed below the abdomen and across the upper thighs. Both the lap and the shoulder straps should be utilized. Both belts should be worn snugly.

Traveling during the last month of pregnancy is discouraged. Labor initiating far from home places the woman in an anxiety-producing situation. Traveling in an automobile long distances while in early labor in an attempt to reach familiar providers is uncomfortable and potentially unsafe. Advise the pregnant woman to stay reasonably close to home in the last few weeks of pregnancy.

Nutrition

Throughout the pregnancy there is an increased need for all the basic nutrients. Nutritional guidelines must be reviewed individually with each pregnant woman. Food preferences as well as activity level must be incorporated into the nutritional plan. Multiple pregnancy alters a nutritional plan. Pregnant adolescents have special nutritional needs. NPs caring for pregnant women should have access to a registered dietitian for patient consultation.

Calories must be sufficient to supply the increased energy and nutrient demands of pregnancy. An extra 300 calories per day is required throughout the pregnancy, a 10%–15% increase over the mother's prepregnancy need. The pregnant woman requires 60 g/day of protein, an increase of 10%–15%. Calcium needs increase 400 mg/day to 1200 mg. Iron needs increase 50% to 30 mg/day. The March of Dimes recommends folic acid in the amount of 0.4 mg/day, citing research indicating that this dose may help prevent neural tube defects. The recommended daily allowance (RDA) standards recommend 70 mg/day of vitamin C, a 10-mg/day increase. The practice of providing vitamin supplementation prenatally has become routine for many health-care providers, even though there is no scientific evidence indicating that there is benefit to either mother or fetus. Extra nutritional requirements can be met with food, with the exception of iron and folic acid. Vitamin and mineral supplementation should not be regarded as a substitute for food.

Management of Common Complaints of Pregnancy

Backache

Backache is a common complaint of pregnancy, particularly during the third trimester.

Etiology: Backache arises from the shift in gravity related to the enlarging uterus, causing muscle strain.

Occurrence: Throughout the pregnancy, but usually third trimester.

Contributing Factors: Pre-existing back pain, excessive weight gain during pregnancy.

Signs and Symptoms: The woman generally reports dull aching back pain that increases throughout the day.

Diagnostic Tests: Physical examination, including neurologic examination and pelvic examination, urine culture and sensitivity, and monitoring of contractions.

Differential Diagnosis: Uterine contractions, pelvic inflammatory disease, urinary tract infection, sciatica, and herniated disk must be ruled out. The woman should not have CVA tenderness or pain with straight leg raises.

Treatment: The woman with backache related to pregnancy should be taught proper body mechanics and techniques for lifting. A regular back exercise program should be encouraged. She should avoid long periods of standing or sitting. A supportive mattress and sleeping in a lateral position may help relieve backache. Massage and relaxation techniques can help to relieve backache. Acetaminophen, 650 mg every 4 hours, may be taken for relief.

Follow-up: As indicated.

Sequelae: None.

Prevention/Prophylaxis: Avoid excessive weight gain during pregnancy.

Referral: Radiologic studies are limited during pregnancy. If sciatica or herniated disk is suspected, referral into the primary care system for further evaluation may be necessary.

Education: Teach the woman to avoid wearing high-heeled shoes. Excessive weight gain during pregnancy should be avoided. Heavy lifting during pregnancy should be avoided. Proper body mechanics and lifting techniques should be reviewed.

Breast Changes

A common complaint during pregnancy relates to the increase in breast size and tenderness.

Etiology: Increased levels of estrogen and progesterone cause the fatty layers of the breast to thicken and also cause the development of milk ducts and glands. As a result, the breasts increase in size and weight and feel tender.

Occurrence: Women frequently complain of breast tenderness in the first trimester of pregnancy.

Contributing Factors: Caffeine.

Signs and Symptoms: Breast enlargement and tenderness.

Diagnostic Tests: Physical examination, including vital signs and breast examination.

Differential Diagnosis: History during first trimester of pregnancy may include breast tenderness, but without pain, redness, fever, injury, masses, or bloody discharge. Physical examination and vital signs should be within normal limits and there should not be any areas of inflammation, masses, dimpling, skin changes, enlarged nodes, or bloody discharge. Mastitis, breast cancer, and breast injury must be ruled out.

Treatment: Reduce caffeine intake. Wearing a supportive bra can be helpful in relieving tenderness.

Follow-up: As indicated.

Sequelae: None.

Prevention/Prophylaxis: Reduce caffeine intake.

Referral: Breast tenderness related to infection or injury should be referred. Symptoms of breast cancer require referral (see Chap. 7).

Education: Explain to the woman that breast tenderness decreases in the second trimester. The woman may find wearing a supportive bra helpful. Caffeine increases breast tenderness and should be avoided. Self breast exam should be conducted throughout pregnancy on a monthly basis.

Constipation

Constipation is a common complaint during pregnancy.

Etiology: Large amounts of circulating progesterone cause decreased contractility of the gastrointestinal (GI) tract, resulting in slow movement through the intestines and increased water reabsorption. The large bowel is also compressed by the growing uterus in the first trimester, and again in the third trimester. Iron taken by mouth during pregnancy increases the likelihood of constipation.

Occurrence: Constipation is a common complaint during pregnancy.

Contributing Factors: Oral iron intake, low-fiber diet, decreased fluid consumption, decreased activity, constipation prior to pregnancy.

Signs and Symptoms: The woman will report difficulty with passing stools and stools that are dry and hard.

Diagnostic Tests: Physical examination including abdominal and rectal examination.

Differential Diagnosis: Preterm labor, appendicitis, and fecal impaction must be ruled out as diagnoses.

Treatment: Bulk-forming laxatives such as Metamucil can be used to relieve constipation. Increasing her fluid intake may relieve the symptoms. A stool softener can be used for relief of constipation. The typical dose is 50 mg; the total dose should not exceed 200 mg/day. Regular exercise and establishing a time of day for defecation decrease constipation. Foods high in bulk such as bran, whole-grain breads and cereal, plus vegetables and fruits should be encouraged. Prune juice and a warm drink at breakfast are helpful for some women. Iron may have to be temporarily eliminated from vitamin and mineral supplementation until constipation is relieved.

Follow-up: As indicated.

Sequelae: Straining with bowel movements can contribute to the formation of hemorrhoids.

Prevention/Prophylaxis: Adequate fluid intake, high-fiber diet, regular exercise.

Referral: None.

Education: Constipation is common during pregnancy. Laxatives other than bulk-forming laxatives should not be utilized during pregnancy.

Dyspepsia

Dyspepsia is a common complaint of the third trimester of pregnancy.

Etiology: The pressure of the uterus against the stomach and intestines causes reflux of gastric contents into the esophagus. Increased levels of progesterone contribute to a decrease in gastrointestinal peristalsis and relaxation of the hiatal sphincter.

Occurrence: Third trimester.

Contributing Factors: Spicy or fatty foods, large meals.

Signs and Symptoms: The woman will report gastric burning, but not chest pain or shortness of breath, upper abdominal pain, diarrhea, or vomiting.

Diagnostic Tests: Physical examination including vital signs.

Differential Diagnosis: Cardiac disease, gallbladder disease, peptic ulcer, and gastroenteritis must be ruled out.

Treatment: Antacids may be taken during pregnancy. Instruct the woman with dyspepsia to follow the package directions for over-the-counter antacids, either calcium-based or aluminum-based. Antacids cannot be taken with tetracycline and should not be taken simultaneously with iron supplementation because they impair iron absorption. The woman should consume small, frequent meals that avoid spicy, fatty, and gas-forming foods. She may need to sleep with her head elevated a few inches to relieve dyspepsia at night.

Follow-up: As indicated to rule out peptic ulcer or gallbladder disease.

Sequelae: None.

Prevention/Prophylaxis: Avoid spicy, fatty foods; alcohol; and coffee.

Education: Reassure the woman that dyspepsia resolves with delivery. Sleeping with the head of the bed elevated may relieve dyspepsia. Instruct the woman not to wear restrictive clothing. The pregnant woman should eat small, frequent meals and avoid excessive weight gain.

Dyspnea

Shortness of breath is a common complaint during the third trimester of pregnancy.

Etiology: An enlarged uterus pressing against the diaphragm prevents full expansion of the lungs and creates dyspnea.

Occurrence: Third trimester prior to descent of the fetal head into the pelvis.

Contributing Factors: Women of short stature experience this symptom more than tall women because of the amount of intra-abdominal space. Poor posture, particularly rounding of the shoulders and leaning forward while sitting or standing, contributes to dyspnea.

Signs and Symptoms: The woman reports feeling short of breath and perhaps light-headed.

Diagnostic Tests: Physical examination including abdominal examination and examination of the heart and lungs.

Differential Diagnosis: Cardiac or respiratory disease including upper respiratory infection.

Treatment: Advise the woman to rest, not to wear restrictive clothing, to keep good posture, and to lie in a lateral position while reclining.

Follow-up: As indicated.

Sequelae: None.

Prevention/Prophylaxis: Adequate rest, good posture.

Referral: None.

Education: Reassure the pregnant woman that the dyspnea will be relieved when the fetal presenting part descends into the pelvis. Sleeping with her head elevated on a pillow or two may relieve nocturnal dyspnea.

Edema

Edema occurs during pregnancy, most often in dependent areas, primarily during the third trimester.

Etiology: The pressure of the uterus alters venous return to the heart from the legs; consequently, fluid passes into the intracellular spaces. Hormone levels during pregnancy increase capillary permeability, contributing to the edema.

Occurrence: Third trimester.

Contributing Factors: None.

Signs and Symptoms: The woman will report mild edema in her hands and feet that worsens as the day progresses. Edema is decreased in the morning and increases throughout the day, particularly during periods of prolonged sitting or standing.

Diagnostic Tests: Physical examination including vital signs. Urine dipstick for protein and measurement of urinary output.

Differential Diagnosis: Generalized edema and facial edema with headache can indicate pregnancy-induced hypertension.

Treatment: Advise the woman with edema related to pregnancy to lie in a lateral recumbent position for resting during the day and sleeping at night. Advise her to decrease prolonged standing or sitting with brief periods of walking. Ask her not to wear constrictive clothing. Have her raise her arms and legs above the level of the heart several times daily to decrease the edema. Her diet should include adequate calories and protein and at least 6–8 glasses of water per day. Salt, sugar, and fats should be consumed in moderation.

Follow-up: As indicated.

Sequelae: None.

Prevention/Prophylaxis: None.

Referral: Refer the woman with symptoms of pregnancy-induced hypertension.

Education: Reassure the client that edema during pregnancy is normal and will resolve after delivery. She should avoid sitting or standing for prolonged periods. Instruct the woman not to wear constrictive clothing with the exception of support hose. Advise the woman to take in adequate calories and drink 6–8 glasses of water per day.

Emotional Lability

Emotional lability is common throughout pregnancy.

Etiology: Hormone levels during pregnancy can create emotional lability. Progesterone has a depressant effect on the nervous system.

Occurrence: Common at any time in the pregnancy or throughout the pregnancy.

Contributing Factors: Fatigue, inadequate support system.

Signs and Symptoms: The pregnant woman may reveal that she has mood swings and cries at times for no apparent reason.

Diagnostic Tests: None.

Differential Diagnosis: Fatigue related to sleep loss or deprivation, fatigue related to iron-deficiency anemia, and emotional psychiatric disorders must be ruled out.

Treatment: Increased time for sleep and rest. Social work referral for an inadequate support system. Adequate distribution of calories throughout the day.

Follow-up: As indicated.

Sequelae: None.

Prevention/Prophylaxis: Adequate sleep and rest, adequate caloric consumption.

Referral: None.

Education: Explain to the woman that emotional lability is common during pregnancy. Taking "time for herself" is essential, as is adequate rest, sleep, exercise, and diet.

Fatigue

Many women report fatigue despite normal amounts of sleep during the first trimester.

Etiology: First-trimester fatigue is probably related to the increased physical demands of pregnancy. Fatigue returns in the third trimester, caused by sleep disturbance, decreased exercise, and the physiologic demand of the pregnancy. Fetal movements and urinary frequency may interfere with sleep.

Occurrence: Fatigue is common in the first trimester of pregnancy. Insomnia in the third trimester of pregnancy commonly leads to fatigue.

Contributing Factors: Demanding work schedules and sleep deprivation.

Signs and Symptoms: Fatigue despite reported 8 hours or more of sleep per 24-hour period.

Diagnostic Tests: Complete blood count to rule out anemia.

Differential Diagnosis: Anemia with hemoglobin less than 11g/dL or depression as measured by history and use of a depression scale.

Treatment: First-trimester fatigue requires adjustment of the woman's schedule to incorporate more sleep. Iron may be prescribed for women with anemia. Amount of oral iron prescribed is dependent upon the blood count results. No sleeping medications should be prescribed for third-trimester insomnia. Describe methods to increase comfort and improve insomnia. Tell patients to avoid exercising in the evening and to avoid caffeine and heavy meals at bedtime. Warm milk may induce sleep.

Follow-up: More frequent prenatal visits may be required for further evaluation of fatigue.

Sequelae: None.

Prevention/Prophylaxis: None.

Referral: None.

Education: Explain to the woman that fatigue is expected during the first trimester. Encourage adequate sleep and rest and assist the woman in arranging her schedule to include additional rest. Discuss methods for decreasing insomnia in the third trimester.

Headache

Headache during the first trimester of pregnancy is a common complaint.

Etiology: Headache during pregnancy is caused by increased circulatory volume, vasodilation caused by high levels of progesterone, and at times low blood sugar.

Occurrence: Headaches are common during pregnancy, particularly in women who have experienced headaches prior to pregnancy.

Contributing Factors: History of headache prior to pregnancy, insufficient caloric intake.

Signs and Symptoms: Mild headache that is frontal in origin occurring less frequently than daily.

Diagnostic Tests: Physical examination including vital signs, ophthalmoscopic examination, and neurologic evaluation.

Differential Diagnosis: History of headaches must include information on frequency, intensity, and duration, as well as a description of the headache. Knowing what triggers the headache and what relieves it is helpful for evaluation. Pregnancy headache history should not include facial edema; changes in level of consciousness; memory changes; motor, visual, or sensory changes; nausea and vomiting with headache; stiff neck; fever; or eye pain.

Headaches during pregnancy can be related to the pregnancy but can also be related to consumption of alcohol, chemical exposure, food allergies, injury, tension, migraine, sinus infection, or fatigue. One of the symptoms of pregnancy-induced hypertension is headache.

Treatment: Small frequent meals, adequate sleep, relaxation techniques, and acetaminophen 650 mg every 4 hours if needed for relief.

Follow-up: Have the client keep a written record of frequency and intensity of headaches. More frequent prenatal visits may be necessary for further evaluation.

Sequelae: None.

Prevention/Prophylaxis: Small frequent meals and sufficient rest and sleep.

Referral: Headache related to migraine, pregnancy-induced hypertension, infection, or injury should be referred for evaluation.

Education: Explain to the woman that physiologic changes are producing the headache and that headaches may resolve in the second trimester. Advise her to avoid triggers for the headaches, such as increased stress or certain foods. Frequent small meals may reduce the incidence of headache. Adequate sleep and rest may reduce the incidence of headache.

Hemorrhoids

Hemorrhoids are a common complaint in the third trimester of pregnancy.

Etiology: Hemorrhoids are varicosities of the rectum. Hemorrhoids are exacerbated during pregnancy by increased intravascular pressure, constipation, and straining at stool.

Occurrence: Third trimester, but may occur at any time during the pregnancy.

Contributing Factors: Constipation.

Signs and Symptoms: The woman complains of swelling, pain, fullness, or bleeding in the rectal area.

Diagnostic Tests: Physical examination including rectal exam, testing of stool for occult blood, hemoglobin levels if bleeding is prolonged or extensive.

Differential Diagnosis: Anal fissures, abscessed or thrombosed hemorrhoids, cancerous lesions, or condyloma. Thrombosed hemorrhoids look like a clot-containing mass, blue or purple in color, near the anus, and are reported as very painful.

Treatment: Hemorrhoids can be relieved with topical anesthetics such as Preparation H during pregnancy. Encourage the woman to avoid constipation, use sitz baths that are warm or cool, and to use Tucks or similar medicated pads.

Follow-up: As indicated.

Sequelae: None.

Prevention/Prophylaxis: Avoid constipation and prolonged standing or sitting.

Referral: Thrombosed hemorrhoids require surgical referral.

Education: Hemorrhoids often resolve after pregnancy. Vaginal delivery exacerbates hemorrhoids, but resolution often occurs during the postpartum period.

Muscle Cramping in the Legs

Muscle cramping in the legs is a common complaint experienced during the second and third trimesters of pregnancy.

Etiology: Cramping occurring in the second and third trimesters is probably related to the pressure of the uterus on the pelvic nerves and blood supply. A calcium imbalance may contribute to the problem.

Occurrence: Cramping occurs most frequently at night and after excessive exercise.

Contributing Factors: Inadequate intake or overconsumption of calcium, excessive exercise.

Signs and Symptoms: Cramping in the calf, usually at night, that resolves spontaneously.

Diagnostic Tests: Physical examination, Doppler flow studies to rule out thromboembolic disease.

Differential Diagnosis: Thromboembolic disease indicated by positive Homan's sign and/or continuous tenderness in the leg and pain on deep palpation; varicosities should be ruled out.

Treatment: During a cramping episode, pressure against the foot as the woman extends her leg hastens the resolution of the cramping. Excessive or inadequate consumption of calcium should be altered.

Follow-up: As indicated.

Sequelae: None.

Prevention/Prophylaxis: Calf-stretching exercises prior to bedtime may be helpful. Adequate calcium intake is necessary for prevention.

Referral: None.

Education: Instruct the woman in calf-stretching exercises.

Nausea and Vomiting

Nausea and vomiting, a common complaint of the first trimester of pregnancy, may or may not be associated with a time of day. Vomiting does not always accompany the nausea.

Etiology: High levels of estrogen and progesterone and the introduction of hCG are probably the cause of nausea and vomiting in the first trimester. Delayed emptying of the stomach is a result of smooth muscle relaxation and hyponatremia. Emotional and dietary factors may also be involved in creating nausea and vomiting.

Occurrence: Over half of all pregnant women in the United States experience these symptoms. The symptoms last until approximately 12–14 weeks of gestation.

Contributing Factors: Ingestion of certain foods, the smell of certain foods, preparing food, heat intolerance, and increased workload can contribute to an episode of nausea and vomiting.

Signs and Symptoms: Nausea with or without vomiting. Women report nausea and/or vomiting in the first trimester that may or may not be limited to a certain time of day. History of nausea and vomiting should exclude fever, pain, diarrhea, bleeding, or head injury, because these are signs of vomiting unrelated to pregnancy and may require medical evaluation. Vital signs will be normal. Uterine size will be appropriate and fetal heart tones audible at 10–12 weeks of gestation. Weight change depends on the severity of the vomiting. If weight loss is greater than 5% of the woman's total weight, hyperemesis gravidarum is suspected and medical evaluation required.

Diagnostic Tests: Urine ketone and specific gravity tests can be used to rule out dehydration.

Differential Diagnosis: Hyperemesis gravidarum, multiple gestation, hydatidiform gestation, gastroenteritis, cholecystitis, inner ear infection, migraine headache, increased intracranial pressure, food poisoning, and eating disorder. Differential diagnoses can be ruled out by history and physical examination, including abdomen examination.

Treatment: Ensure adequate hydration. Intravenous supplementation of fluid may be necessary if the woman is at risk for dehydration. (If the vomiting is severe enough that she cannot retain fluids, she is at risk for dehydration.)

Relaxation techniques may be helpful in relieving nausea. Vitamin B_6 tablets, 50 mg PO at no more than 4 per day, can be helpful in relieving nausea and vomiting. Accupressure applied in the form of wrist bands has been known to be helpful in some women. Eating small, frequent meals and snacks can be effective. Vitamin and mineral supplementation can be discontinued in women with nausea and vomiting until the symptoms have subsided.

Follow-up: More frequent prenatal visits may be required if nausea and vomiting are severe. Hospitalization for hydration is required when dehydration is a risk factor.

Sequelae: If severe and untreated, dehydration can occur, placing both mother and fetus at risk.

Prevention/Prophylaxis: Small, frequent meals. Consumption of food such as dry crackers before rising in the morning helps prevent morning nausea and vomiting. Careful selection of diet, including avoiding foods that induce nausea, may be helpful. Delegation of food preparation to others has been reported as a method that can decrease nausea in prenatal women.

Referral: Any pregnant woman who cannot retain fluids for a 24-hour period requires referral for medical evaluation.

Education: Explain to the woman that nausea and vomiting during pregnancy are usually confined to the first trimester. The woman must remain hydrated. Remind her to drink fluids.

Round Ligament Pain

Pregnant women commonly complain of sharp abdominal pain that is relieved spontaneously and is of short duration. The pain is in the area of the round ligament on one side of the abdomen or the other.

Etiology: Growth of the uterus causes the round ligaments to stretch. The round ligaments attach to the top of the uterus, extend anteriorly and inferiorly through the inguinal canal, and attach to the labia majora.

Occurrence: Usually in the second trimester, the woman reports sharp pain on either side or both sides of the uterus.

Contributing Factors: None.

Signs and Symptoms: The pain can be intense but is short in duration. The pain may be intensified by quick movements and relieved by resting. There should not be evidence of constipation, contractions, or abdominal pain.

Diagnostic Tests: Physical examination including abdominal examination.

Differential Diagnosis: History should not include contractions, flank or abdominal pain, tender lump or lumps in the groin, or constant pain. Evidence of contractions, cervical dilatation, rebound tenderness, or masses indicates that the pain is not related to round ligaments. Preterm labor, ectopic pregnancy (first trimester), constipation, gastroenteritis, and appendicitis must be ruled out.

Treatment: Rest until the pain subsides. Mild heat to the area of the round ligament may provide relief from aching after the painful episode.

Follow-up: As indicated.

Sequelae: None.

Prevention/Prophylaxis: Avoid sudden movements and move from a lying to a sitting position without placing excessive strain on the abdominal muscles.

Referral: None.

Education: Round ligament pain is common during pregnancy. It is frightening to many women because of its intensity. The pain is always of short duration with spontaneous resolution and, at times, with mild aching afterward.

Syncope

Syncope, reported by the pregnant woman as "dizziness," can occur at any time throughout the pregnancy.

Etiology: Pooling of blood in the lower extremities coupled with expanded blood volume can lead to syncope. Syncope can also be related to nausea and vomiting and low blood sugar.

Occurrence: Syncope can occur at any time during a pregnancy.

Contributing Factors: Prolonged standing, inadequate caloric intake.

Signs and Symptoms: The woman will report a light-headed feeling or dizziness that lasts for a brief period of time.

Diagnostic Tests: Physical examination including vital signs, otoscopic examination, complete blood count, and drug screening.

Differential Diagnosis: Orthostatic hypotension, anemia, hypoglycemia, toxicity, substance abuse, and disease of the ear must be ruled out.

Treatment: Advise the woman to lower her head below her heart if feeling faint. Advise her to change positions gradually, especially from lying to standing. Compression stockings may be helpful.

Follow-up: As indicated.

Sequelae: None.

Prevention/Prophylaxis: None.

Referral: None.

Education: A pregnant woman experiencing episodes of syncope must be advised not to drive during episodes of syncope and not to participate in any other activity that may endanger her welfare during an episode of syncope.

Urinary Frequency

Urinary frequency is a common complaint in the first trimester and last trimester of pregnancy. Differentiation between frequency caused by compression of the bladder and urinary tract infection is essential.

Etiology: During the first trimester the enlargement of the uterus compresses the bladder. During the second trimester, as the uterus moves into the abdomen, this symptom improves. During the third trimester urinary frequency is related to pressure on the bladder from the distended uterus.

Occurrence: Urinary frequency is a common complaint in both the first and third trimesters.

Contributing Factors: Consumption of caffeine.

Signs and Symptoms: Increased frequency of urination, sleep disturbance caused by urge to void, involuntary loss of urine.

Diagnostic Tests: Urine dipstick, urinalysis, urine culture and sensitivity, 1 hour post 50-g Glucola serum screening for gestation diabetes, Nitrazine test, and fern test to rule out ruptured membranes.

Differential Diagnosis: History of urinary frequency should not include back pain, fever, hematuria, dysuria, urgency, or pain. Urinalysis and urine culture and sensitivity can be used to rule out urinary tract infection (UTI). The woman reporting urinary frequency should be assessed for polyuria. Polyuria may be a symptom of diabetes, and appropriate screening should be initiated if this is suspected. Nitrazine test and fern test should be performed to rule out ruptured membranes in women who report involuntary loss of fluid.

Treatment: None.

Follow-up: Urine dipstick and examination of the urine with a microscope to rule out UTI at each prenatal visit.

Sequelae: None.

Prevention/Prophylaxis: Reduce intake of caffeine.

Referral: None.

Education: Explain to the woman experiencing frequency of urination the anatomic changes responsible for this symptom. Advise her to maintain an adequate fluid intake (6–8 glasses per day). Water intake can decrease prior to retiring for the night, but overall intake must remain at an adequate level. Remind the woman that alcohol and caffeine increase urinary frequency and should be avoided.

Uterine Cramping

Uterine cramping is a common complaint in the first and third trimesters of pregnancy.

Etiology: Increased vascular congestion in the pelvis may be the reason for a cramping sensation many women report during the first trimester. In the last trimester of pregnancy, the uterus begins painless, irregular contractions known as Braxton Hicks contractions. The contractions are thought to be preparation for labor. The cervix does not dilate in response to Braxton Hicks contractions.

Occurrence: Women during the first trimester of pregnancy report a cramping sensation similar to cramping felt prior to menses. Braxton Hicks contractions are common during the last weeks of pregnancy. The higher the gravida, the more intense the contractions.

Contributing Factors: None.

Signs and Symptoms: Cramping should not be severe, unilateral, abdominal, urinary in origin, or accompanied by bleeding. Physical examination should be within normal limits. There should be no vaginal bleeding, cervical dilatation, adnexal masses, or suprapubic tenderness. With Braxton Hicks contractions, the woman reports a tightening of the uterus that may or may not be accompanied by a sensation of pelvic pressure. The tightening lasts from a few seconds up to a minute. The contractions are not regular and do not increase in intensity over time. The woman does not report regular contractions, leaking membranes, or symptoms of a UTI. Physical exam will be within normal limits. The pelvic exam will not reveal an increase in cervical dilatation or effacement. Timing of contractions does not reveal a regular pattern. The fetus remains active and bowel sounds are normal.

Diagnostic Tests

Serial serum quantitative hCG can be ordered to evaluate progress of an early pregnancy.

Urinalysis and urine culture and sensitivity can be ordered to rule out UTI.

Pelvic examination and the monitoring of contractions will rule out active labor and confirm Braxton Hicks contractions.

Differential Diagnosis: Spontaneous abortion, ectopic pregnancy, and UTI must be ruled out in first-trimester cramping. Preterm labor, labor, and UTI must be ruled out in the last trimester.

Treatment: Rest and relaxation and application of mild warmth to the lower abdomen may relieve cramping.

Follow-up: As indicated by the clinical presentation.

Sequelae: None.

Prevention/Prophylaxis: None.

Referral: None.

Education: Teach the woman the difference between Braxton Hicks contractions and true labor. Advise her that resting in a lateral position or perhaps walking may relieve the contractions.

Varicosities

Varicosities are developed during pregnancy, most commonly in the third trimester.

Etiology: Pressure of the gravid uterus causes increased venous stasis. Many women who develop varicosities have a genetic predisposition.

Occurrence: Anytime during the pregnancy, but most commonly during the third trimester.

Contributing Factors: Prolonged standing, genetic predisposition.

Signs and Symptoms: The women will report aching and sometimes throbbing in the legs and/or vulva. Twisted and swollen veins are visible, with possible mild swelling below the varicosities.

Diagnostic Tests: Physical examination including extremities, testing for Homan's sign, or pain on deep palpation; Doppler flow studies to rule out venous thrombosis or thrombophlebitis.

Differential Diagnosis: Clotting, swelling, redness or tenderness, cyanosis, positive Homan's sign, and/or pain on deep palpation could indicate venous thrombosis or thrombophlebitis.

Treatment: Teach the woman to apply support hose. Instruct her to lie flat and raise her legs to drain the veins. While her legs are elevated, roll on the stockings or pantyhose. She should apply the stockings upon arising in the morning and not remove them until bedtime. She should not cross her legs, wear tight knee-high stockings, or high-heel shoes. She should elevate her legs above the level of the heart at least twice daily (a recliner is perfect for this) and avoid prolonged periods of sitting or standing. Sanitary napkins applied snugly to the vulva may help relieve vulvar varicosities.

Follow-up: As indicated.

Sequelae: None.

Prevention/Prophylaxis: Support hose during pregnancy, rest periods during episodes of prolonged sitting or standing.

Referral: Thrombophlebitis and deep vein thrombosis require referral.

Education: Teach the woman how to apply support stockings. Advise her not to gain excessive weight during the pregnancy.

Management of the Complications of Pregnancy

Diabetes in Pregnancy

Pregnant women with diabetes can be classified into three groups. The first is gestational diabetes, with women developing diabetes for the first time while pregnant. The second is preconceptual diabetes without diabetic sequelae, both insulin- and non–insulin-dependent. The third is preconceptual diabetes with significant diabetic sequelae.

Etiology: Carbohydrate intolerance of varying severity resulting from pre-existing disease or as a consequence of changes in maternal metabolism related to pregnancy.

Occurrence: Gestational diabetes has an incidence of 2%–13% for all pregnant women.

Age: Not significant.

Ethnicity: Not significant.

Contributing Factors: Family history of diabetes, obesity, previous delivery of an infant weighing less than 4000 g.

Signs and Symptoms: Gestational diabetes is usually without symptoms; it has been demonstrated that over one-half of all women diagnosed have no significant risk factors and are under 30 years of age.

Diagnostic Tests: All pregnant women should be screened for gestational diabetes at 24–28 weeks of gestation. Screening for gestational diabetes is a serum glucose measurement 1 hour post 50-g Glucola ingestion drawn at any time of the day. The patient need not be fasting. A serum glucose level greater than 140 mg mandates a 3-hour glucose tolerance test (GTT). Gestational diabetes is diagnosed when two or more values meet or exceed the following: fasting, 105; 1 hour, 190; 2 hours,165; and 3 hours,145 (Fig. 17–2.)

Differential Diagnosis: Inaccurate laboratory diagnosis.

Treatment: Women with pre-existing diabetes, prior to conception, may be insulin-dependent or non–insulin-dependent. All pregnant women with diabetes will require insulin during the pregnancy. Oral hypoglycemics are not utilized

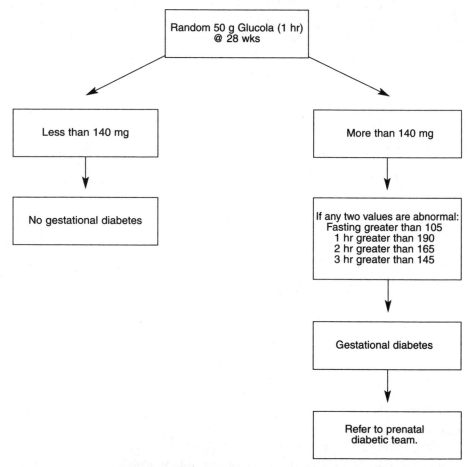

FIGURE 17–2   Diagnosis of gestational diabetes.

during pregnancy. The desired outcome of diabetes and pregnancy is a healthy mother and a healthy baby. The route to that outcome is the maintenance of a maternal environment that is euglycemic throughout the pregnancy. This is maintained with proper diet, insulin therapy, and home glucose monitoring. Antepartum fetal surveillance is an important tool used throughout the pregnancy. Prenatal care for diabetic women is provided by a team consisting of perinatology, endocrinology, obstetrics, neonatology, nutritional therapy, and nursing. An individualized plan of care is designed and carried out by the team.

Follow-up: Care as necessary to achieve diabetic control.

Sequelae: Polyhydramnios, pregnancy-induced hypertension, ketoacidosis, dystocia, congenital anomalies, macrosomia, and urinary tract infection.

Prevention/Prophylaxis: Appropriate prenatal screening and referral.

Referral: Diabetes and pregnancy require referral to a team of health-care providers that includes a perinatologist and an endocrinologist. Pregnancy for the woman with diabetes is substantially risky for both mother and fetus and requires very close and specialized medical and nursing care.

Education: Importance of prenatal care including screening for diabetes. Importance of maternal cooperation and participation in developing a health-care plan that achieves diabetic control.

Ectopic Pregnancy

Etiology: Implantation of a fertilized ovum in a site other than the endometrium of the uterus.

Occurrence: Many early ectopic pregnancies are reabsorbed and undiagnosed. Approximately 1 in 44 pregnancies is ectopic.

Age: Childbearing age.

Ethnicity: Not significant.

Contributing Factors: Risk determinants for ectopic pregnancy include a history of salpingitis, previous tubal surgery, advanced maternal age, postcoital estrogen contraceptives, progesterone-containing intrauterine devices, ovarian hyperstimulation, in vitro fertilization, and previous ectopic pregnancy.

Signs and Symptoms: Signs and symptoms of pregnancy, plus one-sided lower abdominal pain with possible referred shoulder pain. Ectopic pregnancy can occur without any symptoms.

Diagnostic Tests: Laboratory and ultrasonographic testing are the cornerstones of diagnosing ectopic pregnancy. The measurement of hCG is essential to the diagnosis of pregnancy. Measurements of quantitative beta hCG in a serial fashion have been shown to be of diagnostic value for ectopic pregnancy. Levels of serum hCG are known to rise exponentially in early gestation. HCG levels normally increase by at least 66% every 2 days and more than double every 3 days. Pregnancies that deviate from this pattern are typically abnormal. Beyond 6 weeks of pregnancy, the normal rate of increase slows and may take more than 1 week to double. Ectopic pregnancies generally demonstrate a slower rise in levels of beta hCG than is seen in normal pregnancies.

Ultrasound must be combined with serial hCG to diagnose ectopic pregnancy. Using a vaginal probe, visualization of the gestational sac becomes possible at the time of missed menses. The diameter of the sac normally continues to increase daily and by 40 days from last menstrual period approximates 10 mm. A yolk sac normally becomes visible at 5 weeks of pregnancy within the developing gestational sac, confirming the presence of embryonic tissue within the uterine cavity. Deviations from these patterns coupled with adnexal mass and abnormal serum beta hCG level confirms the diagnosis of ectopic pregnancy.

Measurement of serum progesterone is an additional method of evaluation of early pregnancy. Progesterone measurements are commonly depressed in women with abnormal gestations. Measurement of serum progesterone may complement serial hCG and ultrasound measurements (Fig. 17–3).

Differential Diagnosis: Ruptured ovarian cyst, PID, normal pregnancy, irritable bowel syndrome, or appendicitis.

Treatment: Improved detection of ectopic pregnancy allows for greater treatment options. For symptomatic patients in need of acute care, serial examination is not appropriate. In an emergency, rapid urine pregnancy test followed by ultrasound will establish the diagnosis. Laparoscopy is definitive for diagnosis and may be the route for treatment of choice. The choice of surgical technique is determined by condition of the tube, location of the gestation, and size of the gestation. Laparoscopy or laparotomy, linear salpingostomy, segmental resection, or salpingectomy is performed. Linear salpingostomy is the procedure of choice for the treatment of unruptured ectopic pregnancy. Subsequent conception rate following linear salpingostomy is 60% and recurrent ectopic rate is about 13%. Medical therapy, if appropriate, involves the use of methotrexate.

Follow-up: Dependent upon treatment, Rh immunoglobulin to all Rh-negative women.

Sequelae: Ruptured ectopic pregnancy. Subsequent conception rate after linear salpingostomy is 60%, and recurrent ectopic rate is about 13%.

Prevention/Prophylaxis: Avoid contributing factors when possible.

Referral: Ectopic pregnancy requires physician referral for medical or surgical intervention.

Education: Importance of early initiation of prenatal care. Importance of contact with health-care providers in any episode of abdominal pain in early pregnancy.

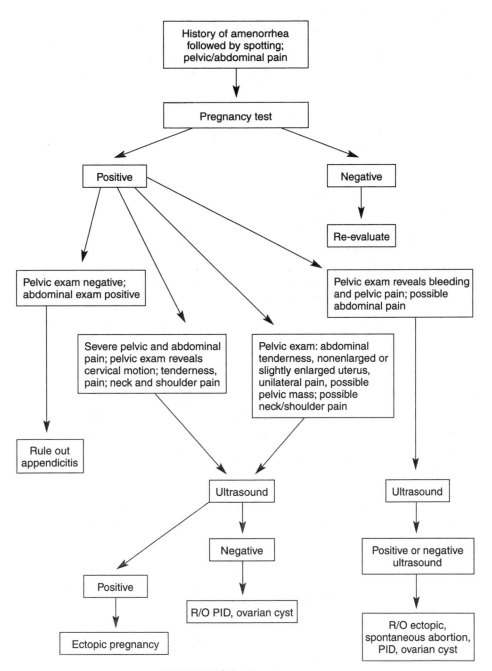

FIGURE 17–3 Ectopic pregnancy.

Placental Abruption

Placental abruption is defined as premature separation of the normally implanted placenta prior to the delivery of the fetus. The degree of separation may be partial or complete.

Etiology: Cause is unknown, but there is an association with hypertension.

Occurrence: Third-trimester bleeding occurs in approximately 4% of pregnancies. Of instances of third-trimester bleeding, 30% are the result of abruptio placenta.

Age: More likely to occur in women older than age 35.

Ethnicity: Not significant.

Contributing Factors: Multiparity, pregnancy-induced hypertension, use of cocaine, and trauma.

Signs and Symptoms: Symptoms can range from minimal vaginal bleeding to severe hemorrhage. Cause is unknown, but there is an association with hypertension. The typical history is that of an acute onset of vaginal bleeding associated with abdominal pain. The degree of bleeding varies. Uterine tenderness is common. Uterine irritability or preterm labor may be evident. Bleeding from abruption can be concealed. This occurs when the edges of the placenta remain attached to the uterine wall so that the bleeding is contained within the retroplacental space and therefore no vaginal bleeding is observed. Diagnosis is made by ultrasound (Fig. 17–4).

Diagnostic Tests: Physical examination reveals vaginal bleeding. Ultrasound confirms placental abruption. Vaginal exam is delayed until placenta previa is ruled out.

Differential Diagnosis: Placenta previa, hematoma, ruptured appendix, ruptured ovarian cyst.

Treatment: Once the diagnosis of abruption has been made, management will be determined by the severity of the abruption. The majority of fetuses are delivered, with the severity of the situation determining the route of delivery.

Follow-up: Dependent upon treatment.

Sequelae: The most common complication of placental abruption is maternal hemorrhage. The blood loss can be significant. There is a risk for disseminated intravascular coagulation (DIC). Abruption is the most common cause of DIC in pregnancy.

Prevention/Prophylaxis: Avoidance or appropriate treatment of contributing factors.

Referral: Physician referral is necessary.

Education: Importance of reporting episode of vaginal bleeding during pregnancy.

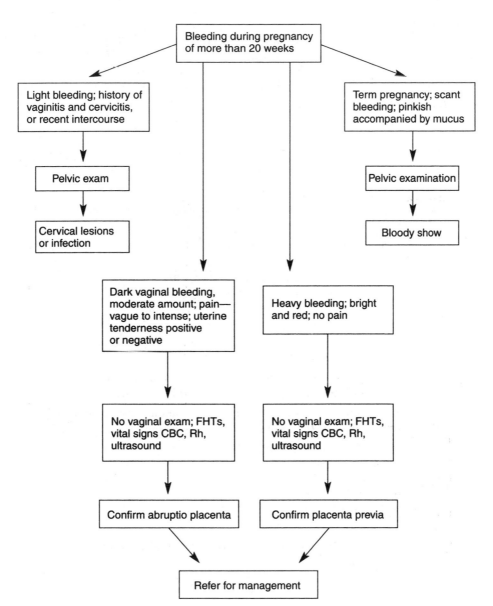

FIGURE 17–4   Bleeding during pregnancy of more than 20 weeks.

Placenta Previa

Placenta previa is defined as the implantation of the placenta over the cervical os. Previa is complete if the placenta totally covers the os and partial if only a portion of the os is covered. "Marginal" is the term used to describe a placenta that extends to the os but does not cover it. If the placental site is in the lower uterine segment but not touching the cervix, the diagnostic term used is "low-lying placenta."

Etiology: Placental implantation in the lower uterine segment.

Occurrence: Once in 200 pregnancies.

Age: Childbearing.

Ethnicity: Not significant.

Contributing Factors: Multiparity, uterine surgical scars.

Signs and Symptoms: The typical symptom of placenta previa is painless vaginal bleeding in the third trimester (see Fig. 17–4).

Diagnostic Tests: Diagnosis is made by ultrasound. Because of the widespread use of ultrasound prenatally, diagnosis of placenta previa in asymptomatic women is common. The diagnosis of previa should be reserved for patients beyond 24 weeks of gestation. Growth of the lower uterine segment results in the appearance of the placenta that is located close to the os "migrating" away from the cervix. If ultrasound performed earlier than 24 weeks shows placenta previa, sonograms should be repeated to validate "migration." Vaginal examination is delayed until ultrasound rules out placenta previa.

Differential Diagnosis: Abruptio placentae; other causes and sources of bleeding, such as rectum, bladder, or genital infection or laceration.

Treatment: Management of previa is decided based upon maternal and fetal stability and gestational age. Route of delivery is determined by the extent of the previa and the maternal and fetal condition.

Follow-up: Serial ultrasounds.

Sequelae: None.

Prevention/Prophylaxis: None.

Referral: Physician consult is required.

Education: Stress the importance of reporting vaginal bleeding during pregnancy to a health-care provider.

Pregnancy-Induced Hypertension

Hypertension during pregnancy is well-recognized as a significant risk for both mother and fetus. Hypertension is the number one cause of maternal death. Perinatal morbidity and mortality are associated with premature delivery, intrauterine growth retardation, and placental abruption related to hypertension.

Pregnancy-induced hypertension (PIH) develops as a consequence of pregnancy, occurs after 20 weeks of gestation, and regresses following delivery. Chronic hypertension is diagnosed prior to pregnancy or is evident prior to 20 weeks of gestation. Chronic hypertension can be superimposed by PIH.

PIH affects the cardiovascular system as well as the coagulation systems, central nervous system, and the hepatic and renal systems.

Etiology: Unknown. Significant family history increases the risk of PIH.

Occurrence: The incidence of PIH ranges from 5%–10%, with a significant increase in primigravidas, multiple gestations, diabetic pregnancies, and in women with pre-existing hypertension of any origin or renal disease.

Age: Adolescents and women over 35 years are at greater risk of PIH.

Ethnicity: Incidence of PIH in all pregnancies is 6%–8%. Incidence of PIH among pregnant African-American women is 15%–20%.

Contributing Factors: Primigravida, diabetes, and multiple gestation.

Signs and Symptoms: Blood pressure (BP) elevated above 140/90 mmHg on at least two occurrences; proteinuria over 300 mg in a 24-hour collection and edema. The women may report headache and/or visual disturbances (Table 17–1).

Diagnostic Tests: There are no specific tests to distinguish chronic hypertension from PIH; therefore, the diagnosis is based on history and physical examination. The diagnostic criteria for PIH are hypertension (BP more than 140/90 or elevation of systolic more than 30 mmHg and diastolic more than 15 mmHg) documented at least twice; proteinuria with a random specimen 1+ or greater or more than 300 mg in 24-hour collection; and nondependent edema, especially of the hands or face.

TABLE 17–1 CLASSIFICATION OF HYPERTENSIVE DISORDERS COMPLICATING PREGNANCY

- Pregnancy-induced hypertension:
  Hypertension develops during pregnancy and resolves postpartum.
  1. Hypertension (without proteinuria and edema)
  2. Hypertension (with proteinuria and edema)
     a. Mild
     b. Severe
  3. Hypertension, proteinuria, edema, convulsions
- Pregnancy-aggravated hypertension
  Underlying hypertension aggravated by pregnancy.
- Coincidental hypertension
- Chronic hypertension that precedes pregnancy and persists postpartum.

PIH is classified as either mild or severe. Severe is diagnosed if any of the following are present: BP greater than 160/110, proteinuria greater than 5 g/24 hours, oliguria less than 20–30 mL/hour, significant visual symptoms or headache, HELLP syndrome (hemolysis, elevated liver enzymes, low platelets), eclampsia, or pulmonary edema.

Differential Diagnosis: Essential or chronic hypertension or HELLP syndrome.

Treatment: Management decisions for PIH include consideration of the severity of the disease and maternal and fetal well-being. Definitive treatment of PIH is delivery. Decision to deliver must consider the risks to the mother of prolonging the pregnancy versus risks to the fetus at delivery. Mild PIH is usually managed with frequent assessment and evaluation of mother and fetus until delivery is determined to be a reasonably safe option. Severe PIH is a difficult management dilemma. Treatment options must be weighed against benefit. The route of delivery is dependent upon the maternal and fetal condition.

Follow-up: Dependent upon severity of symptoms.

Sequelae: None past delivery.

Prevention/Prophylaxis: Unknown.

Referral: Referral to a physician is necessary.

Education: Stress the importance of maintaining a therapeutic plan of care.

Premature Rupture of Membranes

Amnionic and chorionic membranes rupture prior to term pregnancy.

Etiology: The etiology of premature rupture of membranes (PROM) is multifactorial. Factors associated with PROM are cervical incompetence, multiple pregnancy, polyhydramnios, genetic conditions, and exogenous effects on the properties of the membranes.

Occurrence: The incidence of PROM for all pregnancies is 3%–18%.

Age: Less than 17 years or greater than 35 years of age.

Ethnicity: Increased incidence in women of African-American ethnicity.

Contributing Factors: Chorioamnionitis, endometritis, incomplete cervix, and multiple pregnancy.

Signs and Symptoms: Gush of fluid from the vagina or slow fluid "leak" from the vagina.

Diagnostic Tests: Rupture of membranes is diagnosed with history of fluid escaping from the vagina and testing that includes pooling of amniotic fluid, Nitrazine testing, or staining of fetal cells. Initial examination should be performed with a sterile speculum. An amniotic fluid sample is obtained from the posterior vaginal vault. Culture for group B streptococci should also be obtained.

Differential Diagnosis: Leakage of urine.

Treatment: The principle guiding the management of patients with PROM involves attempts to prolong the pregnancy until fetal lung maturity is attained.

Follow-up: Dependent upon medical management.

Sequelae: Preterm birth.

Prevention/Prophylaxis: Treatment of infection.

Referral: Physician referral is required.

Education: Teach the patient the signs and symptoms of preterm labor.

Preterm Labor and Delivery

Preterm delivery, delivery at less than 37 weeks of gestation, is a major cause of neonatal morbidity and mortality.

Etiology: In the United States, 75% of the neonatal deaths result from premature delivery. Approximately one-third of premature delivery is a result of maternal or fetal complications such as hypertension, abruption, or multiple pregnancy. One-third is a result of premature rupture of membranes, and one-third is from unknown causes. Maternal infections outside of the uterus are associated with premature labor, with a special emphasis on infection of the urinary tract. Anatomic variations of the uterus account for a small percentage of premature labor.

Occurrence: 9%–10% of all pregnancies.

Age: Increased risk for women under age 17 or over 35.

Ethnicity: More common in African-American women.

Contributing Factors: Risk factors associated with premature labor are multiple gestation, DES exposure, uterine anomaly, cervical dilatation, previous preterm labor, history of cone biopsy, history of second-trimester abortion, and uterine irritability. Scoring systems have been published and are available for use. Congenital malformations, particularly those associated with oligohydramnios, can result in premature labor. The high frequency of small-for-gestational-age infants among preterm deliveries supports the association of placental insufficiency with preterm labor. Genital tract infection leading to intra-amniotic infection has been proposed as a cause of preterm labor (see Appendix).

Signs and Symptoms: Uterine contractions and cervical change.

Diagnostic Tests: Electronic monitoring, ultrasound, physical examination.

Differential Diagnosis: False labor, urinary tract infection.

Treatment: A woman determined to be at risk for premature labor by use of a scoring system, cervical change, or increased uterine activity must be followed with frequent pelvic exams, have strenuous physical activity limited, and have her work environment altered. Vaginal infection must be identified and treated. Abstinence from sexual intercourse is recommended.

Home uterine activity monitoring is one of the tools available to help the woman identify preterm labor. Telephone transmission of external monitoring for labor awareness is very useful for evaluation. Prophylactic tocolytics may be used. Tocolytic therapy is usually restricted to between 24 and 34 weeks of gestation. Evaluation of fetal maturity is a critical part of the management of preterm labor. The use of steroids to enhance pulmonary maturity has been studied and shows beneficial effect.

Survival rates of preterm infants born in tertiary-care centers are higher than survival rates of those transferred to centers after delivery. Transport to a tertiary-care facility prior to delivery should be initiated when this can be accomplished safely. Method of delivery will be determined by fetal weight, presentation, and establishment of labor.

Follow-up: Dependent upon management.

Sequelae: None past delivery.

Prevention/Prophylaxis: Treatment of infection during pregnancy.

Referral: Physician referral is required.

Education: Stress the importance of prenatal care.

Spontaneous Abortion

Termination of pregnancy before fetal viability is the definition of abortion.

Etiology: Unknown, with genetic abnormalities the most common suspected etiology.

Occurrence: The incidence of spontaneous abortion is approximately 10%. The actual number is difficult to ascertain because many spontaneous abortions are not diagnosed. More than 80% of abortions occur in the first 12 weeks of pregnancy.

Age: Childbearing.

Ethnicity: Not significant.

Contributing Factors: Chromosomal anomalies account for the majority of these terminations, with abnormal development of the zygote, embryo, or early fetus noted. Maternal factors associated with spontaneous abortion include chronic infection, hyperthyroidism, diabetes, progesterone insufficiency, drug use, environmental toxins, autoimmune mechanisms, or uterine defects.

Signs and Symptoms: Hemorrhage and necrotic changes in the tissues usually accompany spontaneous abortion. There may be no visible fetus in the sac on

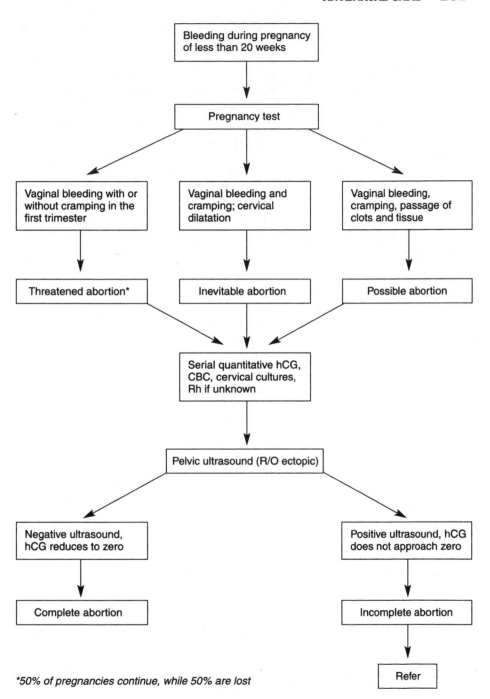

FIGURE 17–5 Bleeding during pregnancy of less than 20 weeks.

ultrasound examination, leading to diagnosis of a blighted ovum. Spontaneous abortion at times involves passing of all of the products of conception with no interference from a provider. Complete abortion can be verified with serial decreasing beta hCG titers. If any products of conception are retained as indicated by pelvic examination and beta hCG titers, dilation and evacuation (D&E) must be performed.

"Threatened abortion" is the term used when vaginal bleeding occurs during the first half of pregnancy. Bleeding can range from slight to heavy. In inevitable abortion, there is rupture of membranes and cervical dilatation. Under these conditions abortion is almost certain. "Missed abortion" is the term used to indicate that products of conception are not viable; however, bleeding and contractions do not follow. Careful palpation and measurement of the uterus at prenatal examinations will reveal no growth of the uterus, and fetal heart tones will be absent. Retained nonviable products of conception, particularly those in the second trimester, can lead to coagulation defects and should be terminated (Fig. 17–5).

Diagnostic Tests: Complete abortion can be verified with serial decreasing beta hCG titers. Threatened abortion requires ultrasound for confirmation of fetal viability and pelvic examination to determine cervical dilatation. In many cases a series of ultrasounds is required to monitor fetal growth and viability.

Differential Diagnosis: Ectopic pregnancy, infection, malignancy.

Treatment: Serial hCG until resolution, D&E, or induction of labor.

Follow-up: According to treatment.

Sequelae: Infection and bleeding if unresolved.

Prevention/Prophylaxis: None.

Referral: Consultation with a physician for management plan is recommended.

Education: Teach the patient to notify the health provider if bleeding during pregnancy occurs.

BIBLIOGRAPHY

Bates, B: A Guide to Physical Examination and History Taking. Lippincott, Philadelphia, 1991.
Gant, N, and Cunningham, F: Basic Gynecology and Obstetrics. Appleton & Lange, Norwalk, CT, 1993.
Olds, S, London, M, and Ladewig, P: Maternal and Newborn Nursing. Addison Wesley, Menlo Park, CA, 1996.
Youngkin, E, and Davis, M: Women's Health. Appleton & Lange, Norwalk, CT, 1994.

CHAPTER **18**

POSTPARTUM CARE

Caring for a woman after delivery primarily consists of observing her body revert to a nonpregnant state. Assessment skills during this transition time are very important. The ability to recognize the usual patterns of recovery versus the abnormal are critical in providing postpartum care.

Assessment

Assessment after Delivery

Uterus

Immediately after delivery the uterus is approximately at the level of the umbilicus and remains there for approximately 2 days, after which it begins a gradual descent into the pelvis. Oxytocin causes the myometrium, the thick muscular walls of the uterus, to contract, thereby compressing exposed placental blood vessels and slowing the uterine bleeding. Uterine bleeding in the postpartum woman is controlled by contraction of the uterus; therefore, careful assessment of the fundus of the uterus immediately following delivery is important. The fundus of the uterus should be palpated for contraction every 15 minutes for the first hour after delivery, every 30 minutes for the next hour, hourly for the next 2 hours, and every 8 hours until discharge to home. The consistency of uterine contraction should be noted, as should the placement of the fundus. (A full bladder can interfere with the placement and contraction of the uterus.) A uterus felt to be "boggy" should be massaged to stimulate contraction. Many factors can interfere with the contraction of the uterus immediately after delivery. These factors are anesthesia, manipulation at birth, multiparity, full bladder, retained placenta, and infection. If the postpartum woman has any of these risk factors, her fundus must be evaluated very frequently immediately after delivery.

If the woman has delivered by cesarean section, anesthesia permits for uterine palpation in the immediate postpartum period. After the effects of anesthesia have ended, palpation of the uterus is performed gently and with guidance from the woman. Lifting of the head tightens abdominal muscles, making palpation even more difficult. Ask the woman to keep her head down during the examination.

Lochia

The lochia in the early postpartum phase, approximately 3 days, is rubra containing blood and deciduous tissue. Exfoliation or sloughing is in process after delivery. In approximately 3 weeks, new endometrium will form. In approximately 6 weeks, the placental site is healed. Healing occurs without scarring. In the immediate postpartum period, the amount of lochia is used as an additional assessment of uterine contraction. Lochia immediately following delivery is heavy, meaning that it would saturate a pad within an hour. It also increases in flow upon arising, with breastfeeding, and with exertion. Clots in lochia serosa may be present but are small in size. Numerous clots, foul smell, and excessive bleeding require further assessment.

Lochia becomes serosa after the first 3 days following delivery. This lochia contains primarily serous fluid, deciduous tissue, leukocytes, and erythrocytes. Its color is pink or brown with a serosanguinous consistency. It should not have a foul odor and should not saturate pads.

Lochia alba appears at approximately day 10 after delivery and consists primarily of leukocytes. It should not saturate pads nor return to red or pink discharge. Lochia alba persists for approximately 2–3 weeks.

Vital Signs

Vital signs should remain stable during the postpartum period. Vital signs are taken simultaneously with assessment of the uterus and lochia. Blood pressure should not alter during the postpartum period; however, slight bradycardia may be present for the first 6–8 days after delivery. Postpartum women are susceptible to orthostatic hypotension because their cardiovascular system adjusts to the nonpregnant state. Temperature elevation up to 100.4°F can be related to dehydration in the first 24 hours after delivery. Persistent or recurrent fever at or above this level could indicate infection.

Vaginal and Perineum

The vagina and perineum are stretched and edematous immediately after vaginal delivery. Bruising may or may not be present. Extensive edema or hematoma requires further evaluation. Ice packs to the perineum in the early postpartum period help to relieve perineal discomfort and decrease edema.

The bladder is edematous and hypotonic following vaginal delivery. The woman experiences decreased sensation and may not recognize the urge to void. The bladder should be palpated for distention frequently during the first postpartum day. If the woman's bladder is distended and she cannot void, pouring warm water over the perineum may be helpful. Catheterization is performed only if necessary. The postpartum woman is susceptible to urinary tract infection, and catheterization increases this risk.

Breasts

Breast engorgement occurs at approximately 48–72 hours following delivery. After delivery, the inhibiting effects of estrogen and progesterone decrease, allowing the luteinizing hormone to initiate lactation. Infant sucking stimulates oxytocin production, allowing the milk to "let down." The breasts are usually soft during the first 2 days after delivery and become substantially larger and firmer on postpartum day 3. Congestion known as engorgement is caused by hormonal change that produces venous stasis and seeping of fluid. When a regular breastfeeding pattern is established, the breasts soften and become more comfortable. Nursing mothers can develop soreness and even cracking and bleeding of the nipples. Engorgement makes "latching on" by the infant more difficult and can result in sore nipples. Breasts should be checked daily while caring for postpartum women. Snug brassieres can help to relieve engorgement. Sore nipples can be relieved with topical medication.

Medication to relieve engorgement is not recommended currently for postpartum women. Women who do not choose to breastfeed should be instructed to relieve engorgement with a tight-fitting bra and no stimulation to the breasts.

In summary, postpartum assessment includes evaluation of vital signs, breasts, uterus, lochia, perineum, incision if present, and legs for thrombophlebitis. Postpartum assessment occurs immediately after delivery, at scheduled intervals over the next few days, and again at 4–6 weeks. Immediate assessment occurs in the hospital or birthing suite. Follow-up assessments can occur in outpatient settings or in the woman's home. Follow-up visits are at more frequent intervals for women who deliver by cesarean section. Follow-up assessment should include the following components: physical exam, laboratory testing, family adjustment, and contraceptive counseling (see Appendix).

Follow-up Assessment

By 4–6 weeks after delivery, the uterus has returned to its nonpregnant state; the lochia is alba containing primarily leukocytes and is scant, and the vagina and perineum are regaining tone. Physical examination includes general health assessment. Vital signs are taken. Extremities are assessed for varicosities. Abdominal exam includes inspection for striae, diastasis, hernias, masses, tenderness, and lymph nodes. If cesarean was the method of delivery, healing of the incision should be assessed.

Breast examination should be performed. The lactating breast will be full without redness or masses. The nonlactating breast should be soft without masses or lymphadenopathy. Milk may discharge from a nonlactating breast for up to 3 months after delivery. External genitalia should be without edema or lesions and the episiotomy, if present, should be well healed. The vagina should have rugae. The cervical os should be closed. The uterus should be 4–6 weeks' size and nontender. The rectum should be free of hemorrhoids and have good sphincter control. Pelvic musculature is evaluated for return to the nonpregnant state. Kegel exercises are suggested to women with relaxed musculature. Schedule a follow-up visit after several weeks of Kegel exercises to re-evaluate strength of pelvic musculature, particularly in the presence of cystocele or rectocele.

Antepartum and postpartum hemoglobin levels should be compared to determine the necessity for continued iron therapy and further testing. Rubella vaccination should be given after delivery to nonimmunized women. Date of next Pap smear should be planned. Glucose tolerance testing for women who were diagnosed with gestational diabetes should be requested.

Family adjustment includes discussion and counseling surrounding the issues of integration of the baby into the family structure, rest and sleep habits, appetite and diet, activity level, exercise program, plans for return to employment, coping ability in caring for the baby, and any problems with the baby.

Resumption of sexual intercourse must be discussed, along with use of contraceptives. Lactation suppresses ovulation, but there is difficulty with determining when ovulation will return. Contraception must be utilized for women who do not desire conception during lactation. Lactation creates a vaginal dryness that must be countered with lubrication during intercourse. Temporary methods of birth control discussed with postpartum women include barrier methods, hormonal methods, and use of spermicidal agents. Oral contraceptives and progestin-only contraceptives can be utilized by lactating women, but a decrease in milk production is possible. This possibility must be discussed with women who desire the use of hormonal contraceptives.

Management of Postpartum Complaints and Complications

Perinatal Loss

Pregnancy loss is an emotionally devastating situation.

Etiology: Early pregnancy loss is related at least 50%–60% of the time to a karyotypic abnormality. As gestation progresses, the proportion of losses arising from genetic factors decreases and those arising from maternal or environmental factors increase. In the third trimester only 5% of stillborns have chromosomal aberrations. When there is a stillborn infant without any obvious cause, a genetic etiology should be sought.

Occurrence: 10%–20% of all pregnancies.

Age: Childbearing.

Ethnicity: Not significant.

Contributing Factors: Maternal infection, anatomic abnormalities of the uterus, maternal chronic disease.

Signs and Symptoms: Delivery of nonviable infant.

Diagnostic Tests: Serial beta human chorionic gonadotropin (BHCG) levels in the first trimester. After second or third-trimester delivery, a thorough examination that includes photographs should be performed. An autopsy should be requested to aid in the diagnosis. Karyotype analysis should be performed.

Differential Diagnosis: Ectopic pregnancy.

Treatment: Bedrest, first trimester: dilation and evacuation (D&E) if BHCG levels do not fall to zero. Second- and third-trimester loss may require cervical ripening and induction of labor (see Appendix).

Follow-up: Dependent upon treatment strategy.

Sequelae: Retained fetal loss increases the risk of an infection and bleeding.

Prevention/Prophylaxis: None.

Referral: Physician referral is required.

Education: Signs and symptoms of infection should be reviewed with the woman.

Postpartum Depression

Etiology: Mood disorder with postpartum onset.

Occurrence: Postpartum depression develops in approximately 10% of all postpartum women. The greatest risk occurs at approximately 4 weeks after delivery.

Age: Childbearing.

Ethnicity: Not significant.

Contributing Factors: Risks for postpartum depression include primiparity, history of postpartum depression, lack of social support, and lack of stable relationships.

Signs and Symptoms: Symptoms of postpartum depression are the same as those of any major depression: sadness, frequent crying, insomnia, appetite change, difficulty concentrating, worthless feelings, inadequate feelings, lack of concern about personal appearance, persistent anxiety, and irritability toward others.

Diagnostic Tests: Patient history of depression.

Differential Diagnosis: The new mother may experience some degree of baby "blues" a few days after delivery. This is the result of many factors, some of which are emotional letdown following delivery, physical discomfort of the immediate postpartum period, fatigue, and anxiety. Mild and transient "postpartum blues" are treated with anticipatory guidance and counseling. If the blues are mild and self-limiting, there is minimal concern. Depression, which is not a normal accompaniment of childbearing, requires investigation. There is no evidence that pregnancy itself causes depression, but it may precipitate underlying disease. Postpartum depression must be identified and treated, preferably through a system that provides a postpartum support group.

Treatment: Hospitalization, medication, psychotherapy.

Follow-up: As per treatment protocol.

Sequelae: Depends on severity.

Prevention/Prophylaxis: None.

Referral: Psychiatric referral.

Education: It is important to report feelings of sadness following delivery to a health-care provider.

Postpartum Hemorrhage

Postpartum hemorrhage has been defined as blood loss of more than 500 mL during the first 24 hours after delivery. This definition is difficult to use since blood loss is estimated at delivery with the estimate often one-half of the actual loss.

Etiology: The two most important causes of immediate postpartum hemorrhage are uterine atony and laceration of the cervix and vagina. The overdistended uterus is likely to be hypotonic after delivery. Thus the woman with a large fetus, twins, or polyhydramnios is prone to postpartum hemorrhage. Labor initiated or augmented with pitocin is more likely to be followed with atony and hemorrhage. Postpartum hemorrhage can also be related to retained placental tissue interfering with uterine contraction. Trauma can lead to postpartum hemorrhage. Examples of trauma can be related to delivery of large infants, midforceps deliveries, and forceps rotations (see Appendix).

Occurrence: Of women delivering vaginally, 5% lose more than 1000 mL of blood. Postpartum hemorrhage is the cause of one-quarter of the deaths from obstetric hemorrhage.

Age: Childbearing.

Ethnicity: Not significant.

Contributing Factors: Delivery of large infant, forceps delivery, multiple gestation, and polyhydramnios. Rarely, postpartum bleeding is related to a coagulation disorder. In women with obstetrical and/or medical complications of pregnancy, disseminated intravascular coagulation (DIC) can occur, resulting in acceleration of the coagulation system and activation of the fibrinolytic system.

Signs and Symptoms: Heavy vaginal bleeding after delivery.

Diagnostic Tests: Retained placental fragments can be diagnosed with ultrasound.

Differential Diagnosis: Vulvar hematoma may cause excruciating pain and is diagnosed with the sudden appearance of a tense and sensitive mass covered by discolored skin or mucous membrane.

Treatment: The cause of the hemorrhage must be determined prior to initiation of treatment. Atony of the uterus should be considered first. If the uterus is "boggy," massage is appropriate, and at times oxytocin must be administered. The role of lacerations in postpartum bleeding must be ascertained. Any lacerations creating excessive bleeding must be repaired. Vulvar hematoma is treated with prompt incision and evacuation of blood with ligation of the bleeding points.

Follow-up: According to therapy.

Sequelae: Anemia.

Prevention/Prophylaxis: Treat causative factor or factors.

Referral: Consultation with a physician is required.

Education: Postpartum women should be taught the normal phases of involution including type and amount of vaginal discharge.

Postpartum Infection

Infection following delivery can occur in the pelvis, breast, or urinary tract. The likelihood of pelvic infection is related to the length of time the membranes were ruptured prior to delivery, the number of examinations the woman had during labor, the amount of manipulation at the time of vaginal delivery, the size and number of incisions and lacerations, and operative method of delivery.

Etiology: Organisms that invade the placental site, incision, and lacerations are typically those that normally colonize the cervix, vagina, and perineum. Most of the organisms are of low virulence and seldom cause infection in healthy tissues. The most common causative agents of postpartum infection are anaerobic streptococci, clostridia, β-hemolytic streptococci, *Escherichia coli,* and *Klebsiella.* Infection of episiotomy and repaired lacerations is unusual considering the degree of bacterial contamination to which the site is exposed.

Occurrence: Unknown.

Age: Childbearing.

Ethnicity: Not significant.

Contributing Factors: Size and number of incisions or lacerations if related to infection. Uterine infection is more common following cesarean delivery, particularly if the cesarean followed long labor with multiple pelvic examinations. Length of time membranes are ruptured is related to infection.

Signs and Symptoms: Postpartum uterine infection involves the decidua, my-ometrium, and parametrial tissues. Symptoms are fever, chills, and abdominal pain. There is bilateral tenderness elicited on bimanual examination and the lochia has a foul odor. If infection of an incision occurs, wound edges become red and swollen and sutures may tear through edematous tissue, causing wound gaping. Drainage may be serous or frankly purulent. Complete breakdown of the repair site may occur. Pain and dysuria are symptoms of episiotomy infection or urinary tract infection (UTI) (Fig. 18–1).

Diagnostic Tests: Culture and sensitivity of urine or wound. Pelvic examination.

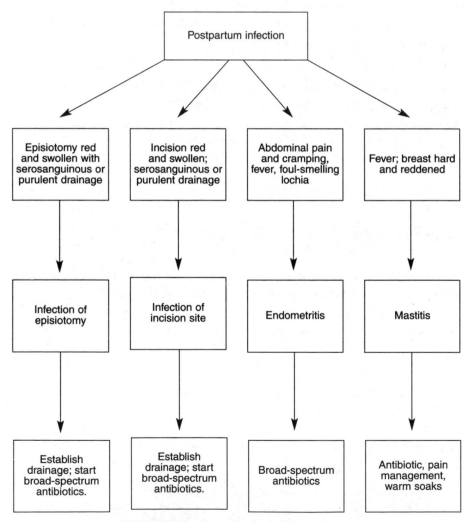

FIGURE 18–1 Diagnosis of postpartum infection.

Differential Diagnosis: Suture irritation, bladder infection.

Treatment: Treatment consists of establishing drainage and administering broad-spectrum antibiotics by oral route or, in the event of severe infection, by intravenous route. Symptoms of endometrial infection rarely occur prior to 5 days after delivery. Urinary tract infection can occur after delivery. Manipulation and use of catheters contribute to this infection. Women experience pain with urination and frequency of urination. Treatment is with broad-spectrum antibiotics after urinary culture and sensitivity to identify the organism involved.

Symptoms of mastitis rarely occur prior to the first week after delivery and as a rule do not occur until the third or fourth week of lactation. Engorgement precedes inflammation. Rise in temperature occurs early in the infection process. The breast becomes reddened, hard, and painful. The most common organism is *Staphylococcus aureus,* the source of which is the infant's mouth and throat. Treatment involves antibiotics, acetaminophen for pain and fever, warm soaks on the affected breast, and frequent nursing on the infected breast.

Follow-up: Repeat culture and sensitivity following resolution of infection.

Sequelae: None after therapy.

Prevention/Prophylaxis: Appropriate management of labor and delivery.

Referral: For unresolved infection, physician referral is required.

Education: Stress to the patient the importance of reporting fever and pain postpartum.

Subinvolution of the Uterus

"Subinvolution of the uterus" is the term utilized when excessive vaginal bleeding occurs in the nonimmediate postpartum period.

Etiology: Prolongation of the involution process.

Occurrence: Unknown.

Age: Childbearing.

Ethnicity: Not significant.

Contributing Factors: Subinvolution accompanied by pain and fever indicates a relationship with endometritis. Multiparity and cesarean delivery may contribute to subinvolution.

Signs and Symptoms: The woman experiences excessive vaginal bleeding with or without fever and pain 1–2 weeks after delivery. The bleeding can be related to retained placental fragments or abnormal involution at the placental site. A subinvoluted uterus will feel "boggy" and tender.

Diagnostic Tests: Complete blood count (CBC), cervical culture, serum human chorionic gonadotropin (hCG), pelvic ultrasound.

Differential Diagnosis: Infection of the endometrium, cystitis, retained placental fragments.

Treatment: The treatment for subinvolution depends on the cause.

Follow-up: Outpatient visits are necessary to ensure resolution.

Sequelae: None.

Prevention/Prophylaxis: None.

Referral: If resolution does not occur in a timely fashion, refer to an obstetric and gynecology physician.

Education: Stress the importance of reporting excessive vaginal bleeding during postpartum period.

Thrombophlebitis

Thrombophlebitis is an infection of the lining of a vessel in which a clot attaches to a vessel wall. Thrombophlebitis may affect the veins in the leg or pelvis after delivery. Thrombophlebitis can be superficial or deep. In superficial, the surface venous system is involved. In deep, changes take place in the deep veins of the calf, thighs, or pelvis. With deep, there is a risk of pulmonary embolism.

Etiology: Thrombophlebitis occurs after delivery and is related to the increased clotting factors during this period.

Occurrence: The incidence is less than 1% of postpartum women, with onset usually between the tenth and twentieth postpartum day.

Age: Thrombophlebitis occurs more frequently with increased maternal age.

Ethnicity: Not significant.

Contributing Factors: History contributing to deep vein thrombosis (DVT) includes obesity, operative delivery, long labor, postdelivery infection, past history of DVT, and varicosities.

Signs and Symptoms: DVT symptoms include positive Homan's sign, elevated temperature, pain in the leg, swelling and tenderness of the leg, and/or groin pain.

Diagnostic Tests: Diagnosis of DVT can be made with Doppler flow studies and with CT or MRI scanning of the pelvis.

Differential Diagnosis: Edema of the leg or leg pain unrelated to thrombophlebitis.

Treatment: Superficial thrombophlebitis is treated with application of continuous moist heat to the extremity and elevation of the extremity. DVT is treated with anticoagulant therapy, bedrest, elevation of the extremity, and analgesia.

Follow-up: As per treatment regime.

Sequelae: Risk of reoccurrence following delivery or surgery. DVT can precede pulmonary embolism. The incidence is 1 in 5000 deliveries.

Prevention/Prophylaxis: Early ambulation after delivery reduces the incidence of thrombophlebitis.

Referral: For diagnostic testing. Refer to a physician if Doppler study is positive.

Education: Stress the importance of reporting signs and symptoms of thrombophlebitis to a health-care provider.

BIBLIOGRAPHY

Gant, N, and Cunningham, F: Basic Gynecology and Obstetrics. Appleton & Lange, Norwalk, CT, 1993.
Quistad, C: How to smooth Mom's postpartum path. RN, 40–49, April 1994.
Youngkin, E, and Davis, M: Women's Health. Appleton & Lange, Norwalk, CT, 1994.

APPENDIX **A**

Resources

ADDRESSES AND TELEPHONE NUMBERS

AIDS Hot Line
Atlanta, GA
800-551-2728

American Cancer Society
Public Information Department
1599 Clifton Road NE
Atlanta, GA
800-227-2345

American Sleep Disorder Association
1610 14th St. NW Suite 300
Rochester, MN 55901
507-287-6006

Bladder Health Council
c/o American Foundation for Urologic Disease
300 W. Pratt St. Suite 401
Baltimore, MD 21201
800-242-2393

Center for Medical Consumers and Health Care Information
237 Thompson St.
New York, NY 10012
212-674-7105

Compassionate Friends
P.O. Box 3696
Oak Brook, IL 60521
708-990-0010

National Association of Area Agencies on Aging
1112 16th St. NW Suite 100
Washington, DC 20036
800-677-1116

274

National Association for Continence
P.O. Box 8310
Spartansburg, SC 29305
800-BLADDER

National Breast Care Cancer Coalition
P.O. Box 66373
Washington, DC 20035
800-935-0434

National Cancer Institute
Cancer Information Service
800-4-CANCER

Women's Health Information Center
Boston Women's Health Book Collective
240 Elm St.
Somerville, MA 02144
617-625-0271

National Women's Health Network
1325 G St. NW
Washington, DC 20005
202-347-1140

Public Citizen Health Research Group
200 P St. NW
Washington, D.C. 20036
202-833-3000

Resolve
1310 Broadway
Somerville, MA 02144-1779
617-623-0744

Simon Foundation for Continence
Box 835
Wilmette, IL 60091
800-23-SIMON

TELEPHONE NUMBERS

Agency for Health Care Policy and Research
800-358-9295

American Red Cross
202-737-8300

Medicare Hot Line
800-638-6833

National Rehabilitation Information
800-346-2742

Salvation Army
703-684-5500

Alcoholics Anonymous
800-443-4525

National Council on Alcoholism and Drug Dependence
800-622-2255

National Institute on Drug Abuse
800-662-4357

American Heart Association
800-242-8721

Planned Parenthood
800-230-7526

CDC AIDS Hot Line
800-342-2437

National Herpes Hot Line
919-361-8488

National STD Hot Line
800-227-8922

WEB SITES FOR WOMEN'S HEALTH NURSE PRACTITIONERS

American Academy of Nurse Practitioners
http://www.aanp.org/

American College of Nurse-Midwives
http://www.midwife.org/

American Nurses Association
http://www.ana.org/

Association of Women's Health, Obstetric and Neonatal Nurses (AWHONN)
http://www.awhonn.org/

Centers for Disease Control
http://www.cdc.gov/

National Association of Neonatal Nurses
http://ww.nann.org/

National Association of Pediatric Nurse Associates and Practitioners
http://www.napnap.org/

National Council of State Boards of Nursing
http://www.ncsbn.org/

National Institutes of Health
http://www.nih.gov/

March of Dimes
http://www.modimes.org/

APPENDIX **B**

Counseling Issues For Adolescents

Adolescence brings changes in physiology, cognition, and personality. Stressors in adolescents often arise from peer pressure, impulsivity, and parental conflicts.

DEFINITIONS

Early adolescence, ages 10 through 14, includes rapid pubertal development. Young girls worry about the size of their hips and breasts. Insecurity about their new bodies make these adolescents self-conscious. They often seek validation for thoughts and feelings from members of the same sex.

Middle adolescence, ages 15 through 17, includes adjustment to new bodies and the acquisition of new cognitive skills. These young women are defiant and self-reliant. "It can't happen to me" is a common position. Dating and experimentation with heterosexual behaviors generally begins in middle adolescence. Intimate relationships tend to be short-lived encounters that help the young women to define themselves in relationship to the opposite sex. Adolescents in this age group are usually serially monogamous, meaning that they have one partner at a time, but change partners frequently.

Late adolescence, ages 18 and 19, includes role seeking and movement into living in an adult society. The peer group and its ideals become less important and influential. Heterosexual relationships become significant, with increasing intimacy and growth in caring and concern for the partner.

COUNSELING ISSUES

Adolescent girls, when stressed, tend to be egocentric. They argue and may refuse to relinquish their viewpoints. The young adolescent girl believes in her own perfection, hence she has difficulty acknowledging her mistakes. Adults, however, have many flaws and adolescents are quick to point them out.

Chronological age alone cannot be used to predict adolescent thinking. Life experience, emotional stability, family support, parental discipline and maturity, and health status all affect the maturity of thinking.

278

Adolescent girls tend to be self-conscious. This concern can inhibit girls from seeking care, or it may influence the tone of a visit.

Anger in adolescent girls is often followed by withdrawal from conflict. Young adolescents tend to be impulsive and use emotion-based strategies in conflict. Older adolescents are better able to focus on and talk about their problems.

Identity, independence, and development of significant love relationships outside the family are the major tasks of adolescents.

Do Not Immunize When . . .

Adult immunization is an important but frequently overlooked part of patient care. High-risk adults should be immunized against vaccine-preventable diseases; travelers may require special vaccines. Adverse reactions to vaccination are rare and are usually local. A history of previous serious allergic reaction is the only absolute contraindication to vaccination in general. However, pregnancy and immunocompromised status may prohibit vaccination.

Likely candidates for adult immunization are:

- Persons with chronic disease
- Immunocompromised patients
- Alcoholics or drug abusers
- Heath-care workers
- Nursing home residents
- Homeless people
- International travelers
- Migrant workers
- Child-care employees
- Institutionalized persons

Factors that are *not* contraindications to vaccination:

- Mild to moderate reaction to a previous vaccination
- Current antibiotic therapy
- Contact with pregnant women
- Recent exposure to illness
- Personal history of allergies
- Family history of allergies

Contraindications to vaccination:

- Influenza—allergy to eggs
- Tetanus-Diphtheria—none
- Polio—pregnancy, compromised immune status, malignancy, HIV infection, or household contact with HIV-infected persons
- Pneumococcal—pregnancy
- Hepatitis A—none

- Hepatitis B—allergic reaction to baker's yeast
- Measles, mumps and rubella—pregnancy, allergy to eggs or neomycin, compromised immune status (should not be given to women who plan to be pregnant within three months of vaccination)
- Varicella—pregnancy, compromised status, receipt of blood products in the last 5 months, allergy to neomycin

---

Adapted from National Coalition for Adult Immunization, 4733 Bethesda Avenue, Suite 750, Bethesda, MD 20814-5228

Flight-or-Flight Response

Common reactions to physical or emotional stress include sweaty palms, tense muscles, blushing, nervousness, insomnia, reduced powers of concentration, queasy stomach, and weak knees. When stress is severe, the nervous system and the hormone-regulating mechanisms produce a fight-or-flight reaction intended to protect the threatened individual. Hans Selye called this response an alarm reaction. This reaction is ideal for escaping as rapidly as possible or for attacking. Following the alarm reaction there is a return to physiologic equilibrium. Long-term exposure to stressful agents produces many alarm reactions and ultimately exhaustion. The body is not designed to sustain the alarm phase for prolonged periods or at frequent intervals.

Physical reactions to stress:

- Tachycardia
- Contraction of blood vessels in the stomach and intestine and along skin surfaces
- Increase in blood pressure
- Increase in blood supply to the large muscles
- Dilation of the pupils
- Secretion of adrenaline from adrenal glands
- Increase in respirations

APPENDIX C

Body Fat Calculations

Locate your ideal weight on the weight chart for a quick estimate of body fat.

1. THE PINCH TEST:

Using the thumb and forefinger, take a fold of skin and subcutaneous tissue in these sites: back of the arm, back below the shoulder blade, thigh, calf, and abdomen. A fold greater than one inch indicates excessive body fat.

2. THE RULER TEST:

The slope of the abdomen between the flare of the ribs and front of the pelvis is flat or slightly concave. A ruler placed on the abdomen along the midline should touch both ribs and the pelvic area.

DESIRED WEIGHTS FOR ADULT WOMEN

Height (feet/inches)	Small Frame	Medium Frame	Large Frame
4'–10"	102–111	109–121	118–131
4'–11"	103–113	111–123	120–134
5'–0"	104–115	113–126	122–137
5'–1"	106–118	115–129	125–140
5'–2"	108–121	118–132	128–143
5'–3"	111–124	121–135	131–147
5'–4"	114–127	124–138	134–151
5'–5"	117–130	127–141	137–155
5'–6"	120–133	130–144	140–159
5'–7"	123–136	133–147	143–163
5'–8"	126–139	136–150	146–167
5'–9"	129–142	139–153	149–170
5'–10"	132–145	142–156	152–173
5'–11"	135–148	145–159	155–176
6'–0"	138–151	148–162	158–179

Weights at ages 25–29 based on lowest mortality weight in pounds according to frame (in indoor clothing weighing 3 lb., shoes with 1" heels).

A Guide to Daily Food Choices

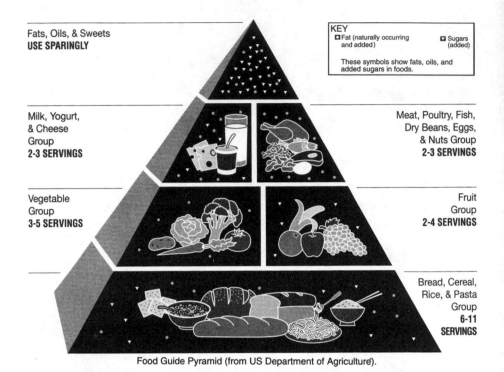

Fats, Oils, & Sweets
USE SPARINGLY

KEY
☐ Fat (naturally occurring   ▨ Sugars
and added)   (added)

These symbols show fats, oils, and
added sugars in foods.

Milk, Yogurt,
& Cheese
Group
2-3 SERVINGS

Meat, Poultry, Fish,
Dry Beans, Eggs,
& Nuts Group
2-3 SERVINGS

Vegetable
Group
3-5 SERVINGS

Fruit
Group
2-4 SERVINGS

Bread, Cereal,
Rice, & Pasta
Group
6-11
SERVINGS

Food Guide Pyramid (from US Department of Agriculture).

Serving Sizes:

Bread, Cereal, Rice, and Pasta:
1 slice of bread
1 ounce of ready-to-eat cereal
1/2 cup of cooked cereal, rice, or pasta

Milk, Yogurt, and Cheese:
1 cup of milk or yogurt
1 1/2 ounces of natural cheese
2 ounces of process cheese

Vegetable:
1 cup of raw leafy vegetables
1/2 cup of other vegetables, cooked or chopped raw
3/4 cup of vegetable juice

Meat, Poultry, Fish, Dry Beans, Eggs, and Nuts:
2–3 ounces of cooked lean meat, poultry, or fish
1/2 cup of cooked dry beans, 1 egg, or 2 tablespoons of
peanut butter count as 1 ounce of lean meat

Fruit:
1 medium apple
1/2 cup of chopped, cooked, or canned fruit
3/4 cup of fruit juice

The Food Pyramid.

GIRLS BIRTH TO 36 MONTHS
HEAD CIRCUMFERENCE FOR
AGE & WEIGHT FOR LENGTH

NAME _____

RECORD # _____

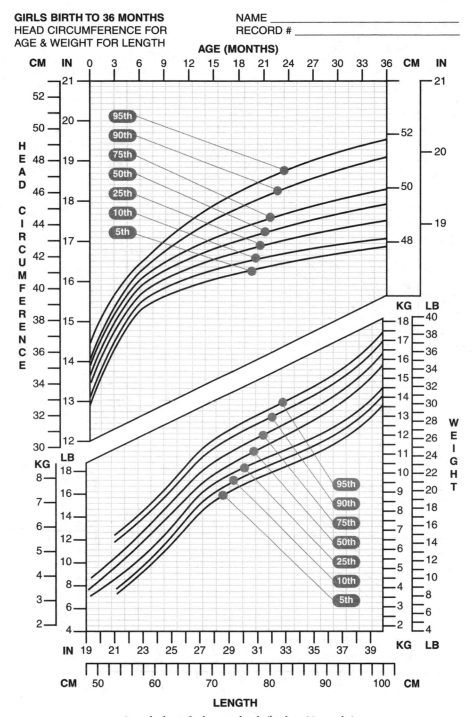

Growth charts for boys and girls (birth to 36 months).

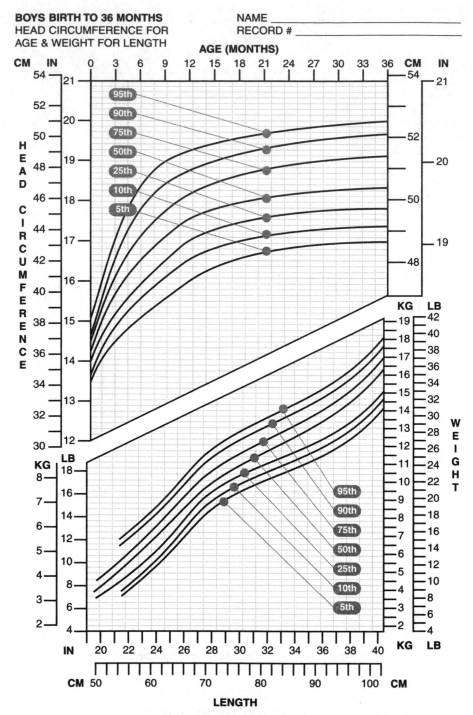

Growth charts for boys and girls *(continued)*.

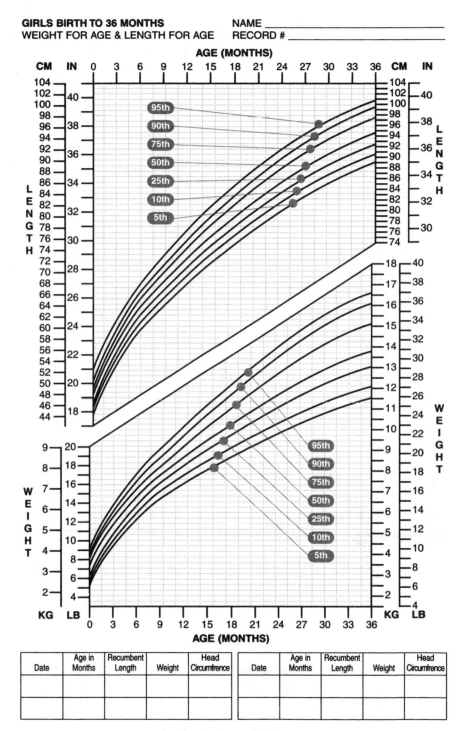

Growth charts for boys and girls *(continued)*.

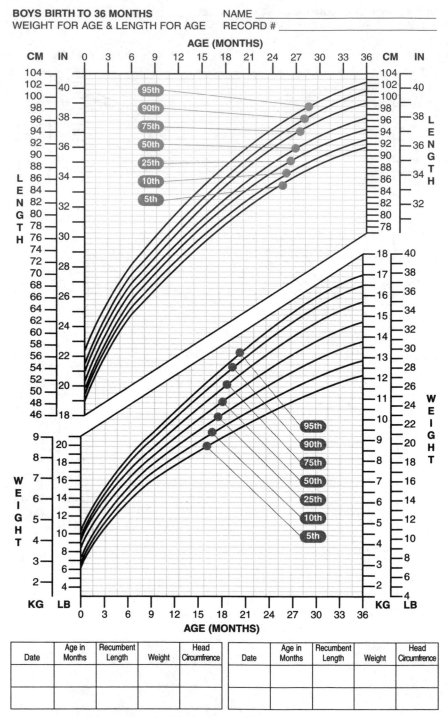

Growth charts for boys and girls *(continued)*.

APPENDIX **D**

Sexual History

Questions about sexual functions or practices are relevant to the patient's history. Sexual questions surrounding the patient's chief complaint or present illness may be asked. Most commonly, the sexual history is obtained during the genitourinary component of the review of systems.

A few introductory comments about why you are asking sex-related questions should begin the discussion. These questions may relate to the woman's complaint, overall health, or chronic illness. Whatever the clinical situation, explanation should be given and consent obtained to go forward with questioning.

POSSIBLE QUESTIONS:

- "Are you sexually active? That is, have you had sex with anyone in the past few months?"
  - If the answer is no, ask "Have you ever been sexually active?" and "Do you have any problems with sexual functioning?"
  - If the answer is yes, ask "Do you have sex with men or women or both?"
  - If the answer is again yes, then proceed to the following questions.
- "Do you have more than one partner?"
- If the woman is of childbearing age, ask "Are you interesting in getting pregnant?"
- "Are you using anything for contraception or doing anything to avoid pregnancy?"
- For every sexually active woman ask "Are you worried about the AIDS virus? Do you think that your partner might have sex with other people, use IV drugs, or do you believe that you have been exposed to the AIDS virus or other infections related to sex?"
- "Do you take any precautions to prevent infections?"
- "Do you have any problems or concerns about sexual functioning?"

Adapted from Bates, B. A Guide to Physical Examination and History Taking, ed 6. JB Lippincott, Philadelphia, 1995.

Women and Work

Since 1950, the labor force participation by women has increased 170%. Today, more than one-half of all women work outside of the home. Nearly one-half of today's work force is made up of women.

Overall, women die of work-related injuries at a lower rate than men do. Industries with the highest work-related fatalities are the same for both men and women: mining, agriculture, construction, and transportation. However, unlike men, almost one-half of women's job-related mortality is caused by homicide.

Considerations for health and working women are numerous. Every workplace should have a health and safety committee as a contact point for concerns about the safety of women at work. The health and safety committee can be a resource for OSHA regulations.

Nurse practitioners (NPs) have concerns for the health of working women in both the reproductive and nonreproductive years. Concerns surrounding safety and work that arise during health interviews with women include:

- Use of chemicals in the workplace
- Ergonomics
- Noise hazards
- Shift work
- Exposure to radiation
- Conditions of extreme temperature (hot or cold)
- Workplace air quality (heavy dust or asbestos)
- Physical stress and strain in the workplace
- Reproductive hazards
- Solvent hazards
- Fire safety

Equal pay has been the law since 1963. But today women continue to be paid less than men. In 1996 women were paid $0.74 for every dollar that a man received. The difference in pay means less money for groceries, housing, childcare and other expenses. Women also have smaller pensions than men.

The picture is even worse for African-American women, who earn only 67 cents for every dollar, and for Latino women, who earn 58 cents for every dollar, that a man earns.

> Women should receive equal pay for equal work.

Adapted from Youngkin & Davis: Women's Health Primary Care Clinical Guide. Appleton & Lange, Norwak, CT, 1994.

Human Female Sexual Response Cycle

EXCITEMENT PHASE

This phase begins with sexual stimulation of some sort. As excitement heightens, blood pressure, pulse rate, and respirations increase. Nipples become erect and breast size increases. A maculopapular rash appears late in the excitement phase. This rash begins in the epigastric region and spreads to include the breasts. Both voluntary and involuntary muscle contraction occurs. The clitoris becomes tumescent and extends out from under the hood. The vagina lubricates, expands and distends, vaginal wall color becomes darker due to vasocongestion. The uterus partially elevates. The labia majora become vasocongested and move slightly laterally away from the midline.

PLATEAU PHASE

If the excitement phase is not interrupted, sexual tension increases. The nipples becomes increasingly turgid and breast size increases. The skin develops a widespread "flush." There is further increase in voluntary and involuntary muscular contraction, and voluntary contraction of the rectal sphincter. Hyperventilation can occur late in the phase. Pulse increases, and blood pressure increases. The clitoris retracts. There is further increase in the width and depth of the vagina as well as full uterine elevation with cervical elevation. The labia majora become more engorged, and there is vivid color change in the labia minora.

ORGASMIC PHASE

Involuntary muscle contractions are concentrated in the clitoris, vagina, and uterus. Skin "flush" continues. There is loss of voluntary control. Involuntary contractions of the rectal sphincter occur. Respiration rate increases as high as 40 per minute, tachycardia can range from 110 to 180, blood pressure rises, systolic 30 to 80 mm Hg and diastolic 20 to 40 mm Hg. Vaginal contractions and uterine contractions occur.

RESOLUTION PHASE

After orgasm, sexual tension is dissipated. Breasts rapidly detumesce. The flush disappears. Respiration, blood pressure, and pulse return to normal. A widespread film of perspiration appears. The clitoris returns to normal position. There is rapid detumescence of the vagina, and the uterus returns to its normal position. The cervical os gaps for up to 30 minutes in the resolution phase. Vasocongestion of the labia resolves.

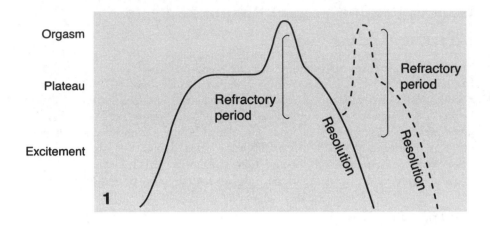

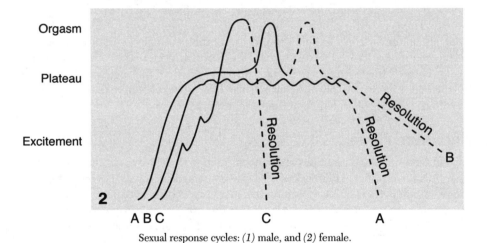

Sexual response cycles: (1) male, and (2) female.

Sample History Form

Identifying data: age, sex, race, place of birth, marital status, occupation, religion

- Source of referral
- Source of history
- Reliability (if relevant)
- Chief complaint (in the woman's own words, whenever possible)
- Present illness

Past history, including:

- General state of health
- Childhood illnesses
- Adult illnesses

- Psychiatric illnesses
- Accidents and injuries
- Operations
- Hospitalizations

Current health status, including:

- Current medications
- Allergies
- Tobacco
- Alcohol, drugs and related substances
- Diet
- Screening tests
- Immunizations
- Sleep patterns
- Exercise and leisure activities
- Environmental hazards
- Use of safety measures (e.g., seatbelts, smoke-detectors)

Family history, including:

- Age and health or age and death of every immediate family member
- Family history of diabetes, heart disease, high blood pressure, stroke, kidney disease, tuberculosis, cancer, arthritis, anemia, allergies, asthma, headaches, epilepsy, mental illness, alcoholism, drug addiction, and symptoms like those of the patient.

Psychosocial history, including:

- Home situation and significant others
- Daily life
- Important experiences
- Religious beliefs
- The patient's outlook

Review of systems, including:

- General
- Skin
- Head
- Eyes
- Ears
- Nose and sinuses
- Mouth and throat
- Neck
- Breasts
- Respiratory
- Cardiac
- Gastrointestinal
- Urinary

- Genital
- Peripheral vascular
- Musculoskeletal
- Neurologic
- Hematologic
- Endocrine
- Psychiatric

Adapted from Bates, B. A Guide to Physical Examination and History Taking, ed 6. JB Lippincott, Philadelphia, 1995

APPENDIX **E**

The Bethesda System For Reporting Cervical/Vaginal Cytologic Diagnosis

FORMAT OF THE REPORT:

A. Statement of the adequacy of the specimen for evaluation
B. A general categorization, which may be used to assist with clerical triage (optional)
C. The descriptive diagnosis

ADEQUACY OF THE SPECIMEN

- Satisfactory for evaluation
- Satisfactory for evaluation, but limited by (specify reason)
- Unsatisfactory for evaluation (specify reason)

GENERAL CATEGORIZATION (OPTIONAL)

- Within normal limits
- Benign cellular changes: See descriptive diagnoses
- Epithelial cell abnormality: See descriptive diagnoses

DESCRIPTIVE DIAGNOSES

Benign cellular changes

- Infection
  - Trichomonas vaginalis
  - Fungal organisms morphologically consistent with *Candida* spp
  - Predominance of coccobacilli consistent with shift in vaginal flora
  - Bacteria morphologically consistent with *Actinomyces* spp
  - Cellular changes associated with herpes simplex virus
  - Other

Reactive changes

- Reactive cellular changes associated with:
  - Inflammation (includes typical repair)
  - Atrophy with inflammation ("atrophic vaginitis")

293

- Radiation
- Intrauterine contraceptive device
- Other

Epithelial cell abnormalities

- Squamous cell
  - Atypical squamous cells of undetermined significance: Qualify°
  - Low-grade squamous intraepithelial lesion encompassing human papil-lomavirus°° or mild dysplasia/ CIN°°°1
- High-grade squamous intraepithelial lesion encompassing
  - Moderate and severe dysplasia
  - CIS/CIN2 and CIN3
  - Squamous cell carcinoma
- Glandular cell
  - Endometrial cells, cytologically benign, in a postmenopausal woman
  - Atypical glandular cells of undetermined significance: Qualify°
  - Endocervical adenocarcinoma
  - Endometrial adenocarcinoma
  - Extrauterine adenocarcinoma
  - Adenocarcinoma, not otherwise specified (NOS)
- Other malignant neoplasms: Specify
- Hormone evaluation (applied to smears only)
  - Hormone pattern compatible with age and history
  - Hormone pattern incompatible with age and history: Specify
  - Hormone evaluation not possible due to: Specify

°Atypical squamous or glandular cells of undetermined significance should be further qualified as to whether a reactive or a premalignant/malignant process is fa-vored.

°° Cellular changes of human papillomavirus—previously termed koilocytosis atypia, or condylomatous atypia—are included in the category of low-grade squa-mous intraepithelial lesion.

°°° CIN indicates cervical intraepithelial neoplasia.

Hormone Replacement Therapy Guidelines

Hormone replacement therapy (HRT) protects against cardiovascular disease and osteoporosis. It also treats menopausal symptoms. When treating a woman with es-trogen, the uterus must be protected from endometrial carcinoma by the addition of progesterone.

Counseling women regarding hormone replacement therapy should include the following information:

- Endometrial carcinoma—unopposed estrogen appears to increase the risk of uterine cancer by four to eight times. By adding progesterone, the risk is reduced to the same as, or less than women not receiving estrogen.

- Ovarian carcinoma—a relationship between estrogen replacement therapy and ovarian cancer has not been demonstrated.
- Breast cancer—There is an increased risk of breast cancer in women who use estrogen replacement. The risk is unclear and current data confusing.
- Cholelithiasis—There may be a slight increase in the incidence of gallstones in women who receive estrogen (controversial).
- Thromboembolic disease—There is no evidence that estrogen therapy increases the risk of thrombosis.
- Hypertension—Estrogen therapy modestly lowers blood pressure in some women and increases blood pressure in others.

Contraindications to HRT:

- Unexplained vaginal bleeding
- Active liver disease
- Chronic impaired liver
- Recent vascular thrombosis
- Carcinoma of the breast
- Carcinoma of the endometrium

Relative contraindications to HRT:

- Seizure disorder
- Very high levels of triglycerides and lipids
- Migraine headaches
- Atraumatic thrombophlebitis
- Current gallbladder disease

A dose of 0.625 mg of estrogen daily is thought to provide protection against cardiovascular disease and osteoporosis. A progestin must be added to protect the uterus. A daily dose of 2.5 mg of progesterone is adequate to provide this protection.

Estrogen and progesterone may be given in a cyclic fashion. Administration in a cycle produces withdrawal bleeding. The majority of menopausal women do not desire withdrawal bleeding; therefore, estrogen and progesterone are given on a daily basis.

Contraindications adapted from ACOG Guidelines for Women's Health, 1996.

Physical Examination

Vital signs

Temperature_____ Respiration_____ BP (L) Arm (R)
_____ Supine _____
_____ Sitting _____
_____ Standing _____

Height _____ Weight _____

General

Skin, hair, nails, mucous membranes

Head

Scalp _____
Face _____
(CNs V, VII) _____
_____
Sinus areas _____
Nodes _____
Cranium _____

Eyes

Visual acuity _____
Visual fields _____
Ocular movements (CNs III, IV, VI) _____
Corneal light reflex _____
Lids, lacrimal organs _____
Conjunctiva, sclera _____
Cornea (CN V) _____
Lens _____
Pupils: Pupillary reflexes (CN III) _____
Light, direct and consensual _____
Fundi (CN II) _____

Ears

External structures _____
Canal _____
Tympanic membranes _____
Hearing (CN VII) _____

Adapted for use from Malasonos, Health Assessment, ed 2. CV Mosby, St. Louis.

Nose

Septum _____

Mucous membranes _____

Patency _____

Olfactory sense (CN I) _____

Oral cavity

Lips _____

Mucous membranes _____

Gums _____

Teeth _____

Palates and uvula (CNs IX and X) _____

Tonsillar areas _____

Tongue (CN XII) _____

Pharynx _____

Voice _____

Neck

General structure _____

Trachea _____

Thyroid _____

Nodes _____

Muscles (CN XI) _____

Breasts and area nodes

_____

_____

_____

Chest, respiratory system

Chest shape _____

Type of respiration _____

Expansion _____

Fremitus _____

General palpation _____

Percussion _____

_____ Diaphramatic excursion: (R) _____cm (L) _____cm

Breath sounds _____

_____

_____

_____

Adventitious sounds _____

_____

Sample physical examination form *(continued)*.

Cardiovascular system

Rate and rhythm: Radial (palpation) _____

Apical (auscultation) _____

Precordium: Inspection _____

Palpation _____

Auscultation _____

S_1 _____

S_2 _____

S_3 _____

S_4 _____

Extra sounds _____

Murmur(s): Systolic _____

Diastolic _____

Carotids _____

Juglar venus pulse and pressure _____

_____

Description of peripheral pulses

	Brachial	Radial	Femoral	Popliteal	Dorsal pedal	Post. tibial
R						
L						

Abdomen and inguinal areas

Contour, tone _____

Scars, marks _____

Auscultation _____

_____

Liver _____

Spleen _____

Kidneys _____

Bladder _____

Hernias _____

Masses _____

Palpation _____

Percussion _____

Genitalia and area nodes

External genitalia _____

Vagina _____

Cervix _____

Uterus _____

Adnexa _____

Rectovaginal exam _____

Rectal examination

_____

Sample physical examination form *(continued)*.

Musculoskeletal system

Gait _____

Deformities _____

Joint evaluation _____

_____

Muscle strength _____.

_____

Muscle mass _____

Range of motion _____

Spine

Contour _____

Position _____

Motion _____

CVA tenderness _____

Nervous system

Mental status _____

Language _____

Cranial nerves (summarize) _____

Motor; Coordination: Upper extremities _____

Lower extremities _____

Involuntary movements _____

Deep tendon reflexes:

Note: +s denote finger jerks, brachioradialis, biceps, triceps, reflexes, 4-quadrant abdominal scratch reflexes, patellar Achilles reflexes, and plantar reflexes. Abdominal reflexes are recorded as 0 or +. Scale: 0–4 (++++); normal = 2 (++).

Sensory

Light touch _____

Pain (pinprick) _____

Vibration _____

Position _____

Sample physical examination form *(continued)*.

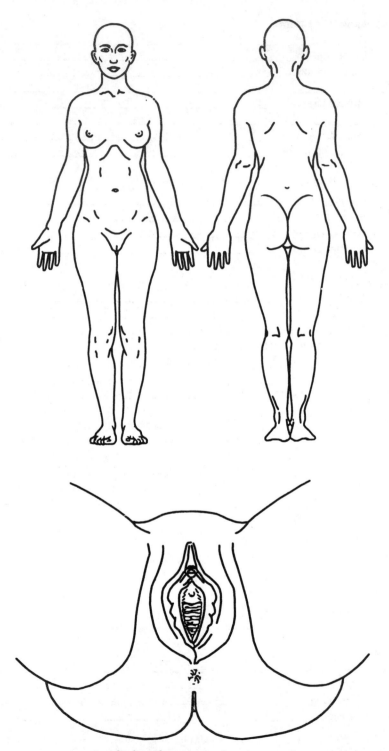

Sample physical examination form *(continued)*.

APPENDIX F

Factors Contributing to Heart Disease in Women

MODIFIABLE RISK FACTORS FOR HEART DISEASE

LDL and HDL Cholesterol

Low-density lipoprotein (LDL) is the major carrier of cholesterol in the blood. Too much LDL can build up within the walls of the arteries that feed the heart and brain. Together with other substances, it can form plaque, a thick, hard, deposit. The formation of a clot in the region of a plaque can block the flow of blood. A high level of LDL, therefore, is associated with stroke and heart disease.

About one-third to one-fourth of blood cholesterol is carried by high-density lipoprotein (HDL). HDL removes excess cholesterol and thus slows the formation of plaques.

Cholesterol comes from two sources. It is made by the liver and it is found in foods. The American Heart Association recommends that the average daily cholesterol intake be less than 300 milligrams.

Physical Inactivity

Physical inactivity has been established as a major risk factor for heart disease. Even mild or moderate activities, if done daily, reduce the risk of heart attack. Examples of daily activities include walking for pleasure, gardening, yard work, housework, dancing, and home exercise programs.

Cigarette Smoking

Smoking is a major risk factor for heart disease. Smoking has been shown to lower HDL cholesterol.

Obesity

Obesity is a major risk factor for coronary heart disease. Obesity raises blood cholesterol, lowers HDL, raises blood pressure and can induce diabetes.

Breast Tenderness

Suggestions for women with breast tenderness:

- If tenderness is related to oral contraceptives or hormone replacement therapy, reduce the estrogen dose, if possible, without interfering with the desired effect of the medication.
- Ask the woman to support her breasts with a brassiere (may be worn at night as well).
- Applying ice packs to the tender areas of the breast may be helpful.
- Restricting sodium intake may reduce tenderness.
- Abstaining from caffeine and chocolate reduces tenderness.
- Vitamin E 400 IU twice daily is effective in reducing breast tenderness.
- Relief can be obtained with salicylates or anti-inflammatory medication.

APPENDIX **G**

IUD Consent Form

Before you give consent to have an IUD, be sure that you understand the information we have given you. If you have any questions, we will be happy to answer them. Your consent is entirely voluntary.

Place your initials next to each statement to indicate that you have read and understand, and agree to the statement.

INITIALS

_____ I have received a brochure containing information on the use, effectiveness, and benefits and risks of the available birth-control methods. I have read the brochure, understand it, and have had my questions answered.

_____ I have been given, have read, and understand the information contained in the manufacturer's brochure about the IUD I will have inserted.

_____ I have been told how to get care in case of a medical emergency, including heavy vaginal bleeding or continuous, lower abdominal or pelvic pain.

_____ I have been instructed and understand that medication will be given prior to insertion of the IUD.

_____ My IUD is due for removal or replacement in _____.

_____ I understand how to check my IUD string.

_____ I understand that I should use another method of birth control for the first month of IUD use.

_____ I will make an appointment to see a health-care provider if my period is late or missed, if I have unusual vaginal bleeding, if I am unable to feel the IUD string, if I want the IUD removed, or the IUD is expelled.

_____ I understand that the IUD should be used with caution in women who have a history of tubal infection, cervical infection, infertility, multiple sex partners, or HIV infection. The IUD should be used with caution in women who are diabetic, anemic, taking a corticosteroid on a regular basis, at risk for bacterial endocarditis, or have large fibroid tumors.

Adapted from standard forms currently in use by Planned Parenthood Association of Bucks County, PA.

Norplant Informed Consent

Please read this form carefully. You will be asked to sign your name once you *understand* this information *completely.*

Before giving your consent, be sure that you understand both the advantages and the disadvantages of using the Norplant system. This form outlines possible problems that can occur with Norplant, warning signs you should watch for, and side effects that some women experience. If you have any questions as you read this, please ask. We will answer any questions you have.

Also, remember that your consent is entirely voluntary. You can change your mind any time before Norplant is inserted. Once Norplant is inserted, you can have it removed any time that you want.

As you read, please initial each section.

HOW NORPLANT WORKS

The Norplant system consists of six soft, thin rubber (Silastic) capsules that are placed in your upper arm. Each capsule contains 36 milligrams of levonorgestrel, a hormone similar to progesterone produced by the ovaries. Levonorgestrel is released through the walls of the capsule to provide a steady flow of hormone at a low dose.

_____ The Norplant hormone is the same hormone used in several brands of birth-control pills; the Norplant dose, however, is much lower.

_____ Norplant prevents pregnancy by interfering with ovulation. It also causes your cervical mucus to be thick and sticky so that sperm have trouble reaching your uterus. Because the dose of hormone is steady, the Norplant system provides extremely good birth-control protection. No other birth control method for women is as effective except having your tubes tied. Fewer than 1 woman in 1000 using Norplant will become pregnant each year. The Norplant system provides steady protection for 5 years. Norplant does not protect against sexually transmitted infections. You will need to use condoms or avoid intercourse and other sexual contact if there is any risk of infection from a sex partner.

WHO SHOULD USE NORPLANT

_____ Norplant is not a wise choice for women with certain medical problems:
- Thrombophlebitis (blood clots in vein) or embolism (clots in lung, eye, brain)
- Abnormal vaginal bleeding that has not been diagnosed
- Pregnancy or suspected pregnancy
- Severe active liver disease or liver tumors
- Breast cancer

_____ Before having Norplant inserted, be sure to *discuss* with your clinician any serious medical condition you may have. Some examples include: diabetes, high blood pressure, high cholesterol, migraine or severe headaches, epilepsy, depression, gallbladder, heart or kidney disease. Norplant may not work as well for women taking epilepsy drugs such as Dilantin or Tegretol or the antibiotic Rifampin.

WHAT TO EXPECT

_____ *Almost all* women using Norplant have *irregular periods or bleeding* especially during the first year after it is inserted. You could have many bleeding days, spotting, or irregular periods. Some women skip periods or have very light periods. Overall, the total amount of blood loss is usually less than with normal periods, but the *timing is not as predictable.* These problems tend to decrease after the first year or can sometimes be treated with additional hormone medication.

POSSIBLE PROBLEMS

_____ In the first week after insertion, be alert for itching, pain, pus, or bleeding at the Norplant insertion site. Let your clinician know about any of these problems.

While using Norplant, you will need to watch for *warning signs of serious problems* such as high blood pressure inside your skull, stroke, liver disease, breast cancer, thrombophlebitis, embolism, depression, or accidental pregnancy. If you become pregnant or develop one of these problems, Norplant may need to be removed. Report any warning signs *right away:*

- No period after having a period every month
- Sudden weakness or numbness on one side
- Norplant comes out
- Shortness of breath
- Severe depression
- Coughing blood
- Headache(s)—persistent, more frequent, or more severe than usual
- Severe pain in the stomach or abdomen
- Blurry or double vision or loss of vision
- Unusual swelling or pain in the legs or arms
- Visual sparks or flashes
- Yellowing of the skin or eyes
- Ringing sound in ears
- Heavy bleeding from the vagina
- Feeling dizzy or fainting
- Lump in breast
- Sharp or crushing chest pain

_____ Although pregnancy is very unlikely while using Norplant, you must have a pregnancy test if you have symptoms of pregnancy or if you go more than 6 weeks with no menstrual bleeding. Tubal (ectopic) pregnancy can occur with Norplant. These problems with Norplant are *uncommon:*

- Headache
- Nausea or dizziness
- Ovary enlargement

- Dermatitis or acne
- Appetite change
- Weight gain
- Breast pain or discharge
- Increased body hair growth
- Hair loss from scalp
- Skin discoloration over implants
- Difficulty removing implants
- Numbness in hand or forearm of Norplant arm
- Nervousness

_____ If they do occur, these problems usually go away when Norplant is removed.

INSERTING AND REMOVING NORPLANT

_____ The six Norplant capsules, each about 1/8 inch wide and 1 inch long, will be inserted just under the skin of the upper arm through a 1/8-inch incision. Local anesthetic is used before insertion to make the skin temporarily numb. A lot of bruising usually occurs in the insertion area but should disappear within a few weeks. The incision will be protected with a bandage for the first few days. The site will usually heal quickly. No stitches are required, and the scar will be small. You will be able to feel the Norplant capsules, and they may be visible under the skin. After you have used Norplant for 5 years, or sooner if you choose, the implants will need to be removed because all the hormone may be used up. Removal will require local anesthesia and one or more small incisions. There is usually an additional medical fee for removal.

YOUR CONSENT

I have read this Informed Consent summary, and have discussed my questions with my clinician. I also understand the risks and benefits of other methods of birth control, including birth-control pills, the IUD, the diaphragm, cervical cap, condoms, spermicide, and sterilization surgery. I have thought about all these factors. I *voluntarily choose* to have the Norplant system inserted. I have received a copy of the Norplant system booklet from the manufacturer.

Date _____   Signature_____

Witness_____

Used with permission from The Nurse Practitioner 19(4):97, © Springhouse Corporation.

Female Sterilization Consent Form

COUNSELING PRIOR TO OBTAINING CONSENT

Presterilization discussions and decision making should take place well in advance of the operation and consent forms should be signed prior to admission for the procedure. This is particularly important if the sterilization is to be performed after childbirth or after a termination or loss of pregnancy.

Emphasize that sterilization is permanent. Despite what the woman may have heard about reversals, reanastomosis is not a frequently done procedure and is only 70%–80% successful. The prospects for successful reversal depend on the condition of the tubes after sterilization.

Involve both partners in the decision and discuss both male and female sterilization.

Discuss sterilization in the context of all contraceptive methods. Give full explanations of each method and emphasize the long-term, reversible contraceptives available.

Inform the patient of failure rates associated with sterilization and the risk of ectopic pregnancy. Suspected pregnancy should be ruled out as soon as possible.

Emphasize that sterilization affords no protection from sexually transmitted diseases, including HIV.

Screen candidates for indicators of poststerilization regret. Women most likely to regret having the procedure are:

- Young
- Had sterilization at the time of abortion
- Had sterilization at the time of delivery

Discuss the surgical methods appropriate for the woman, including side effects, failure rates, and recovery time. Explain in detail:

- Surgical procedure
- Preoperative instructions
- Surgical site
- Timing of the procedure
- Type of anesthesia
- Length of recovery
- All medical benefits and risks including
  - General surgical risks
  - Risk of failure to complete the surgery
  - The possibility of unrelated changes in menstruation

Answer all questions.
Discuss the lack of change in sexuality.
Provide printed material that the woman and her partner can review.

INFORMED CONSENT

Informed consent is a voluntary decision made by a person who has been fully informed about a surgical procedure. The procedure must be explained in a language that the person can understand. Informed consent for sterilization must include:

- Type of operation, including risks and benefits
- Availability of other methods for birth control
- The fact that the operation, if successful, will prevent the client from having any more children
- Intended permanence of sterilization
- Acknowledgment that reversal is possible, but that it is expensive, requires a highly technical and major surgery, and that results cannot be guaranteed
- Possibility of failure (pregnancy) after the procedure
- Option to decline surgical contraception without loss of medical or financial benefits.
- Signature of both the patient and the surgeon

Adapted from: Contraceptive Technology, ed 16, Irvington Publishers, New York, 1994, and Grimes, D and Wallach, M: Modern Contraception, Emron, NJ, 1997.

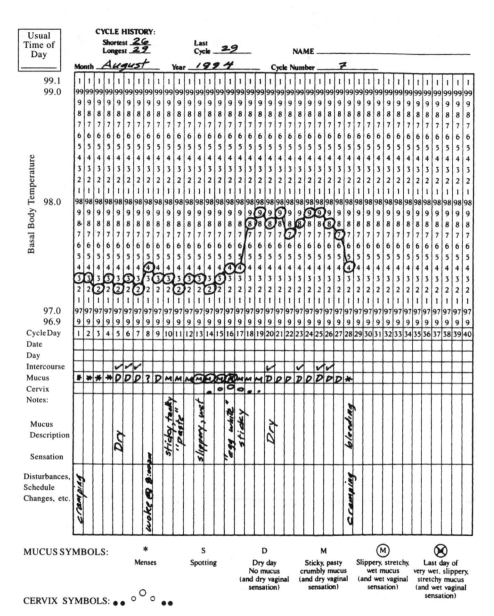

Sample basal body temperature (BBT) form. Adapted from the Fertility Awareness Manual: An Instructional Guide for Clients. James Bowman: San Francisco.

APPENDIX **H**

Kegel Exercises

The Kegel exercise is designed to strengthen the muscle group that forms the pelvic floor. The exercise is prescribed for women who have stress incontinence, experience pelvic relaxation, have recently delivered a child vaginally, or have poor vaginal muscle tone.

In order to perform the exercise, the woman must first locate the muscle group. There are two ways to identify the muscle group. One involves stopping the flow of urine by contracting the muscle. The other involves placing a finger or fingers into the vagina and squeezing those fingers with the muscle. These techniques should be used only to identify the muscle, not to perform the exercise itself.

Once the muscle has been identified, the woman contracts the muscle; holds it contracted for a least the count of one, two; and then relaxes the muscle for the count of five to ten. This exercise requires concentration so that the muscles being contracted are the correct ones and not the abdominal or the gluteal muscles. Breath-holding is not a part of this exercise.

At the start of an exercise regimen, Kegels should be performed 10 times at least twice daily. In time, the length of time the muscles are held contracted can be increased and the number of repetitions and sessions per day can be increased.

APPENDIX **I**

Bone Densitometry Testing (Osteoporosis)

COUNSEL ALL WOMEN ON RISK FACTORS FOR OSTEOPOROSIS

Risk factors for osteoporotic fracture include:

Nonmodifiable:

- Personal history of fracture as an adult
- History of fracture in a first-degree relative
- Caucasian race
- Advanced age

Modifiable:

- Cigarette smoking
- Low body weight
- Estrogen deficiency
- Low calcium intake
- Alcoholism
- Recurrent falls
- Inadequate physical activity

CLINICAL GUIDELINES

- Perform evaluation for osteoporosis using bone densitometry on all postmenopausal women who present with fractures.
- Recommend densitometry testing for all women over age 65, regardless of risk factors.
- Recommend bone densitometry testing for postmenopausal women under age 65 who have one or more additional risk factors for osteoporosis.

- Women who are considering medication for the prevention of osteoporosis may find testing helpful in decision making.
- Advise all women to obtain adequate calcium intake.
- Recommend regular weight-bearing exercise.
- Advise women to avoid tobacco smoking and to limit alcohol intake.

BONE MINERAL DENSITY

Measurements of bone mineral density (BMD) at any skeletal site have value for indicating fracture risk. BMD is expressed as a relationship to two norms: the expected BMD for the patient's age and sex and/or the norm for a "young normal" adult. The difference between the patient's score and the norms will be reported.

BMD testing techniques:

- Dual energy x-ray absorptiometry (DEXA) can be used to measure BMD in spine, hip, or wrist. Scanning is completed in a few minutes with radiation exposure one-tenth that of a standard chest x-ray.
- Single energy absorptiometry measures BMD in the forearm or finger and sometimes the heel.
- Radiographic absorptiometry (RA) is a technique used in a standard x-ray of the hand.
- Quantitative computed tomography measures trabecular and cortical bone density at several sites in the body. It may be used as an alternative to DEXA scanning for vertebral measurements.
- Ultrasound densitometry assesses bone in the heel, tibia, patella, or other sites where bone is relatively superficial. Ultrasound measurements are not as precise as DEXA or single scans but accurately predict fracture risk.

APPENDIX J

Thyroid Lab Values

TOTAL SERUM T$_4$ (THYROXINE)

Measures both free T$_4$ and bound T$_4$. The normal level is 5 to 12 µg/dL. The level is increased by pregnancy, estrogen therapy, and hypothyroidism.

TOTAL SERUM T$_3$

Normal is 80 to 200 ng/dL.

THYROID STIMULATING HORMONE (TSH)

Monoclonal antibody TSH assay is useful in testing for both hypo and hyperthyroidism; normal value is 0.4 to 4.8 mLU/L.

RADIOACTIVE IODINE (RAI) UPTAKE

A tracer dose of RAI is given and a count is taken over the thyroid gland hours later. The value of this test is to determine whether a thyroid nodule is active or inactive.

Anorexia and Bulimia

ANOREXIA

Anorexia nervosa usually appears in early or middle adolescence. A girl begins to starve herself and sometimes exercises compulsively as well. Her weight falls and her health deteriorates. She may conceal her weight loss and discard food instead of eating it. She may believe that she looks fat. Her refusal to eat does not involve appetite. Her appetite is normal. The refusal of food remains a mystery.

According to the American Psychiatric Association's *Diagnostic and Statistical Manual of Mental Disorders, Fourth Edition* (*DSM-IV*), a woman is suffering from anorexia, not just fasting or dieting, when her weight falls to 15% below the normal range and she has not menstruated for at least three months.

313

Additional symptoms include:

- Drowsiness, and lethargy
- Skin, nails, and hair that are dry and brittle
- Lanugo on the limbs
- Constipation, anemia, and swollen joints

Possible long-term consequences include:

- Death
- Low heart rate and blood pressure
- Low serum potassium
- Osteoporosis
- Kidney damage

BULIMIA

Bulimia can develop at any age from early adolescence until age 40, but is usually the most clinically serious in late adolescence. Bulimic women binge eat followed by vomiting or purging (use of laxatives or diuretics). Binge eating may alternate with compulsive exercise and fasting. Many anorectic women also indulge in eating binges and one-half of anorectic women make a transition to bulimia; 40% of severely bulimic women have a history of anorexia.

Bulimia is defined as two or more episodes of binge eating (rapid consumption of a large quantity of food—up to 5000 calories) every week for at least three months.

Additional symptoms include:

- Fatigue and weakness
- Constipation
- Fluid retention
- Swollen salivary glands
- Erosion of dental enamel
- Sore throat from vomiting
- Scars on the hand from inducing vomiting

Long term consequences can include:

- Dehydration
- Decreased serum potassium
- Tearing of the esophagus

APPENDIX **K**

Depression Symptom List

Symptoms

- Loss of interest in things that used to be enjoyed, including sex
- Feeling sad, blue, or down in the dumps
- Feeling slowed down or feeling restless and unable to sit still
- Feeling worthless or guilty
- Changes in appetite or weight loss or gain
- Thoughts of death or suicide; suicide attempts
- Problems concentrating, thinking, remembering, or making decisions
- Trouble sleeping or sleeping too much
- Loss of energy or feeling tired all the time

Other symptoms include:

- Headaches
- Aches and pains
- Digestive problems
- Sexual problems
- Feelings of pessimism or hopelessness
- Being anxious or worried

Adapted from AHCPR Publications Clearing House, P.O. Box 8547, Silver Spring, MD 20907.

Suicide Risk Assessment

Suicide is almost impossible to predict. There is no test sensitive enough to identify which people are going to kill themselves without intervention. Suicide is now the eighth leading cause of death in the United States. The actual number of suicides, however, is difficult to determine. Statistics are compiled from death certificates, but at times ruling out homicide gets more priority than does establishing suicide. When death is due to falls, automobile accidents, or drug or alcohol overdose, it is very difficult to establish suicide as the motive.

FACTORS THAT CONTRIBUTE TO SUICIDE

- Suicide rates are highest in old age. 40% of suicides are over age 60. After age 75, the rate is three times higher than the average. The suicide rate in the elderly declined from 1950 to 1980 but has been rising since that time.
- The age group of 15 to 24 now accounts for 20% of male suicide and 14% of female suicide. The rate in this age group has quadrupled since 1950. Suicide attempts are a common reason for hospital admission in people under the age of 35.
- People who have never been married are twice as likely to take their own lives as are currently married people. The highest rate of all is among divorced or widowed people. Suicide is lower in rural areas than in cities. People with strong religious conviction have a lower suicide rate than average. Doctors have a higher rate of suicide and psychiatrists have a higher rate than any other medical specialty.
- The great majority of suicides are in people with mental or emotional disorders. The most common associated diagnosis is depression. One-third of schizophrenic patients attempt suicide; 5%–10% succeed.
- Substance abuse can be an instigator of suicide. About 20% of suicides are in alcohol abusers. A drinking binge can lead to suicide, even in nonalcoholics. Illicit drug abusers have a high suicide rate.
- Rates of suicide are high in men who are abusers. Murderers commit suicide. Men who kill women are at particular risk. A "lover's suicide pact" is often murder and suicide.
- Among the elderly who commit suicide, one-half or more suffer from a chronic physical illness. Among adolescents who commit suicide, it is often associated with alcoholism, drug abuse, and family disorganization. Adolescents who commit suicide often suffer from child abuse and neglect. Separation, unemployment, imprisonment, and death are common in families of adolescents who attempt suicide.

WARNING SIGNS OF SUICIDE

- Eight out of 10 people who commit suicide give some sign of intention. People who talk about suicide, threaten to commit suicide, or call suicide hot lines are 30 times more likely to kill themselves than people who do not.
- Suicide attempts are by the far the best indicator of a risk for suicide.
- No suicide threat or attempt should be treated casually.

REFERRAL FOR PEOPLE THREATENING SUICIDE

Threatening suicide is important. Failure to see the danger in a suicidal threat, failure to take preventive action, or incorrect treatment are each bases for malpractice. Take all suicide threats seriously.

Adapted from: Philip Long M.D., Internet Mental Health, www.mentalhealth.com.

Posttraumatic Stress Disorder

Physical harm occurs when something or someone assaults the body. Posttraumatic stress disorder (PTSD) occurs when the mind and emotions as assaulted. The American Psychiatric Association has recognized PTSD as a psychiatric diagnosis since 1980.

The cause of PTSD is defined as an event or series of events that involves actual or threatened death or serious injury or a threat to physical integrity. It might be a natural disaster, accident, or a human action. Examples include fire, earthquakes, floods, assault, rape, child abuse, and torture. The immediate response to such an event is intense fear, helplessness, or horror. The event may be witnessed rather than directly experienced. The response may begin immediately or may emerge days, weeks, months, or even years later. The symptoms of PTSD include:

- Hyperalertness—defined as being irritable, easily startled, or constantly on guard. Victims sleep poorly, are agitated easily, and have difficulty concentrating
- Involuntary reexperiencing of the event in the forms of memories, nightmare, and flashbacks. Reexperiencing can be triggered by anything that resembles or recalls the event.
- Emotional numbing—defined as a need to avoid feelings, thoughts, and situations reminiscent of the event.

The risk for the development of PTSD is high when the stress is sudden, unexpected, severe, prolonged, and repetitive and when it causes physical harm, threatens life, humiliates the victim, or destroys the victim's community and social-support system.

Nearly one-half of the people with PTSD also suffer from major depression and more than one-third from phobias and alcoholism.

APPENDIX **L**

Preterm Labor and Delivery

RISK FACTORS FOR PREMATURE LABOR

Demographic Risks

- Age under 17 or over 34
- Low socioeconomic status
- Unmarried
- African-American race
- Low education level

Medical Risks

- Parity of 1 or more than 4
- Genitourinary anomalies/surgery
- Previous low birth weight, preterm labor
- Multiple spontaneous abortions
- Low weight for height

Risks in Current Pregnancy

- Multiple gestation
- Hypertension
- First- or second-trimester bleeding
- Spontaneous rupture of membranes
- Anemia or hemoglobinopathy
- Fetal anomalies
- Hyperemesis gravidarum
- Short interpregnancy interval
- Oligohydramnios
- Isoimmunization
- Incompetent cervix

Environmental Risks

- Smoking
- Alcohol or substance abuse
- High altitude
- Poor nutritional status
- Exposure to toxic compounds

Adapted from Youngkin and Davis, Women's Health: A Primary Care Clinical Guide, Appleton and Lange, 1994.

POSTPARTUM ASSESSMENT

Area Assessed	Findings Day 1	Findings Day 2–3
Normal Findings		
Vital Signs		
Temperature	Elevated (100.4)	Normal
Pulse rate	40–70 beats per minute	Bradycardia or normal
Blood pressure	Normal	Normal
Involution		
Uterus	Fundus at umbilicus	1–2 cm below umbilicus
Lochia	Rubra	Rubra to serosa
Abdomen		
	Soft	Soft
Perineum		
	Edematous	Less edema
Breasts		
Consistency	Soft, colostrum	Firm, large, warm
Nipples	Intact	May be reddened, sore
Lactation	Colostrum	Milk
Legs		
	Pretibial, pedal edema	Edema minimal
Elimination		
Voiding	Up to 3000 mL	Decreasing amount
Defecation	None	Bowels move
Discomfort		
	Perineum aching, Hemorrhoid pain, Generalized aching	Less perineal pain, less hemorrhoid pain
Energy Level		
	Fatigued	Tired

Area Assessed	Findings Day 1	Findings Day 2–3
Normal Findings		
Appetite		
	Often thirsty	Very hungry
Emotional State		
	Euphoric, excited	Happy, concerned

Postpartum Hemorrhage

The causes of postpartum hemorrhage are:

- Uterine atony
- Lacerations
- Retained placenta
- Coagulation disorders

Uterine atony must be carefully observed for in the immediate postpartum period. Bleeding must be checked frequently, and the fundus must be palpated for position and firmness.

Blood pressure must be closely watched as an indicator for hidden bleeding.

Hematomas can be large and create pain as well as bleeding.

Lacerations can create bleeding.

Retained placental fragments prevent uterine contraction and therefore create excessive bleeding.

Perinatal Loss

The loss of a pregnancy leaves a woman struggling to regain her emotional balance at the same time her body is healing. The following is a list of suggestions for emotional support for women who have experienced the loss of a pregnancy.

Love of a child cannot be measured by time the parent has with the child. There is no less right to grieve for infants than for older children.

The parent will never be "over it." The pain never completely leaves. Grieving continues throughout life for the child that could have been with us. The death of a child at any age or under any circumstances is a tragic, life-changing event. Time eases the pain, but it never goes away.

Sleeping pills or alcohol do not help resolve the pain. Grieving is delayed by medication. The work of grieving should not be delayed.

Having another baby does not decrease the grief. Another child never replaces the lost child. Another baby can add more pressure to the grieving process. Women should be careful not to become pregnant too soon after the death of a child.

Support groups can be helpful. People who understand the depth of the pain are those who have experienced it. Support groups are a safe place for parents to go and share their pain with others who have experienced the same feelings.

Many couples find rituals helpful in mourning. Ceremonies can help bring the grief out into the open, allowing people to share their feelings. People choose different kinds of ceremonies, depending on their belief system. Some people find comfort in traditional religious services while others prefer quiet meditation or the symbolism of planting a tree.

Many people who have experienced the death of a child feel like they are "going crazy." The intensity and array of emotions can be overwhelming and frightening. Some people find work impossible. Others become overly absorbed in work. Reassurance that grieving people are not crazy people can be helpful.

RESOURCES:

Resolve HelpLine: 617-623-0744
http://www.resolve.org
Compassionate Friends HelpLine: 708-990-0010

ACOG ANTEPARTUM RECORD

DATE _____

NAME _____
　　　LAST　　　　　FIRST　　　　　MIDDLE

HOSPITAL OF DELIVERY _____

ID# _____　　REFERRED BY _____　　FINAL EDD _____

NEWBORN'S PHYSICIAN _____

| BIRTH DATE | AGE | RACE | MARITAL STATUS | ADDRESS |
| Mo　Day　Yr | | | S　M　W　D　Sep | Zip　　Phone　　(H)　　(O) |

Insurance Carrier/Medicaid#

OCCUPATION

EDUCATION
(Last Grade Completed)

□ Homemaker

□ Outside Work _____ Type of Work _____

□ Student

EMERGENCY CONTACT _____　RELATIONSHIP _____　PHONE _____

| Total Preg | Full Term | Premature | Abortions Induced | Abortions Spontaneous | Ectopics | Multiple Births | Living |

MENSTRUAL HISTORY

LMP □ Definite □ Approximate (month known)　MENSES MONTHLY □ Yes □ No　FREQUENCY: Q ___ days　MENARCHE ___ (age onset)

　□ Unknown □ Normal Amount/Duration　PRIOR MENSES ___ Date ___　On BCP's at Concept □ Yes □ No　hCG+ ___/___/___

Sample pregnancy history and physical examination form.

PAST PREGNANCIES (LAST SIX)

Date Mo/Yr	GA Weeks	Length of Labor	Birth Weight	Type Delivery	Anes	Place of Delivery	Perinatal Mortality Yes/No	Treatment Preterm Labor Yes/No	Comments/ Complications

PAST MEDICAL HISTORY

	O Neg + Pos	Detail Positive Remarks Include Date & Treatment		O Neg + Pos	Detail Positive Remarks Include Date & Treatment
1. Diabetes			15. Alcohol		
2. Hypertension			16. Rh Sensitized		
3. Heart Disease			17. Tuberculosis		
4. Rheumatic Fever			18. Asthma		
5. Mitral Valve Prolapse			19. Allergies (Drugs)		
6. Kidney Disease/UTI			20. Gyn Surgery		
7. Neurologic/Epilepsy			21. Operations/Hospitalizations (Year & Reason)		
8. Psychiatric			22. Anesthetic Complications		
9. Hepatitis/Liver Disease			23. History of Abnormal Pap		
10. Varicosities/Phlebitis			24. Uterine Anomaly		
11. Thyroid Dysfunction			25. Infertility		
12. Major Accidents			26. In Utero DES Exposure		
13. History of Blood Transfus.			27. Street Drugs		
	Amt/Day Prepreg	Amt/Day Preg	#Yrs Use	28. Other	
14. Tobacco					

COMMENTS: _____

Sample pregnancy history and physical examination form *(continued)*.

ACOG ANTEPARTUM RECORD (CONT'D.)

GENETICS SCREENING

INCLUDES PATIENT, BABY'S FATHER, OR ANYONE IN EITHER FAMILY WITH:

	YES	NO
1. Patient's Age ≥ 35 years		
2. Thallassemia (Italian, Greek, Mediterranean, or Oriental Background) MCV < 80		
3. Neural Tube Defect (Meningomyelcele, Open Spine, or Anencephaly)		
4. Down Syndrome		
5. Tay-Sachs (eg, Jewish Background)		
6. Sickle Cell Disease or Trait		
7. Hemophilia		
8. Muscular Dystrophy		
9. Cystic Fibrosis		

	YES	NO
10. Huntington Chorea		
11. Mental Retardation If Yes, Was Person Tested for Fragile X?		
12. Other Inherited Genetic or Chromosomal Disorder		
13. Patient or Baby's Father Had a Child with Birth Defects Not Listed Above		
14. ≥3 First Trimester Spontaneous Abortions or a Stillbirth		
15. Medications or Street Drugs Since Last Menstrual Period If Yes, Agent(s)		
16. other significant family history (see comments)		

COMMENTS: _____

INFECTION HISTORY	YES	NO
1. High Risk AIDS		
2. High Risk Hepatitis B		
3. Live with Someone with TB or Exposed to TB		

	YES	NO
4. Patient or Partner Have History of Genital Herpes		
5. Rash or Illness Since Last Menstrual Period		
6. History of STD. GC. Chlamydia. HPV. Syphilis		
7. Other (See Comments)		

COMMENTS: _____

_____ INTERVIEWER'S SIGNATURE _____

Sample pregnancy history and physical examination form *(continued)*.

INITIAL PHYSICAL EXAMINATION

Date ____/____/____ Prepregnancy Weight _____ Height _____ BP _____

1. Heent	□ Normal	□ Abnormal		12. Vulva	□ Normal	□ Condyloma	□ Lesions	
2. Fundi	□ Normal	□ Abnormal		13. Vagina	□ Normal	□ Inflammation	□ Discharge	
3. Teeth	□ Normal	□ Abnormal		14. Cervix	□ Normal	□ Inflammation	□ Lesions	
4. Thyroid	□ Normal	□ Abnormal		15. Uterus	□ Normal	□ Abnormal	□ Fibroids	
5. Breasts	□ Normal	□ Abnormal		16. Adnexa	□ Normal	□ Mass		
6. Lungs	□ Normal	□ Abnormal		17. Rectum	□ Normal	□ Abnormal		
7. Heart	□ Normal	□ Abnormal		18. Diagonal Conjugate	□ Reached	□ No	_____ CM	
8. Abdomen	□ Normal	□ Abnormal		19. Spines	□ Average	□ Prominent	□ Blunt	
9. Extremities	□ Normal	□ Abnormal		20. Sacrum	□ Concave	□ Straight	□ Anterior	
10. Skin	□ Normal	□ Abnormal		21. Arch	□ Normal	□ Wide	□ Narrow	
11. Lymph Nodes	□ Normal	□ Abnormal		22. Gynecoid Pelvic Type	□ Yes	□ No		

COMMENTS (Number and explain abnormals): _____

_____ EXAM BY _____

_____

_____

Sample pregnancy history and physical examination form *(continued)*.

ACOG ANTEPARTUM RECORD (CONT'D.)

INITIAL LABS	DATE	RESULT	REVIEWED	COMMENTS/ADDITIONAL LAB
Blood Type	/ /	A B AB O		
Rh Type	/ /			
Antibody Screen	/ /			
HCT/HGB	/ /	%____ g/dl		
Pap Smear	/ /	Normal / Abnormal / ____		
Rubella	/ /			
VDRL	/ /			
GC	/ /			
Urine Culture/Screen	/ /			
HBsAg	/ /			

8–18 WEEK LABS (WHEN INDICATED)	DATE	RESULT		
Ultrasound	/ /			
MSAFP	/ /	____ MOM		
AMNIO/CVS	/ /			
Karyotype	/ /	46. xx or 46. xy / Other ____		
Alpha-Fetoprotein	/ /	Normal ____ Abnormal ____		

Sample pregnancy history and physical examination form (*continued*).

ACOG ANTEPARTUM RECORD (CONT'D.)

PLANS/EDUCATION   (Counseled ☐)

☐ Anesthesia Plans _____
☐ Toxoplasmosis Precautions (Cats/Raw Meat) _____
☐ Childbirth Classes _____
☐ Physical Activity _____
☐ Premature Labor Signs _____
☐ Nutrition Counseling _____
☐ Breast or Bottle Feeding _____
☐ Newborn Car Seat _____
☐ Postpartum Birth Control _____
☐ Environmental/Work Hazards _____

☐ Tubal Sterilization _____
☐ VBAC Counseling _____
☐ Circumcision _____
☐ Travel _____

REQUESTS _____
_____
_____
_____

TUBAL STERILIZATION   **DATE**   **INITIALS**

Consent signed   ____ / ____ / ____   _____

AA128   1   / 2

Sample pregnancy history and physical examination form *(continued)*.

24–28 WEEK LABS (WHEN INDICATED)	DATE	RESULT	REVIEWED	COMMENTS/ADDITIONAL LAB
HCT/HGB	/ /	___% ___ g/dl		
Diabetes Screen	/ /	___ 1 Hr.		
GTT (If Screen Abnormal)	/ /	FBS ___ 1 Hr. / ___ 2 Hr. ___ 3 Hr.		
Rh Antibody Screen	/ /			
Rhig Given (28 weeks)	/ /	Signature ___		
32–36 WEEK LABS (WHEN INDICATED)	DATE	RESULT		
Ultrasound	/ /			
VDRL	/ /			
GC	/ /			
HCT/HGB	/ /	___% ___ g/dl		
OPTIONAL LABS (HIGH RISK GROUPS)	DATE	RESULT		
HIV	/ /			
HGB Electrophoresis	/ /	AA AS SS AC SC AF TA$_2$		
Chlamydia	/ /			
Other	/ /			

Sample pregnancy history and physical examination form *(continued)*.

NAME _____

LAST   FIRST   MIDDLE

DRUG ALLERGY: _____

ANESTHESIA CONSULT PLANNED   □ YES   □ NO

MEDICATION LIST:	Start date	Stop date
1.		
2.		
3.		
4.		

PROBLEMS/PLANS

1. _____

2. _____

3. _____

4. _____

EDD CONFIRMATION

Initial EDD:

LMP ____/____/____ = _____ = EDD ____/____/____

Initial Exam ____/____/____ = _____ wks = EDD ____/____/____

Ultrasound ____/____/____ = _____ wks = EDD ____/____/____

Initial EDD ____/____/____   initialed by _____

18–20-WEEK EDD UPDATE:

Quickening ____/____/____ + 22 wks = ____/____/____

Fundal HT at umbil. ____/____/____ + 20 wks = ____/____/____

FHT w/fetoscope ____/____/____ + 20 wks = ____/____/____

Ultrasound ____/____/____ = ____ wks = ____/____/____

Final EDD ____/____/____   initialed by _____

(cont'd)

Sample pregnancy history and physical examination form *(continued)*.

ACOG ANTEPARTUM RECORD (CONT'D.)

32–34-WEEK EDD—UTERINE SIZE CONCORDANCE (±4 OR MORE CM SUGGESTS THE NEED FOR ULTRASOUND EVALUATION)

Visit Date (year ___)											
Weeks gest. (best est.)											
Fundal height (cm)											
FHR present F = fetoscope D= doptone											
Fetal movement (+ = present; 0 = absent)											
Prematurity: Signs/symptoms* (+ = present; 0 = absent)											
Cervix exam (DIL./EFF./STA.)											
Blood pressure inital repeat											
Edema (+ = present; 0 = absent)											
Weight (prepreg: ___)											
Cumulative weight gain											
Urine (glucose albumin/ketones)											
Next appointment											
Provider (initials)											
Test reminders CVS/AMNIO/MSAFP	8–18 weeks GLUCOSE SCREEN/Rhig						24–28 weeks				

COMMENTS: _____

*For example: vaginal bleeding, discharge, cramps, contractions, pelvic pressure.

Sample pregnancy history and physical examination form *(continued)*.

CHAPTER 1 HANDOUTS

Managing Menses

The age at which menses appears has declined in recent years; the average time at which menses begins is now age 12 or 13 years. In a small number of normal girls menses may occur as early as 10 years of age or as late as 16 years of age. Puberty is a broad term meaning the entire transition from childhood to sexual maturity. The appearance of menses is just one sign of puberty.

The time between the start of menses is usually 28 days, although there is considerable variation among women. Different variations do not indicate infertility (inability to get pregnant).

The menstrual flow usually lasts from 4–6 days, but duration between 2 and 8 days is considered normal. In each woman, the duration of flow usually remains similar from cycle to cycle. The menstrual discharge consists of shed fragments of the lining of the uterus mixed with blood. Usually the blood is liquid, but if the rate of flow is excessive, blood clots of various sizes may be seen. The amount of blood loss per cycle is about ½–1 cup.

There are five main stages to the menstrual cycle. They are as follows:

1. Menstruation
2. Postmenstrual reorganization under the influence of estrogen
3. Ovulation—rupture of an egg
4. Secretion of glands under the influence of estrogen and progesterone
5. Preparation for menses

Menses can produce a cramping feeling. Ibuprofen is very effective for relieving the discomfort in most women.

Suggestions for tampon use:

- Avoid deodorant tampons.
- Avoid "superabsorbent" tampons.
- Do not use more than one tampon at a time.
- Avoid tampon use at "the end" of a period when the flow is light and the vaginal walls are drier.
- Reduce overall tampon use by using sanitary pads some of the time—perhaps at night.
- Women who experience a high fever, vomiting, or diarrhea from using tampons should not use them.

Adolescent Nutrition

With adolescence comes increased demand for calories, protein, vitamins, and minerals.

CALORIES

The demands of growth plus energy expenditure require calories. Adolescent girls need about 2200 calories per day and boys about 2500 to 3000 calories per day.

PROTEIN

Adolescent growth requires increases in protein. Protein can be found in eggs, milk, fish, beef, rice, peanuts, oats, wheat, corn, soybeans, sesame seeds, and peas.

VITAMINS

The B vitamins are required in increased amounts during adolescence. Supplementation with B-complex vitamins is recommended. Vitamins C and A are also needed. 60 mg of vitamin C and 800 μg of Vitamin A are needed daily. In girls, a lack of folic acid can lead to anemia. Supplementation of 400 μg daily is recommended.

MINERALS

Calcium requirement for all adolescent girls is 1200 mg daily. Adolescence is a crucial time for developing bone mass. In menstruating girls, iron may require supplementation, at 15 mg daily.

Women Aging in America

Positive health has become a key concept for women aging in America. Strategies for attaining and maintaining positive health include education, health screening, disease-prevention activities, and psychosocial support.

EDUCATION

Myths of aging need to be dispelled. When women become aware of what to expect with the passage of time, they can take responsibility for their own lives and engage in behavior that will have a positive impact on their present and future health. Education is an important tool in women's health.

Education about self-care measures, such as sleeping 7–8 hours per day, controlling weight, eating a well-balanced diet, drinking 6–8 glasses of water per day, exercising, limiting alcohol intake, and eliminating smoking can produce better health and increase longevity. Classes or readings on safe driving and stress reduction can alter women's behavior in a positive way.

HEALTH SCREENING

- Breast self-examination and mammography are important screening tools for women.
- Pap smears and pelvic examinations, cholesterol screening, blood pressure screening, and glaucoma testing are all important to the health of women.
- Flu shots and immunizations, as recommended by the practitioner, should be obtained.
- Regular hearing and vision screening can prevent illness.
- Regular screening examinations that include cancer testing should be scheduled by health-care practitioners.

DISEASE-PREVENTION ACTIVITIES

- Osteoporosis can be prevented with regular exercise, calcium intake, and vitamin D supplementation.
- Prevent heart disease, stroke, and obesity with regular physical activity. Physical activity creates a greater sense of well-being, and it maintains strength and range of motion.
- Stop smoking. Seek an individual or group plan to help you stop smoking.
- Discuss the benefits of estrogen replacement therapy with your practitioner.

PSYCHOSOCIAL SUPPORT

Many women are caregivers rather than care receivers. Sources of support must be explored. Seeking support from family or friends is valuable. Communities also provide valuable support services.

CHAPTER **2** HANDOUTS

Factors to be Considered Prior to Pregnancy

IMMUNIZATIONS

Appropriate and timely immunizations should be received prior to pregnancy. Rubella, a major cause of birth defects, can be immunized against prior to pregnancy. Women should wait several months to become pregnant after rubella vaccination.

NUTRITION

- Adequate protein intake
- Adequate calories
- Adequate calcium intake
- Adequate iron
- Additional folic acid: 400 µg daily

RH FACTOR

An Rh-negative woman must prevent "sensitization" with the Rh factor. Sensitization is prevented through a drug called RhoGam. RhoGam must be given after the birth of every child, after every miscarriage, and after every abortion.

INFECTION

Sexually transmitted diseases can create scar tissue within the pelvis that can prevent pregnancy.

Certain viral infections can cause congenital defects. Proper hand washing, particularly for those who work with urine, saliva, and respiratory secretions, can help prevent these infections.

Prior to pregnancy, screening for cytomegalovirus (CMV) and human immunodeficiency virus (HIV) should be performed.

ENDOMETRIOSIS

Early treatment of endometriosis reduces difficulty with conception.

RADIATION

Exposure to radiation may affect an early pregnancy. Radiation to the pelvis should be avoided by shielding the abdomen during x-rays. If the pelvis must be exposed, a pregnancy test should be performed prior to testing.

MEDICATIONS

Drug use—both street and prescription drugs—can affect fertility and can severely affect developing embryos.

Any prescription medication taken on a regular basis should be evaluated by an obstetrician or midwife prior to conception. Some medications affect conception, and some affect the developing fetus. Substitute medications and changes in dose should be considered in these cases.

Avoid over-the-counter (OTC) drugs unless absolutely necessary. If you use an OTC drug, use one with a single ingredient.

ALCOHOL AND DRUGS

Women who consume alcohol run the risk of delivering a baby with fetal alcohol syndrome. Reduction in consumption of alcohol should occur prior to pregnancy.

Avoid marijuana, cocaine, and other illicit substances entirely *prior* to pregnancy. Illicit drugs affect fertility and can lead to serious growth and development problems and birth defects for the unborn baby.

SMOKING

Smoking affects the developing fetus in a negative way. Smoking creates lower birth weight and a reduction in oxygen available to the developing fetus. The effects are dose-dependent. Stop smoking prior to pregnancy.

CONTRACEPTION

Any woman taking the pill should use an alternate method of birth control for at least one cycle prior to conception.

EMPLOYMENT

Many women face hazards in their occupations. The most hazardous jobs for women related to pregnancy are nurses, x-ray technicians, hairdressers, and lab personnel.

Avoid exposure to potentially hazardous substances prior to pregnancy. Agents that can affect pregnancy are anesthetics, carbon monoxide, ethylene oxide, lead, mercury, pesticides, radiation, and solvents. If possible, avoid these substances. If this is impossible, use protective garb including gloves, masks, gowns, and ventilation hoods. Wash hands meticulously. Discuss how to reduce the risk of exposure with your obstetrician or midwife prior to pregnancy.

Benefits of Stress Management

Various factors contribute to the stressors that women experience and the ways in which women cope with the stressors. Women have practical problems related to everyday existence that men do not experience. Employment, inequities in earning power, and changing family patterns are all stressors for women. Stress can be related to role change, women's changing bodies, minority status, discrimination, and low income.

Women cope with stress by evaluating the situation, examining the available resources, and problem solving (coping). The ability to solve or cope with the stressor depends upon the woman. At times, stressors can be avoided or removed. At other times, stressors cannot be "dealt with" or removed but must be "lived with."

When a stressor cannot be removed, coping strategies are necessary. These strategies can include:

Learning about the body: Through health-care providers and/or through reading materials, women becoming more aware of their bodies and their function can help themselves to deal with physical stressors. Learning about the mind's connection with the body can help women to deal with some psychological stressors.

Stress management techniques: These exercises have been designed to assist women in reducing tension in their bodies.

Counseling: Counseling can help the woman examine issues within her psyche that can help in dealing with real-life dilemmas.

Support groups: These groups can be helpful in assisting women in crisis. The groups are a source of emotional support and they are avenues for discussion about the stressor.

Relaxation Techniques

GUIDED IMAGERY

Guided imagery is a way to employ your imagination to create relaxation. Guided imagery focuses on images to put you into a relaxed state and is designed to relieve tension and stress. The elements of guided imagery include finding a comfortable position, closing your eyes, focusing on your physical sensations, and practicing deep breathing. Listen and allow yourself to follow the directions. Don't force the issue, let it flow freely.

Leave the room and the cares of the day behind . . . You find yourself walking on a path in beautiful meadow . . . It's a bright and sunny day, and a gentle breeze is blowing. As you walk along, find a little path to walk on. Let the gentle breeze blow against your body, see the beautiful flowers blowing . . . As you walk along, find a spot to sit in and put down your stress, all the things that cause you tension, all your worries. Give these tensions shapes and colors. Now set them down on the side of the path. Continue to walk on your path until you come to a big beautiful blue lake. Walk long the sandy beach, feel the warm sand on your feet, feel the warm breeze blowing. Look out across the lake. What do you see? Find yourself a comfortable spot by the lake. Look around, tell yourself that this is your very special place to relax and that you can come here anytime you need to relax. Now come back to the room.

PROGRESSIVE RELAXATION

Progressive relaxation is essential in learning the difference between a muscle that is tense and one that is relaxed. The basic principle used is that when a muscle or group of muscles is tensed, the opposite energy difference is relaxation. Because immediately relaxing the muscle is difficult to do, it is beneficial to begin with tensing a muscle, as a person would do when exercising, and then performing the opposite relaxing response. To obtain an even deeper relaxed state, it is important for you to be aware of the difference in the feeling of your muscles when tensed in contrast to the feeling when they are relaxed. This should give you a better mental understanding of the relaxed state you should obtain.

Take three deep breaths, inhaling as deeply as possible through your nose and exhaling as much air as possible out of your mouth. Then allow your body to breathe at will.

Feet, ankles, and lower legs: Point your toes away from you and feel the areas of tension. Now point your toes toward your head and feel the areas tense. Now relax and allow the lower legs to go limp. Notice how your feet tend to point outward as you relax and allow them to do so. Repeat two times

Knees and adjoining muscles: Push your heels away from you; feel the tension in the muscle areas. Now relax. Note the difference. Repeat two times.

Thighs and buttocks: Tense your thighs by tensing your complete leg and tightening your buttock muscles. Feel the tension. Now relax. Repeat two times.

Pelvic area and buttocks: Again tighten your buttocks and tense the pelvic area. Feel the tension. Now relax. Repeat two times.

Stomach and lower back: Tense this area by bearing down, but don't strain yourself. Now relax. Repeat two times

Chest, shoulders, and upper back: Squeeze your upper arms toward your body and slightly arch your back. Feel the tension. Now relax. Repeat two times

Shoulders: Raise your shoulders toward your head and press them backward. Feel the tension. Now relax. Repeat two times.

Upper arms: Tense your upper arms by bending your arms toward your head. Hold that tension. Now relax. Repeat two times.

Lower arms: Press your hands flat down against whatever surface you are lying on. Feel the tension. Now relax. Repeat two times.

Hands: Make a fist in both hands. Then spread your hands open as far as you can. Now make a fist again. Hold the tension. Now relax. Repeat two times.

Face, jaw, and neck: Bite down with your jaw, push your tongue up toward the roof of your mouth, and press your chin forward against your chest. Now press your lips together and squint your eyes. Feel the tension. Now relax. Repeat two times

Eyes and forehead: Squint your eyes, make a frown, and wrinkle your forehead. Feel the tension. Now relax.

Complete body tension: Press your head backward, push your heels downward, and press your hands flat against the floor. Tense your complete body. Feel the tension. Now relax. Do not repeat; instead, take three deep breaths, inhaling through your nose and exhaling through your mouth. Try not to move any other parts of your body. Just allow yourself to feel completely relaxed.

Source: Griffith-Kennedy, J: Contemporary Women's Health. Addison-Wesley Publishing Co., Menlo Park, Calif., 1986, with permission.

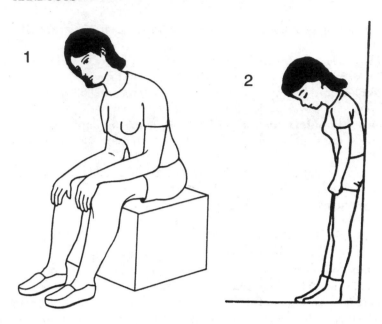

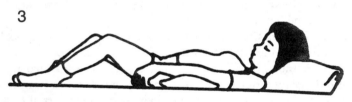

General Rules for Achieving Relaxation

Set aside a time for relaxation each day.
Have a relaxed atmosphere in a quiet room.
Maintain a comfortable position–loosen tight clothing.

Patient Instructions for Relaxation Positions

Sitting
1. Place your feet flat on the floor; sit with your forearms on your thighs.
2. Relax the muscles of the shoulders and neck. Breathe slowly (do not force respirations).

Standing
1. Place your feet about 6 in from the wall.
2. Lean back against the wall. Let your arms hang loosely at your side.

Lying
1. Lay on the bed with your head supported with a pillow.
2. Place pillow under each arm for support. Flex the knees slightly (pillows underneath the knees). Breathe slowly.

Illustrations adapted from Blodgett, DE: Manual of Pediatric Respiratory Care Procedures. JB Lippincott, Philadelphia, 1982.

Signs of Cancer

Cancer's seven warning signals, according the American Cancer Society, are:

C   hange in bowel or bladder habits
A   sore that does not heal
U   nusual bleeding or discharge
T   hickening or lump in the breast or elsewhere
I   ndigestion or difficulty in swallowing
O   bvious change in wart or mole
N   agging cough or hoarseness

If you have a warning sign, make an appointment with a practitioner.

Vulvar Self-Examination

HOW TO PERFORM VSE

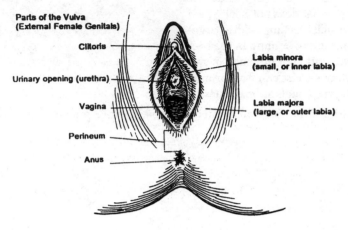

Vulvar self-examination.

WHERE TO LOOK

Position: Find a comfortable, well-lighted place to sit, such as a bed or a carpet. Hold a mirror in one hand. Then, use the other hand to separate and expose the parts of the vulva surrounding the opening to the vagina. Once you have a good viewing position, examine the main parts of the vulva as follows:

- Check the "mons pubis" (the area above the vagina around the pubic bone where the pubic hair is located). Carefully look for any bumps, warts, ulcers or changes in skin color (pigmentation, especially newly developed white, red, or dark areas). Then, use the finger tips to check any visible change and to sense any bump just below the surface you may feel, but not see.
- Next, check the "clitoris" and surrounding area (directly above the vagina) by looking and by touch.
- Next, examine the "labia minora" (the smaller folds of skin just to the right and left of the vaginal opening). Look and touch by holding the skin between thumb and forefinger.
- Then look closely at the "labia majora" (the larger folds of skin just next to the labia minora). Examine both right and left just as you did the labia minora.
- Move down to the perineum (the area between the vagina and the anus) Check thoroughly.
- Finally, examine the area surrounding the anal opening as before by looking and touching.

Important note: Every woman should know the parts of the vulva (see illustration). You should also talk about the VSE with your physician or nurse practitioner, who can note what is "normal" for your individual anatomy. This is a good time to ask questions.

Remember the basic rule: "Vulvar diseases are most easily safely and successfully treated when discovered early." Now you know . . . and now you have yet another good way to help protect your own health . . . the vulvar self-examination.

Source: Lawhead, R, and Allen Jr, M.D:. What Every Woman Should Know: Your Guide to the Benefits of Vulvar Self examination." 1990.

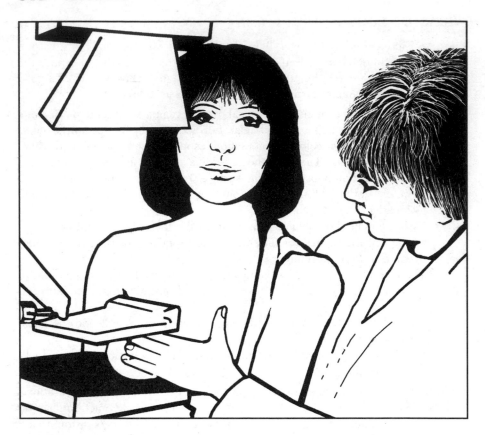

How is a mammogram done?

You will stand in front of a machine. The person who takes the x-rays will gently place your breast between two plastic plates.

These plates will make your breast flat. This may be uncomfortable for a minute, but it helps make any breast changes or lumps easier to see.

What if the mammogram finds a lump?

Your doctor will help decide if you need more tests.

If cancer is found and treated early, most women can be cured. In many cases, only the small lump will need to be taken out, often saving the breast.

Mammogram.

Mammogram

WHAT IS A MAMMOGRAM?

A mammogram is a low-dose x-ray of the breasts. This procedure detects tumors that are too small to be felt by breast self-examination. Mammograms are performed in an outpatient setting, such as a radiology center or a doctor's office. A technician who has been trained in mammography performs a mammogram, and a radiology physician interprets the results.

WHAT CAN I EXPECT DURING A MAMMOGRAM?

You are asked to undress from the waist up, remove necklaces, and wear an examination gown that opens in the front. You are then asked to stand in front of a mammogram machine. Two plastic plates are used to compress one breast at a time while films are taken. Compression is used to enhance the films taken and to reduce radiation exposure. After the films are taken, you are asked to wait a few minutes before dressing while the technician develops the films to make sure that they can be read by the radiologist. Results of the mammogram can be given shortly after the test. In some settings, results will not be forwarded to you until several days after the test.

HOW DO I PREPARE FOR A MAMMOGRAM?

To prepare for a mammogram, do not to apply powder, cream, or deodorant on the day of the test. These substances may appear on the x-ray film and lead to false diagnosis of a problem.

There is temporary discomfort with the compression needed to perform the test. To minimize the discomfort, the test should be performed during the week after menses when breasts are least tender. Discomfort occurs only with compression. Discomfort ceases as soon as the plates are removed.

WHEN SHOULD I HAVE A MAMMOGRAM?

Your first mammogram should be performed between the ages of 35 and 40. Mammograms should then be performed every year or every other year until age 50 and once a year thereafter.

CHAPTER **3** HANDOUTS

Nutrition for Women

Diet plays an important role in health. Studies have shown that coronary artery disease, stroke, diabetes, and some types of cancer have nutrition-related risks. Proper nutrition and weight control are important preventive health measures.

Recommendations from the U.S. Department of Agriculture, the U.S. Department of Health, and the U.S. Surgeon General are as follows:

- Eat a variety of foods.
- Maintain a healthy weight.
- Choose a diet low in fat and cholesterol.
- Eat adequate vegetables, fruits, starch, and fiber.
- Use sugar in moderation.
- Avoid excessive salt.
- Consume no alcohol or alcohol in moderation.

Approximately 2200 calories per day is needed by the average nonpregnant woman. Total fat intake should not exceed 30% of the diet.

Calcium requirements are 1200 mg daily for adolescent girls, at least 800 mg daily for adult women, 1200 mg daily for pregnant women, and 1200 to 1500 mg per day for menopausal and postmenopausal women.

Menstruating women should include iron-rich food in their diet and take an iron supplement daily.

Cancer research provides the following dietary recommendations for women:

- Avoid obesity.
- Decrease fat intake.
- Increase intake of whole-grain foods.
- Increase intake of dark green, deep yellow, and orange vegetables.
- Eat smoked and cured foods in moderation.
- If alcohol is used, use it in moderation.

Guidelines for Adding Calcium to Your diet

The typical American diet includes 600 mg of calcium daily. About 75% to 80% of calcium consumed in American diets is from dairy products. Before menopause, healthy women need 1200 mg of calcium daily. After menopause, they need 1200 to 1500 mg daily.

SOURCES OF CALCIUM

- Milk   300 mg per 8 ounce serving
- Yogurt   400 mg per 8 ounce serving
- Cheese   200 mg per 1 ounce serving
- Sardines   370 mg per 3 ounce serving
- Oysters   270 mg per cup
- Canned salmon   160 mg per 3 ounce serving
- Tofu   120 mg per 3 ounce serving

VITAMIN D

Vitamin D plays a major role in calcium absorption and bone health. Vitamin D is found in vitamin D–fortified milk (400 IU per quart) and cereals (50 IU per serving), egg yolks, saltwater fish, and liver. A regular intake of 400 to 800 IU daily is recommended for bone health.

MEDICATIONS

Drugs that interfere with calcium absorption are anticonvulsants, steroids, tetracycline, diuretics, and aluminum-containing antacids.

CALCIUM SUPPLEMENTS

Calcium carbonate has the highest amount of calcium per tablet—40%. Calcium lactate and calcium gluconate have only about 10% of each tablet containing calcium.

Guidelines for Adding Iron to Your Diet

Foods high in iron content:

MEATS, POULTRY, FISH, DRY BEANS, EGGS, NUTS

Beef liver
Clams
Oysters
Beef
Black-eyed peas
Chickpeas
Lentils
Lima beans
Pinto beans
Soybeans

SUGAR

Molasses, black
Sugar, brown

VEGETABLES

Avocado
Potato (baked with skin on)
Spinach

FRUITS

Dried figs
Prunes
Raisins

BREADS, CEREALS, RICE, PASTA

Bran flakes
Cream of wheat
Enriched pasta
Wheat flakes

CHAPTER **6** HANDOUTS

Genital Herpes

Genital herpes is caused by a virus. There are two different types of the virus, but both are spread by direct skin contact, including genital-to-genital contact and mouth-to-genital contact. Anyone who is sexually active can get herpes. You can get it if you have only one partner who happens to be infected. Many people do not know that they have herpes, so that they infect others without realizing they are doing so. Using a condom can prevent the spread of genital herpes and other sexually transmitted diseases.

The only way to tell for sure that you have herpes is to visit a health-care provider. Herpes can look like many things, including simple irritation. It is important to report to the practitioner any redness or sores in the genital area.

A first outbreak of genital herpes can occur in 2–21 days after sex with an infected partner. Some women have severe symptoms whereas others have mild symptoms. Herpes symptoms include:

- Pain or itching in the genital area or buttocks
- Burning during urination
- Unusual vaginal discharge
- Swelling and reddening
- Small bumps in the genital area
- Bumps become painful sores that open up, crust over, and eventually heal
- Fever, chills, muscle aches, tiredness, headache

Without treatment, a first outbreak can last for about 3 weeks. Most people experience repeated outbreaks that are less severe and last for a shorter time. The interval between outbreaks varies from woman to woman.

Once infected with the virus, it remains with a person for life. There is no cure, but it can be treated and outbreaks reduced.

Genital Warts

WHAT ARE GENITAL WARTS?

Genital warts are small growths that appear on or inside the genitals of both men and women. They are spread from person to person by close physical contact during vaginal, anal, or oral sex.

WHERE DO THEY APPEAR?

Genital warts look and feel like bumps. They are usually painless but can cause itching and burning. In women, they occur inside and outside the vagina and on the cervix (the opening to the uterus). They can also occur on the rectum (anus) and in the throat.

The warts can be seen and/or felt if they are on the outside of the body. Warts inside the vagina and on the cervix can only be detected by a health-care provider. An abnormal Pap smear may mean that you have genital warts.

WHAT CAUSES GENITAL WARTS?

A virus causes genital warts. The virus is contagious and can be passed to someone else during sex. Warts can take weeks to appear after the virus has been contracted. The virus remains in the body even after the warts are removed.

HOW ARE GENITAL WARTS TREATED?

Treatment depends on how many warts are present and if they are inside or outside of the body. Some warts can be removed with a medicine that is applied to them. Some can be frozen or burned off. Some need to be removed by surgery. Warts can return after they have been removed because the virus remains in the body.

There are several "wart" viruses. Most are not associated with cancer, but a few are associated with cancer of the cervix. If genital warts are discovered on the cervix, follow-up Pap smears are very important.

WHAT ABOUT MY SEX PARTNER(S)?

Your partner should be examined and treated when you are diagnosed with genital warts.

HOW DO I PREVENT GETTING GENITAL WARTS?

- Examine your partner before having sex.
- Use latex condoms every time you have sex. Condoms can protect you from sexually transmitted diseases, including genital warts.
- Do not have sex with a person you think might have a sexually transmitted disease.
- Do not use drugs or alcohol before having sex.

Pubic Lice

WHAT ARE PUBIC LICE?

A species of human lice causes this common sexually transmitted disease. Another name for pubic lice is "crabs." Body and head lice do not usually affect the pelvic area. Pubic lice, however, have been found in beards, eyelashes, and eyebrows.

HOW DO I GET PUBIC LICE?

The crab louse requires human blood to survive. Off the body, the lice die quickly. Direct contact must occur for lice to be "caught."

Itching is the primary symptom. Itching leads to scratching, redness, and irritation.

HOW DO I GET RID OF PUBIC LICE?

Lice are treated with over-the-counter or prescription medication. Some medications may not be used during pregnancy. Follow the manufacturer's directions for use carefully.

Wash with hot water, dry-clean, or run through the dryer all contaminated clothing, towels, and bedclothes to destroy the lice.

Spray couches, chairs, and items that cannot be washed or dry-cleaned with an over-the-counter product.

Sexual partner(s) should be treated simultaneously.

CHAPTER **7** HANDOUTS

Women and Heart Disease

The three major risk factors for heart attack are elevated blood cholesterol, cigarette smoking, and high blood pressure.

Blood cholesterol levels should be tested every 5 years for every woman over age 20. High levels should be reduced with changes in diet.

Blood pressure above 140/90 mmHg increases the risk for stroke and heart attack. High blood pressure should be controlled by diet and/or medication.

Women who smoke a pack a day have twice the risk of heart attack as non-smokers. Women who smoke more than a pack of cigarettes a day have three times the risk. Cigarette smoking is the most preventable cause of heart attack. If you smoke, quit!

Other factors that contribute to heart attack include:

- Previous heart attack
- Family history of heart disease
- Diabetes
- Obesity

Good control of diabetes is very important for the health of the heart.

Obesity should be reduced by diet and regular exercise.

CHAPTER **8** HANDOUTS

Vaginal Infections

BACTERIAL VAGINOSIS

The most common form of infection of the vagina is bacterial vaginosis (BV). This infection is caused by a bacterium. Recent research suggests a nonsexual mode of transmission. BV does occur in sexually active women, however, and is related to premature labor and pelvic infection. BV can be found in male partners, but males do not develop a disease per se.

Women with BV may be without symptoms, or they may have vaginal discharge that smells badly. Often women report a foul odor from the vagina, which is most noticeable after intercourse.

BV is treated with an antibiotic. There is no need for sexual partner(s) to be treated.

YEAST INFECTION

Candida albicans, or a "yeast" infection, is a common vaginal infection that is not related to sexual activity. An upset in the balance in the vagina leads to yeast infection. This upset can be related to use of antibiotics, pregnancy, or diabetes.

Yeast infection creates vaginal itching, burning, and irritation. Burning when urine hits the inflamed tissue is common. Vaginal discharge is white and thick. Symptoms frequently worsen prior to a period.

Yeast is treated with an antifungal medication. There is no need to treat sexual partner(s).

TRICHOMONIASIS

Trichomoniasis is a vaginal infection caused by an organism. The organism can live in both women and men. It is transmitted during intercourse. Trichomoniasis creates a foul-smelling, yellow-green, sometimes frothy vaginal discharge. This infection is treated with an antibiotic. Sexual partner(s) should also be treated.

GENERAL RULES FOR WOMEN WITH VAGINAL INFECTION

- Do not douche when you have a vaginal infection.
- Keep clean by showering or bathing.
- Do not use feminine hygiene deodorant sprays.
- Take the entire course of medication as prescribed.
- Do not use tampons if medication is applied into the vagina because they will absorb the medication.
- Soak your diaphragm or cervical cap in a 70% alcohol or a Betadine solution for 30 minutes.
- Avoid intercourse for a least 1 week after treatment.

Sexually Transmitted Diseases

Anyone who is sexually active is at risk for acquiring a sexually transmitted disease (STD). The best approach to STDs is prevention. There is currently an epidemic of STDs in America, specifically in the 15- to 34-year-old age group. Chlamydia, gonorrhea, herpes, syphilis, genital warts, and HIV/AIDS are all STDs with related health risks. Safe sex protects against STDs including AIDS.

WHAT IS SAFE SEX?

Safe sex means preventing the exchange of body fluids during sexual contact. It also means basic hygiene practices such as urinating and washing after sex. Safe sex means choosing your partners wisely and not being afraid to discuss the use of condoms before sexual contact. The following guidelines will help to reduce the risk of developing an STD:

- Limit the number of sexual partners ideally to one partner who is faithful to you.
- Be sure that a partner uses a condom, particularly one containing spermicide.
- Remember that the pill does not prevent STD.
- Do not engage in sexual activity with anyone who has symptoms of an STD.
- Talk to a partner about STD before sexual contact.
- Avoid high-risk activities that include exchanging body fluids with new partners. High-risk activities are unprotected vaginal intercourse, oral sex, and anal sex.
- Check your body frequently for signs of infection
- Have regular Pap smears and checkups.

WHAT ARE THE SYMPTOMS OF SEXUALLY TRANSMITTED DISEASES?

The symptoms of STDs are:

- Abnormal vaginal discharge
- Pain with urination
- Burning or itching around the vagina
- Warts in the genital area
- Rashes, blisters, bumps, or sores in the pelvic area
- Pain in the pelvic area, fever, and chills
- Vaginal bleeding that is not your period
- Pain with intercourse

Sexual activity has *two* risks: pregnancy and STDs. If you believe that you have an STD, seek help; most county health departments have a special STD clinic.

IF A SEXUALLY TRANSMITTED DISEASE IS DIAGNOSED . . .

- Take all of the medication prescribed.
- Tell your sex partner(s).
- Return for follow-up care.

Endometriosis

A woman has endometriosis when small pieces of displaced tissue act like the tissue from inside the uterus so that every month or so it thickens and bleeds just as it would during menstruation. The displaced pieces of tissue can be found on the ovaries and fallopian tubes, on the rectum, on the outside of the uterus, and on the bladder. The bleeding from the pieces of tissue cannot leave the body via the vagina as menstrual blood does; it remains in the body and forms cysts and scars.

SYMPTOMS OF ENDOMETRIOSIS

Pain is the most common symptom—painful periods, painful sex, backache. Belly pain and pains with bowel movements are also common. The pain is worst at the start of menses (periods). The amount of pain does not always indicate the seriousness of the problem. Some women have little pain and some have severe pain. The amount of pain is not reflective of the amount of displaced tissue. Periods may be heavy, frequent, or irregular.

Difficulty conceiving may be the first sign of endometriosis.

DIAGNOSIS OF ENDOMETRIOSIS

The only way to be sure that you have endometriosis is to see a doctor. He or she may schedule a test performed in the operating room to confirm that you have the displaced tissue inside the pelvis.

TREATMENT

Treatment for endometriosis includes:
- Pain-killing drugs
- Hormone drugs including birth control pills
- Surgery to remove scar tissue and displaced tissue

Fibroids

Uterine fibroids are benign (not malignant) tumors of the uterus. They can create pelvic pain, abnormal vaginal bleeding, urinary frequency, constipation, pelvic pressure, and pain with intercourse. They most commonly occur during a woman's fertile years. They usually shrink during menopause.

The diagnosis of uterine fibroids is made with a test called an ultrasound. An ultrasound is performed in the x-ray department or in the doctor's office and provides a picture of the uterus.

Treatment of fibroids includes medication or surgery. Medication can reduce the size of the fibroid. Surgery can remove the fibroid only or the entire uterus. Sometimes, treatment involves waiting and watching for growth or shrinkage of the fibroid. Fibroids may be watched without the fear of cancer developing. Treatment will depend upon the symptoms the fibroid(s) are producing. Uterine fibroids do not appear to interfere with the ability to conceive.

Infertility

Infertility is the failure to conceive after adequate attempts to become pregnant for 1 year. Some 10%–15% of couples are infertile. Half of infertility is related to the female partner, 30% to the male partner, and the rest to factors in both.

The evaluation for infertility is complex and involves both partners. Evaluations are performed in the doctor's office; rarely is hospitalization required.

The major factors causing infertility are:

- Inadequate sperm
- Lack of ovulation (egg production)
- Altered cervical (opening to the uterus) mucus
- Closure of the tubes that deliver the egg from the ovary
- Presence of pelvic adhesions (scar tissue in the pelvis of the woman)

The "work-up" for infertility depends on these factors. Testing includes:

- Analysis of semen (fluid containing sperm)
- Ovulation prediction tests and recording of body temperature to indicate ovulation
- Test to determine the patency (opening) of the tubes
- Test to rule out endometriosis that causes scarring in the pelvis
- Test to observe cervical mucus at the time of ovulation

Treatment for infertility depends on the cause.

Contraceptive Options

Method	Advantages	Disadvantages	Effectiveness
Female sterilization	Continuous protection No need to remember daily	Permanence Surgery required	99%
Male sterilization	Continuous protection No need to remember daily Some health benefits	Permanent Surgery required	99%
Birth control pills	Continuous protection Reversible	Need to remember daily Risks, esp. for smokers Side effects	99%
Subdermal implants	Protection for 5 years Reversible No need to remember daily	Minor surgery required Some side effects	99%
DMPA	Protection for 3 months No need to remember daily	Quarterly injections Some side effects Delayed return to fertility	99%
IUD	Protection for up to 10 years No need to remember daily	Expulsion possible Increased risk of infection	99%
Condom	STD prevented Easy to obtain Best used with spermicide	Less spontaneity Reduction in sensation possible Breakage possible	88%–99%
Diaphragm with spermicide	Insertion up to 6 hours before intercourse	Insertion required Increased risk of bladder infection	82%–94%
Cervical cap	Insertion prior to intercourse	Insertion required	82%–94%
Periodic abstinence	No intervention	Planning and motivation required Method not for women with irregular cycles	80%–99%
Spermicide	Easy to obtain Good results when used with condom or diaphragm	Insertion necessary Messy Reapplication with each intercourse needed	79%–97%
Withdrawal	No other intervention	Control required Sperm leaks prior to ejaculation	72%

DMPA = Depo-medroxyprogesterone acetate; IUD = intrauterine device.

How to Use a Male Condom Correctly: Instructions for Women

- Make sure that your partner uses a new condom every time you have sex. Never reuse a condom.
- Do not open the condom package until you are ready to use the condom (the condom can dry out and possibly tear during use).
- Handle condom carefully. Avoid damaging it with teeth or fingernails.
- Have you partner put the condom on his penis after it is erect, but before it touches your body.
- Make sure that there is adequate space left between the end of the condom and the tip of the penis.
- Check to make sure that no air is trapped in the tip of the condom.
- Lubricate the condom if desired after it is put on. Use only water-soluble lubricants such as K-Y jelly. Do not use oil-based lubricants such as Vaseline, cooking oils, or massage lotions.
- Make sure you are adequately lubricated for intercourse.
- Use a spermicidal foam, cream, or jelly.
- Make sure that your partner holds the condom firmly against the base of his penis when pulling out so that the condom does not slip off. He should withdraw his penis when it is still erect to be sure that no semen leaks out of the top of the condom.

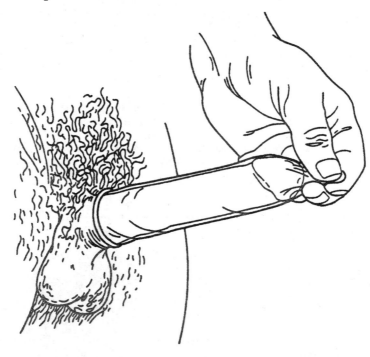

Using a male condom. Leave a half-inch empty space at the tip. Adapted from standard forms currently in use by Planned Parenthood Association of Bucks County, PA.

Using a Female Condom

- A female condom has been approved by the Food and Drug Administration and is now available in drugstores. The female condom is a thin polyurethane sheath that lines the vagina and has a ring at both ends.
- The female condom is inserted much like a tampon or diaphragm. Squeeze the inner ring at the closest end of the pouch and insert it into the vagina, placing the ring behind the pubic bone so that it covers the cervix.
- Carefully follow the manufacturer's directions for insertion.
- The female condom can be inserted up to 8 hours before intercourse, during foreplay, or prior to intercourse.
- You do not have to use spermicide with the female condom, but you may if you like.
- Female condoms are prelubricated.
- Like the male condom, it can be used for only one act of intercourse.
- Unlike the male condom, it can be used only for vaginal sex.
- Unlike the male condom, it is available in only one size.

Like the male condom, maximum prevention of pregnancy and STDs depends upon correct use.

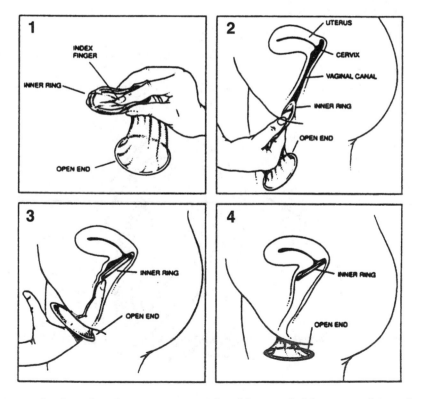

Using a female condom: Four-step insertion. Adapted from standard forms currently in use by Planned Parenthood Association of Bucks County, PA.

Using a Cervical Cap

INSTRUCTIONS FOR INSERTION AND REMOVAL

- Spermicide may be placed in the cap prior to insertion. If utilized, the spermicide should fill approximately one-third of the cap.
- Choose a position for insertion—stand with one foot on a chair, lying down or squatting.
- Locate your cervix with one finger.
- Squeeze the cap rim and insert the cap while separating the labia with the other hand.
- Slide the cap into the vagina and push it up onto the cervix.
- Place the rim around the cervix, creating a suction. Sweep a finger around the cap to make sure that the cervix is completely covered.
- The cap must stay in place for 8 hours after intercourse.
- To remove the cap, push the rim away from the cervix to break the suction and pull the cap out.
- Do not leave the cap in place for longer than 48 hours.
- Do not use the cap during menses.

GUIDELINES FOR USE

Cervical caps may not be for all women. For some, their cap size is unavailable or insertion is too difficult. Women with abnormal Pap smears cannot be fitted with a cap until the reason for the abnormal test result is resolved. Women with a history of toxic shock syndrome should not use a cervical cap. Inflammation of the cervix or previous surgery to the cervix may make fitting impossible.

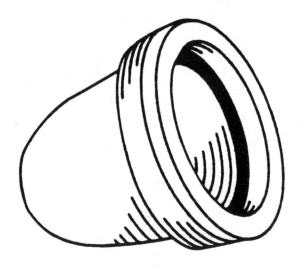

Cervical cap.

Contact the nurse practitioner if any of the following occur:

- Sudden high fever with vomiting and diarrhea, weakness, a sunburn-like rash
- Pain or burning with urination
- Discomfort when the cap is in place
- Unusual vaginal discharge
- Irregular vaginal spotting or bleeding

Source: Text adapted from standard forms currently in use by Planned Parenthood Association of Bucks County, PA. Illustration from Contraceptive Technology, ed 16, Irvington Publishers, New York, 1994.

Using a Diaphragm

INSTRUCTION FOR INSERTION AND REMOVAL

- Urinate prior to inserting the diaphragm.
- The diaphragm may be inserted up to 2 hours prior to intercourse.
- Place approximately 1 teaspoon of contraceptive jelly or cream designated for use with a diaphragm in the center of the diaphragm and around the rim. The contraceptive cream or jelly is placed in the diaphragm on the side that will be next to the cervix.
- Choose a position for inserting—standing with one leg on a chair, lying down, or squatting.
- Pinch the rim of the diaphragm together with the cream or jelly inside. Separate the labia with the other hand and insert the diaphragm into the vagina.
- Push the diaphragm up and as far back as possible, making sure that the cervix is covered.
- Feel for your cervix covered by the dome of the diaphragm.
- Leave the diaphragm in place for 6–8 hours after intercourse.
- Urinate after intercourse, leaving the diaphragm in place.
- If intercourse is repeated or occurs more than 2 hours after insertion, leave the diaphragm in place and insert another application of contraceptive cream or jelly.
- To remove the diaphragm, pull the diaphragm down and out using one finger.
- Do not leave the diaphragm in place for more than 24 hours.

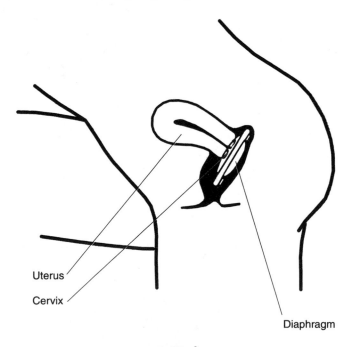

Uterus

Cervix

Diaphragm

Diaphragm.

GUIDELINES FOR USE

Diaphragms should be refitted after a full-term pregnancy, pelvic surgery, or weight gain or loss of 10 pounds or more. Women who have poor vaginal muscle tone or a history of toxic shock syndrome or bladder infection should use diaphragms with caution.

Contact the nurse practitioner if any of the following occur:

- Sudden high fever with diarrhea and vomiting, weakness, a sunburn-like rash
- Pain and burning with urination
- Discomfort when the diaphragm is in place
- Unusual vaginal discharge
- Irregular vaginal spotting or bleeding

Source: Adapted from standard forms currently in use by Planned Parenthood Association of Bucks County, PA.

Norplant Information

Norplant is six thin tubes made of a soft material that have a man-made hormone in them. After insertion of the tubes into the body, usually the arm, a small amount of the hormone is released into the body all the time. Norplant works by keeping eggs from being released and making the mucus from the cervix (opening to the uterus) thick. Norplant prevents pregnancy. For every 100 women who use Norplant, there will be less than one pregnancy per year.

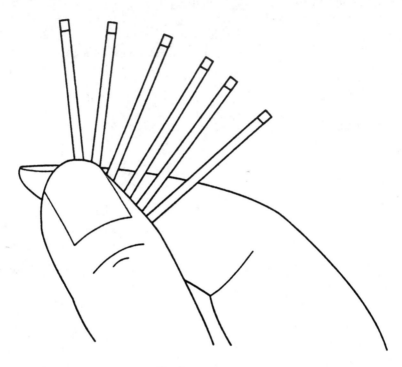

Norplant system.

CHAPTER 8 HANDOUTS **371**

Norplant lasts for 5 years. There is no medicine to take every day, and there is nothing to do before sex to prevent pregnancy.

Norplant should *not* be used if you are pregnant or have serious liver disease, bleeding from the vagina that is not menses, cancer of the breast, or had recent blood clots in the legs or lungs. Discuss the use of Norplant with your practitioner if you have heart disease or stroke, diabetes, abnormal liver tests, depression, or epilepsy.

Some women have experienced one or more of the following problems when they use Norplant:

- Acne, skin rash
- Weight gain
- Change in coloring of the skin over the implant site
- Cysts of the ovaries
- Depression
- Hair loss or increased hair
- Nausea and dizziness
- Nervousness
- Sore breasts

The danger signs to watch for when using Norplant are:

- Sudden severe headache
- Dizziness, fainting, numbness
- Sharp, crushing chest pain
- Pain in the arm or calf of the leg
- Severe pain in the stomach or belly
- Yellowing of the skin or eyes
- Severe depression
- Unusually heavy vaginal bleeding
- No period after a period every month
- Lump in the breast
- Pus, bleeding, or pain at the insertion site
- Norplant coming out

Call your practitioner if any of these signs occur.

Norplant Instructions

- For a few days you may notice tenderness and swelling of the skin around the implants. Bruising and discoloration of the skin may last a week or two.
- Try not to bump the area for a few days. Keep the area clean and dry. Keep the bandage on for 24 hours. Keep the tape on for 3 days.
- You can do normal activities right away. Do not lift heavy objects for a few days.

After healing, do not worry about bumping the area. You can touch or wash the area as usual.

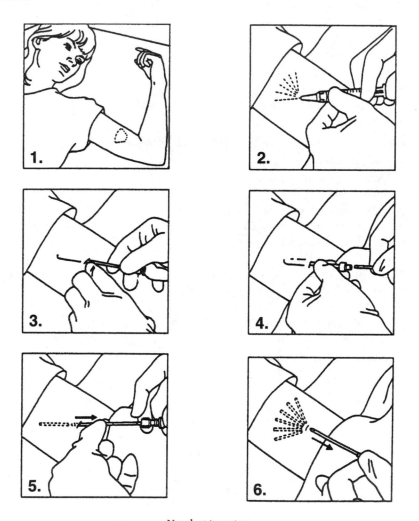

Norplant insertion.

Return to the office:

- In 72 hours
- In 3 months
- Once a year for checkups

Call the office if you:

- Have questions about Norplant
- Think that you might be pregnant
- Want the Norplant capsules removed

or if you:

- Have a delayed period after having regular periods
- Experience unusually heavy bleeding
- Have arm pain
- Observe pus or bleeding at the insertion site
- Notice a capsule has come out
- Experience severe headache

Source: Adapted from standard forms currently in use by Planned Parenthood Association of Bucks County, PA.

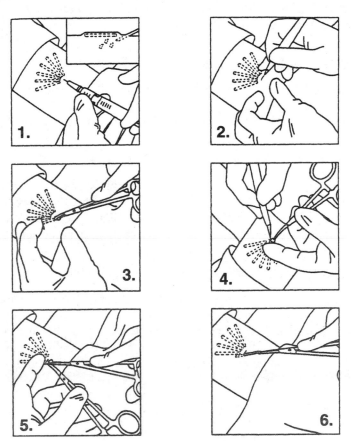

Norplant removal.

Intrauterine Devices

WHAT IS AN INTRAUTERINE DEVICE?

An intrauterine device (IUD) is a small plastic device that is inserted into the uterus to prevent pregnancy.

ARE THERE DIFFERENT TYPES OF INTRAUTERINE DEVICES?

Yes, many different kinds of IUDs are used all over the world. Two types of IUDs are currently available in the United States: one has copper and the other contains the female hormone progesterone. Both are shaped like the letter "T" and are about 1¼ inches tall. Each IUD has a thread or string on the end, which allows you to check that the IUD is in place; it also makes it easier for the practitioner to remove the IUD.

The copper IUD has copper wire coiled around the stem and arms. The copper IUD can be used for up to 10 years. The progesterone device has a hollow stem that contains the hormone progesterone. The hormone is continuously released into the uterus and acts locally, so there are no hormonal effects throughout the body. This IUD must be replaced once a year.

HOW DOES THE INTRAUTERINE DEVICE WORK?

All the ways an IUD can prevent pregnancy are not fully understood. The most recent studies suggest that IUDs work mainly by preventing fertilization, interfering with the normal development of the egg and the sperm's ability to reach the egg.

HOW EFFECTIVE ARE INTRAUTERINE DEVICES?

IUDs are the most effective form of nonpermanent birth control. The copper IUD is about as effective in preventing pregnancy as sterilization. For every 100 women using the copper IUD, fewer that one per year will get pregnant. With the hormone-containing IUD, about three women per year will get pregnant.

ARE THERE SIDE EFFECTS?

With the copper IUD, the most common side effects are increased menstrual flow and cramps. Cramps can be relieved by the use of over-the-counter pain medication such as ibuprofen. These side effects usually lessen after the first few months as the uterus gets used to the IUD. With the hormonal IUD, bleeding may also occur between menstrual periods, although total blood loss and painful periods are reduced.

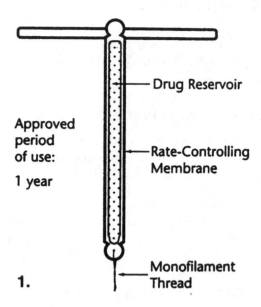

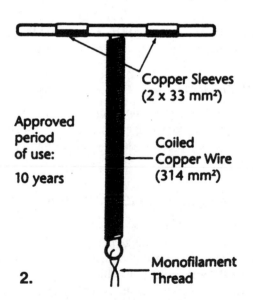

IUDs: (1) Progesterone T IUD and (2) Copper T 380A IUD. Adapted from standard forms currently in use by Planned Parenthood Association of Bucks County, PA.

ARE INTRAUTERINE DEVICES SAFE?

Intrauterine devices are a safe and effective method of birth control when used by the right women. Although one of the early IUDs used in the 1970s was associated with an increased risk of pelvic infection, this IUD has been off the market for over 25 years.

WHO CAN USE AN INTRAUTERINE DEVICE?

Women at low risk of STDs are good candidates for using IUDs. The IUD is best for a woman who is in a steady and faithful relationship with a partner who is faithful and who does not have any sexually transmitted infections.

Intrauterine devices do not protect against STDs. STDs can increase a woman's risk of becoming infertile. If you are using an IUD and believe you may be at risk of getting an STD, use a latex condom to help protect yourself. You may also want to discuss with your doctor or nurse whether the IUD is still a good choice for birth control.

WHAT ARE THE BENEFITS OF INTRAUTERINE DEVICES?

IUDs are safe, effective, easy to use, and less expensive than most other forms of contraception over the long run. There is no need to remember to use the method every day or with every act of sex. The copper IUD can last for up to 10 years. In addition, because any hormone in the IUD does not affect the entire body, women do not get side effects such as nausea, breast tenderness, or headache.

WHAT IF I GET PREGNANT?

Overall, the copper IUD protects women against having a pregnancy outside the uterus compared with women not using contraception. However, if you are using an IUD and suspect you are pregnant, you should see a practitioner promptly to rule out ectopic pregnancy.

HOW MUCH DOES AN INTRAUTERINE DEVICE COST?

Prices for IUDs themselves vary, but range between $100 and $300. The clinic or health-care provider also charges for the medical visit and insertion of the device. About 90% of Planned Parenthood family planning clinics in the United States offer the IUD. In government-funded family planning clinics, about 50% offer the IUD to low-income women. Your insurance policy may or may not cover the cost of the IUD and the insertion visit. Check your health plan.

Source: The Contraceptive Report, November 1998, with permission.

Emergency Contraception

WHAT IS EMERGENCY CONTRACEPTION?

Emergency contraception refers to birth control options that can be used after unprotected intercourse to help prevent pregnancy. In the United States, women have the option of using hormonal emergency contraception (birth control pills) or having an intrauterine device inserted. Emergency contraception can be used after forced sex (if you've been assaulted), or if you have forgotten to use your birth control method, or if the method fails (for example, if a condom breaks)

Hormonal contraception is often the first choice rather than the IUD. Your practitioner will discuss which option is best for you. Most women choose the birth control pills for emergency contraception. Be sure to discuss regular birth control with your practitioner.

Use of Emergency Contraceptive Pills

IS EMERGENCY CONTRACEPTION THE SAME THING AS THE MORNING AFTER PILL?

The morning after pill, which consists of several tablets of birth control pills, is one type of emergency contraception. However, the name morning after pill is misleading, since it can be used up to 72 hours (3 days) after sex, not just the next morning.

DO I HAVE TO SEE MY DOCTOR TO GET EMERGENCY CONTRACEPTIVE PILLS?

No, you do not always have to see a health-care provider to get emergency contraception. A new program in the state of Washington allows pharmacists to sell emergency contraception directly to women without requiring a doctor's prescription.

If you've forgotten to use your birth control, or a condom has broken, or your diaphragm has become dislodged during sex, you should call your health-care provider. Your regular practitioner may prescribe the pills over the phone or may ask you to come into the office. If you're already using birth control pills for contraception, you will probably be told the correct number of pills to take over the telephone. Talk with your practitioner during your regular visit before you need emergency contraception. If you have been a victim of sexual assault, then you should go to an emergency department to be treated and examined.

HOW DOES THE EMERGENCY CONTRACEPTION WORK?

Most birth control pills contain two hormones—estrogen and progestin. When used as emergency contraception, these hormones disrupt the natural hormone patterns necessary for pregnancy. The hormones also are thought to interfere with the release of an egg and or fertilization of the egg by the sperm. Some evidence also suggests that hormones change the lining of the uterus.

HOW DO I USE EMERGENCY CONTRACEPTION?

Call you clinician to discuss emergency contraception as soon as possible after unprotected intercourse. If you use birth control pills, the number you take will depend on the type of pills that you have been prescribed. Your clinician will tell you how many to take. Then, 12 hours later, you will take the same number of pills for the second time.

HOW SAFE IS EMERGENCY CONTRACEPTION?

Emergency contraception pills are very safe. In 1997, the Food and Drug Administration reviewed the evidence and concluded that the treatment is safe and effective.

ARE THERE WOMEN WHO SHOULDN'T USE EMERGENCY CONTRACEPTIVE PILLS?

The World Health Organization lists confirmed pregnancy as the only reason not to use emergency contraceptive pills.

ARE THERE SIDE EFFECTS OF EMERGENCY CONTRACEPTIVE PILLS?

The most common side effects are nausea and vomiting. About one-half of women have nausea and about one-quarter vomit; however, your clinician may give you some medicine to take to reduce the nausea and vomiting.

Some medications are available over-the-counter in the drug store that help decrease the nausea and vomiting. Usually the medicine is taken about 1 hour before you take the emergency contraception pills. You may want to ask your clinician to recommend or prescribe an antinausea drug.

If you vomit within 1 hour of taking the birth control pills, you may need to repeat the dose of emergency contraception (take it again). Refer to your written instructions or call your practitioner if you have questions.

USE OF THE INTRAUTERINE DEVICE AS EMERGENCY CONTRACEPTION

The IUD is another type of emergency contraception. The IUD works by changing the lining of the uterus. In addition, the IUD is believed to interfere with the sperm fertilizing the egg and with the ability of the sperm to reach the egg. The IUD can be inserted up to 5 to 7 days after unprotected intercourse. If the IUD is used, you will need to see a practitioner to have it inserted.

Call your practitioner within 3 weeks for a pregnancy test if your period has not returned.

INFORMATION ON EMERGENCY CONTRACEPTION

A toll-free emergency contraception hotline provides 24-hour automated information on emergency contraceptive methods and a national directory of providers who offer the treatment.

The toll-free number is 1–888-NOT-2-LATE.

For information on emergency contraception available through the Internet, see the Emergency Contraception Website @ http://opr.princeton.edu/ec/.

Remember. . .

Emergency contraception is not as effective in preventing pregnancy as using regular birth control. Do not rely on this treatment for ongoing birth control. If you are at risk for an STD, use latex condoms to protect yourself. Don't stop taking or using your birth control method on your own. Always call a practitioner and talk things over.

Source: The Contraceptive Report, May 1998, with permission.

Voluntary Sterilization

Healthy women are fertile until ages 50 to 51. Healthy men are fertile throughout their life. Because many couples have their children before they naturally end their reproductive capabilities, they seek sterilization. Voluntary sterilization is a very popular method of birth control in America. It is a very safe and cost-effective method to prevent pregnancy.

Ideally, a couple should consider both vasectomy and female sterilization. They are both comparable in effectiveness, and both are intended to be permanent. If both are acceptable to the couple, vasectomy is the medically preferred procedure.

FEMALE STERILIZATION

Sterilization for women involves mechanically blocking the fallopian tubes to prevent the sperm and the egg from uniting. This is a safe procedure with a low failure rate. Sterilization can be performed without increasing the risk after the delivery of a baby.

Female sterilization involves the application of clips or bands or burning of the fallopian tubes (the tubes that carry the egg from the ovary to the uterus). The tubes are reached via the abdomen using a small incision, or at the time of cesarean birth or abdominal surgery.

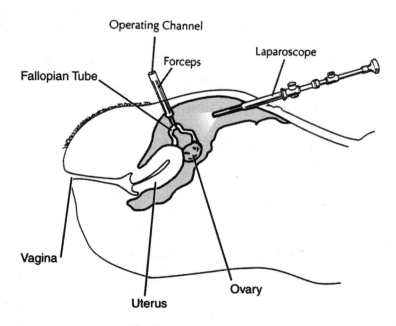

Female sterilization.

Advantages of female sterilization:
- Permanence
- Effectiveness
- Cost-effectiveness (over time)
- Nothing to buy or remember
- No long-term side effects
- No interruption in lovemaking

Disadvantages of female sterilization:
- Permanence
- Reversibility difficult and expensive
- Surgery required
- Expensive when performed
- Low failure rate, but failure can mean a pregnancy in the tube
- No protection against sexually transmitted diseases

MALE STERILIZATION

Vasectomy is male sterilization through surgery. This operation blocks the tubes that carry the sperm into the ejaculatory fluid. Vasectomy is very effective. Male sterilization involves exposing the tubes that carry sperm and cutting or burning them.

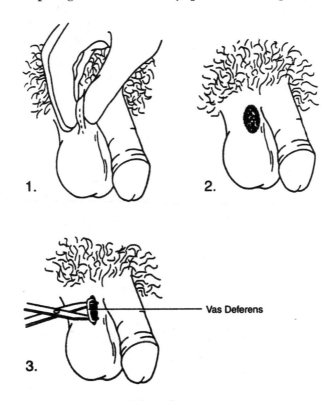

Male sterilization.

Advantages of male sterilization:

- High effectiveness
- Inexpensive over time
- Permanence
- Safety
- Quick procedure

Disadvantages of male sterilization:

- Protection for the male, not the female who can become pregnant
- Surgery required
- Expensive in the short term
- Permanence
- No protection against sexually transmitted diseases

COMPARISON OF MALE AND FEMALE STERILIZATION

Characteristic	Male	Female
Effectiveness	Highly effective	Highly effective
Safety	Safest	Very safe
Location	Doctor's office	Hospital or outpatient surgery
Anesthesia	Local	General
Typical cost	$500	$2500
Recovery time	2–3 days	2–3 days
Number in United States each year	500,000	640,000

CHAPTER **9** HANDOUTS

Menopause

Symptom	Cause	Medication	Herbs	To Do
Hot flashes	Sudden loss of estrogen	Hormone therapy Vitamin E 800 IU daily	Black cohosh Ginseng Dong quai	Regular exercise Keep the house cool Dress in layers Do not overeat Avoid caffeine Avoid alcohol Stop smoking
Breast tenderness	Change in hormones	Vitamin E 400 IU daily	Primrose oil	Stop smoking Decrease caffeine
Vaginal dryness	Lack of estrogen	Hormone therapy Vitamin E supplement Estrogen cream	Black cohosh Dong quai Chaste berry Primrose oil Ginseng	Use water-soluble lubricants Kegel's exercises Increase zinc in the diet
Heavier menses	Change in hormones	Hormone therapy Ibuprofen Iron supplements	Chaste tree	Restrict activity Keep a menstrual record Stop alcohol, nicotine, and caffeine use
Mood swings	Change in hormones	Vitamin B$_6$ Calcium supplements	St. John's wort Valerian root Chamomile	Regular exercise

WHAT IS MENOPAUSE?

Menopause is when menstrual periods cease. The ovaries no longer produce eggs and the female hormones decrease. Menopause marks the end of the childbearing years. Menopause is a normal process that can take place over 2 or 3 years.

WHEN DOES MENOPAUSE OCCUR?

The average age for menopause is 50–51 years. The age at which menopause occurs does appear to run in families. Your periods will likely end around the same age your mother's did.

WHAT ARE THE SIGNS OF MENOPAUSE?

Lack of menses: For some women, menstruation stops abruptly. For others, there is gradually diminishing flow. For most women, the periods become irregular. The number of days of flow and the length of time between periods varies, with no pattern seen.

Vaginal dryness: With the decrease in estrogen, the vaginal walls become thinner, dryer, and less elastic. Lubrication for intercourse is not produced as easily during sexual stimulation. Intercourse can become painful.

Increased urination: The urethra (where the urine comes from) may become thinner, and women may need to urinate more often.

Hot flashes: A hot flash is an intense feeling of heat that generally starts at the waist and moves up to the head. You may or may not perspire with a hot flash. Some women experience hot flashes at night, "night sweats," and are awakened from sleep, finding themselves wet with perspiration. Hot flashes are not harmful but are annoying.

Other symptoms of menopause: Nervousness, sadness, insomnia, breast tenderness, heavier menses, weight gain, forgetfulness, and lack of interest in sex are all symptoms of menopause.

WHEN CAN I STOP USING BIRTH CONTROL?

Keep using your birth control method until 1 year has passed without a menstrual period.

WHAT CAN I DO TO STAY HEALTHY?

- Examine your breasts every month and have a mammogram as recommended by your health-care provider.
- Maintain good dental health.
- Eat a healthy diet that is high in carbohydrates and low in fat.
- Supplement your diet with calcium.
- Begin a daily exercise routine to strengthen your bones, heart, and lungs. Walking for 30 minutes 3–5 times weekly is a common exercise routine.
- Keep your pelvic muscles strong with Kegel exercises.
- If you smoke, stop.
- Have regular pelvic examinations and checkups.
- Minimize alcohol consumption.

Hormone Replacement Therapy

WHAT IS HORMONE REPLACEMENT THERAPY?

Hormone replacement therapy (HRT) gives a woman female hormones after menopause. Hormones are often prescribed to relieve the symptoms of menopause and to prevent osteoporosis. There is also evidence to suggest that hormone replacement reduces the risk of heart disease.

WHO SHOULD USE IT?

- Women whose menopausal symptoms are serious enough to disturb their quality of life
- Women in whom relief of menopausal symptoms does not occur with diet, vitamins, exercise, or stress reduction
- Women at risk for osteoporosis
- Women at risk for heart disease

IS THERE ANY DANGER IN USING HRT?

Some women should not use HRT: women who have liver disease, unexplained vaginal bleeding, a history of breast cancer or cancer of the uterus, recent blood clots, or fibroids.

WHAT ARE THE POSSIBLE SIDE EFFECTS?

- Breast tenderness
- Abdominal bloating
- Nausea
- Headache
- Abnormal vaginal bleeding

WHAT ARE THE WARNING SIGNS OF POTENTIAL PROBLEMS FOR WOMEN USING HRT?

- Leg pain
- Chest pain
- Difficulty breathing
- Abnormal bleeding
- Headache

Nutrition and Menopause

VITAMIN AND MINERAL DAILY REQUIREMENTS

Calcium—1200–1500 mg daily
Vitamin D—400–800 IU daily
Vitamin E—200–600 IU daily
B-complex vitamin—daily

NUTRITIONAL GUIDELINES

Breads and grains—6–11 servings/day
Fruits and vegetables—5 servings/day
Protein—2–3 servings/day
Dairy products—2–3 servings/day
Low fat consumption

Some foods have been associated with hot flashes and night sweats. They are:

- Garlic
- Onions
- Cayenne
- Oranges
- Grapefruit
- Tomatoes

CHAPTER **10** HANDOUTS

Bladder Infections in Women

Urine is sterile—that is, without any bacteria—in the normal state. The urethra (the opening where the urine comes from), the bladder, or the kidneys can be infected with bacteria. The bacteria will be apparent in the urine when the bladder or kidneys are infected. Bladder infections are experienced by 10% to 25% of women.

WHERE DO THE BACTERIA COME FROM?

Bacteria normally reside in the bowel. Many infections of the bladder in women are caused by bacteria normally found in the intestinal tract.

Sexual activity places women at risk. The risk for infection of the bladder increases specifically with vaginal intercourse. Any manipulation of the urethra through oral sex or masturbation can also increase the risk. The vagina is not sterile and houses organisms that can produce bladder infections.

WHAT ARE THE SYMPTOMS OF BLADDER INFECTION?

- Frequency of urination
- Urgency (must urinate urgently) of urination
- Pain (burning) with urination

HOW CAN I AVOID BLADDER INFECTIONS?

- Void after intercourse.
- Avoid intercourse with a partner who has burning on urination.
- Do not delay urinating when the urge occurs.
- Drink 6 to 8 glasses of water per day.
- Avoid the use of a diaphragm for birth control.

HOW ARE BLADDER INFECTIONS TREATED?

Bladder infections must be treated promptly with an antibiotic. It is possible for bladder infection to progress to kidney infection, a more serious illness.

Urinary Incontinence

Urinary incontinence is the involuntary passing of urine. It can affect both men and women, especially middle-aged and elderly persons. It frequently goes untreated because people are too embarrassed to seek treatment and/or assume that incontinence is part of the aging process. Television ads can reinforce the idea that incontinence is part of the aging process.

Incontinence in women occurs when the pelvic muscles have been damaged or stretched or when pressure is applied to the bladder. There is an "urge" to urinate and an inability to reach a toilet "in time." Urine can be lost during laughing, coughing, sneezing, or lifting heavy objects.

Urinary incontinence can be a symptom of an underlying problem such as urinary tract infection or neurologic disease. Urinary incontinence can be a result of medication. It can be a result of pregnancy and childbirth or deterioration of the pelvic muscles. In women, an age-related decline in estrogen levels can contribute to urinary incontinence.

If you have problems holding your urine, you should talk to your health-care provider. To help your health-care provider determine the cause of the problem and devise a treatment plan, collect the information requested below before your appointment and bring it along to the visit.

- When did the urine loss start?
- Does it happen during the day, night, or both?
- Does it happen when lying down or sitting still?
- Do you feel a sense of urgency before losing urine?
- When you use the toilet, how much urine do you release?
- Do you have difficulty starting or stopping the flow of urine?
- Do you have pain when urinating?
- Do you lose urine when coughing, sneezing, or straining?
- When you lose urine, how much do you lose?
- Have you had pelvic or bladder surgery?
- Do you have a neurologic disease?
- Are you taking any medications? (If so, take them with you to the visit.)

Ask your health-care provider about available treatments for incontinence. Treatments may include bladder training, Kegel exercises, biofeedback, medication, or surgery. The first step in curing the problem is to discuss it with a health-care provider.

Hepatitis

Hepatitis A, or infectious hepatitis, is a viral inflammation of the liver. Hepatitis A causes fatigue, nausea, vomiting, fever, and yellowing of the skin and eyes. Hepatitis A virus is the causative organism. The virus is transmitted by hand, after touching diapers or linens of an infected individual. Infection can occur from common household items such as glasses and eating utensils. Symptoms of hepatitis A have a rapid onset and last for about 1 week. A vaccine for hepatitis A does exist, and medication to relieve symptoms is available.

Hepatitis B, or serum hepatitis, results in a disease that can affect the liver mildly or very seriously. Hepatitis B is the causative organism and can be contracted through sexual activity, via intravenous drug use, or from pregnant woman to infant. Symptoms of hepatitis B are fatigue, weight loss, nausea, vomiting, diarrhea, and aching. The onset of symptoms is gradual and their resolution slow. A vaccination for Hepatitis B is available, and treatment of the disease is necessary to relieve symptoms and prevent complications.

Hepatitis C occurs primarily after transfusion and can be transmitted from mother to infant. Symptoms are similar to hepatitis B infection. Medication is available for treatment.

CHAPTER **11** HANDOUTS
Osteoporosis

WHAT IS OSTEOPOROSIS?

Osteoporosis is the most common human bone disease. Osteoporosis means low bone mass, deterioration of bone leading to fragile bones, and an increased risk of fractures (breaks). Osteoporosis affects many women; it is estimated that between 13% and 18% of all women who have experienced menopause have osteoporosis. The consequence of osteoporosis can be a fracture (break) of a bone. The most serious of these is fracture of the hip.

Osteoporosis is preventable and treatable, but there are no warning signs until fracture occurs. Osteoporosis is a silent disease.

HOW DO I PREVENT OSTEOPOROSIS?

Ensure adequate calcium absorption: All women should maintain an adequate intake of calcium; 1200 mg should be consumed daily, using supplements if necessary. Women at risk for osteoporosis (i.e, elderly, chronically ill, homebound, or institutionalized women) should also consume vitamin D at a level of 400 to 800 IU daily. Calcium and vitamin D reduce the risk of fracture.

Perform regular weight-bearing and muscle-strengthening exercises: Muscle strengthening improves agility, strength, and balance, thus reducing the risk of falls. Weight-bearing exercise increases bone density. Weight-bearing exercise includes walking, jogging, stair climbing, dancing, and tennis.

Avoid tobacco smoking and reduce alcohol intake: The use of tobacco has a negative effect on health in general and on bones in particular. Alcohol is detrimental to bone health if consumed at more than a moderate level.

HOW IS OSTEOPOROSIS DIAGNOSED?

Osteoporosis is diagnosed by bone densitometry testing. All women should be screened for osteoporosis after menopause. Women with low body weight, estrogen deficiency, low calcium intake, alcoholism, and a history of recurrent falls or of fractures should also be tested.

Bone density can be measured anywhere on the skeleton. Bone densitometry testing is done by scanning portions of the skeleton. It is not painful and can be completed in a few minutes, with total radiation exposure much less than that of a chest x-ray.

HOW IS OSTEOPOROSIS TREATED?

Osteoporosis is treated with hormone replacement therapy, calcium supplementation, and medications that prevent bone loss and thereby reduce the risk of fracture.

CHAPTER **12** HANDOUTS

Women and Lipids

Cholesterol is a soft, fatlike substance found in all body cells. Cholesterol is produced by the body and is found in certain foods. It is an important part of the body, responsible for the formation of cell membranes and hormones. But too much cholesterol increases your risk for heart attack.

Cholesterol travels through the bloodstream to the cells of the body. Cholesterol has to be carried to the cells by proteins. The "bad guys" are low-density lipoproteins (LDLs), which circulate in the bloodstream and can, along with cholesterol, form a thick, hard coating that clogs arteries. A level of LDL that is too high indicates a risk for heart attack. The "good guys" are high-density lipoproteins (HDLs), which tend to carry cholesterol away from the arteries and back to the liver. A high level of HDL tends to protect against heart attack.

Blood cholesterol levels should be checked approximately every 5 years, beginning at about age 20. The total blood cholesterol, plus the LDL and HDL levels, will be reported. Total blood cholesterol should be below 200 mg/dL. LDL cholesterol levels of more than 160 mg/dL indicate an increased risk of heart attack. In the average women, HDL cholesterol levels are from 50 to 60 mg/dL. Calculating the risk for heart disease requires professional expertise. Total cholesterol, HDL and LDL levels, as well as medical history, are used to establish risk.

The average American woman consumes 320 mg of cholesterol daily. The American Heart Association recommends that the daily consumption be less than 300 mg. It is relatively easy to reduce cholesterol in the diet. Plants don't contain cholesterol. All dietary cholesterol comes from animal products. Egg yolk and organ meats contain the most cholesterol, but cholesterol is found in all meats, fish, poultry, and animal fats. To reduce cholesterol, eat fewer high-fat foods and eat more low-fat foods. This means eating more fruits, vegetables, and grains and fewer fatty meats and bakery goods. Eat lean meats, such as poultry with the skin removed, instead of fatty meats, and drink skim milk rather than whole milk. Save butter, cream, and ice cream for special occasions. Limit egg consumption. Eat low-fat cheeses, such as cottage cheese, mozzarella, and ricotta, rather than high-fat cheeses such as cheddar. Reduce consumption of processed meats such as bologna and hot dogs. These meats are high in calories and fat.

Sometimes reducing cholesterol in the diet is not enough. When this is the case, medication to lower cholesterol levels can be prescribed.

CHAPTER **13** HANDOUTS

Premenstrual Syndrome

Premenstrual syndrome (PMS) refers to a variety of symptoms that a woman may have prior to her period. The most common symptoms of PMS are tension and irritability, weight gain, headache, and depression. Other symptoms include breast tenderness, lower abdominal cramping, fatigue, and anxiety.

PMS always occurs prior to menses and improves once the period has started. The timing of the symptoms is central to distinguishing between PMS and other disorders. In PMS, the symptoms are followed by at least one symptom-free week, and the pattern of symptoms tends to remain constant from month to month.

Keeping a careful daily diary of symptoms is important to the diagnosis of PMS. This record of symptoms should be kept for at least three cycles. The diary or symptom calendar should be discussed with a health-care provider familiar with the diagnosis and treatment of PMS. Many treatment options exist. Medications that target the most bothersome symptoms can be prescribed.

Treatment for PMS that can initiated without a practitioner is as follows:

- Try to minimize stressful situations during the time that you have PMS.
- Reduce refined sugar in your diet during PMS.
- Avoid caffeine found in coffee, tea, chocolate, and cola.
- Take daily B_6 supplements, up to 50 mg.
- Get regular outdoor exercise.

A visit to a health-care provider is needed for further treatment options.

Month _____

Name _____ Date of Birth _____ LMP _____

Symptom	1	2	3	4	5	6	7	8	9	10	11	12	13	14	15	16	17	18	19	20	21	22	23	24	25	26	27	28	29	30	31
1																															
2																															
3																															
4																															
5																															
6																															
7																															
8																															
9																															
10. Weight each day																															

Day 1 is the first day of menstrual bleeding.

Directions: Write in symptoms in the column labeled 1–10. Mark with either a X or ✔ under the day of the cycle that the symptom occurs. At the end of the cycle, circle the days that each symptom was the most distressing.

Mestrual cycle diary.

Eating Disorders and Women

Symptoms indicating an increased risk for an eating disorder:
- Inability to maintain a recommended weight
- Engaging in secretive eating
- Self-induced vomiting
- Use of laxatives and diet pills
- Spitting out food after chewing
- Lack of menses
- Mood change around eating
- Frequent weighing
- Expressed dissatisfaction with appearance
- Fear of weight gain
- Comments from others regarding weight, eating, or exercise behavior

GETTING HELP

Eating disorders can be treated with a combination of medications and counseling. Most women with eating disorders have good recovery. Women with symptoms should seek treatment from a professional trained to deal with eating disorders as soon as possible.

CHAPTER **14** HANDOUTS

Symptoms of Depression

Depression is more than having a bad day. It should not be confused with the "down" days or "blues" we all have. Depression is an illness that affects your body, your mood, and your thoughts.

Depression can occur at any age and at any time. Depression occurs twice as often in women as in men. Depression can be mild, moderate, or severe. Mild depression usually occurs after a trauma in your life. Moderate depression leaves you feeling less energetic and enthusiastic. Job productivity goes down and you wonder if life is worth living. Severe depression creates suffering such that you can hardly function. There is no joy in life and you feel completely powerless to change. Feelings of hopelessness and worthlessness prevail.

Depression can accompany serious medical illnesses. It can also be related to medication. People who are most likely to suffer from depression are those who have suffered from depression previously, have attempted suicide in the past, have recently delivered a child, or are substance abusers.

SYMPTOMS OF DEPRESSION

- Feelings of sadness and irritability that don't go away
- Loss of interest or pleasure in activities you used to enjoy
- A change in weight or appetite
- Sleep disturbances
- Feelings of guilt, lack of self-worth, or helplessness
- Decreased ability to concentrate
- Fatigue
- Restless or slowed activity
- Thoughts of life not being worthwhile or about suicide or death

Depression can be treated. Depression is not a personal weakness or flaw. Several treatment options are available to those who suffer from depression. Seek help if you have symptoms of depression. Assist someone who is displaying symptoms of depression in seeking help.

Women and Alcohol

Although women currently use, abuse, and become dependent on alcohol and other drugs at a rate less than men, use is quickly becoming similar to that of men. Women experience more devastating physical, emotional, psychological, and social responses and consequences than men do.

Alcohol abuse has a range of presentations, from social drinker to the person who uses alcohol in excess when under stress.

Social drinker: This person consumes alcohol in amounts and circumstances that seem socially acceptable. There may be a problem if social occasions are a reason for overindulging in alcohol.

Heavy social drinker: This is someone who drinks in socially appropriate circumstances but seeks out situations in which to drink and drinks excessively. At least two drinks per day are consumed, and the amount increases over time. This person's work and social routines do not seem to be affected.

Problem drinker: This person engages in heavy drinking and gets drunk on occasion; consequences of alcohol can be seen in the medical, legal, or social arena. Functioning varies and denial of a problem is common.

Alcohol-dependent drinker: This is someone who consumes the same amount of alcohol regardless of mood or situation. Alcohol is given top priority in all situations, including work and social situations. Tolerance to alcohol develops, and withdrawal symptoms can be seen. Drinking at lunch and "happy hour" is needed to relieve symptoms.

Severely deteriorated drinker: This person maintains a constant state of intoxication, undergoes hospitalization for detoxification, and has medical problems related to alcohol use.

GETTING HELP

Help for alcohol problems requires a combination of medical interventions, counseling, health education, life skills, and social service. Treatment can be in an inpatient center that deals with women with alcohol problems or on an outpatient basis with a team that works with women to achieve full recovery.

Domestic Violence

QUESTIONS TO ASK

Are you in a relationship in which you are physically hurt or threatened by your partner?

Does your partner ever destroy things that you care about?

Has your partner ever threatened to injure or kill you or your children?

Does your partner abuse your children?

Does your partner abuse your pets?

Has your partner ever forced you to have sex when you didn't want to?

Do you feel afraid of your partner?

Has your partner ever prevented you from leaving the house?

Do you have guns in your home? Has your partner ever threatened to use them?

If the answer to any of these questions is Yes, ask for help. Call a domestic violence hotline at anytime of the day or night; a counselor will help you to make a plan to end the violence.

The toll-free number of the nationwide hotline is 800-799-SAFE.

Sexual Assault

WHO IS AT RISK FOR SEXUAL ASSAULT?

Any woman is a risk for sexual assault regardless of age, race, socioeconomic status, or education. Women between the ages of 15 and 24 are at the highest risk. Sexual assault can occur in women, children, and men. Anyone can be forced to have unwanted sex by a stranger, friend, relative, or partner.

WHAT ARE THE WARNING SIGNS?

- Men who see women as sex objects and do not indicate respect for women
- Men who resent women in positions of authority
- Men who continue to touch women even after they have been asked to stop touching
- Men who act aggressively
- Men who expect relationships with women to be on their terms only

HOW CAN I PREVENT SEXUAL ASSAULT?

- Sexual assault cannot always be prevented.
- Communicating desires and limits *clearly* may help to prevent sexual assault by an acquaintance.
- If you are feeling uncomfortable in a situation with a man, pay attention to that feeling.
- Be alert for warning signs.
- Using alcohol or drugs increases the risk for sexual assault. For many young women who report rape, alcohol and/or drug use by the victim and the perpetrator was involved.

IF I AM THREATENED WITH SEXUAL ASSAULT, WHAT SHOULD I DO?

- Try to stay calm.
- Be assertive.
- Try leaving the situation.
- Trust your feelings about the situation. Sometimes submission will decrease the chance of injury.

IF I AM SEXUALLY ASSAULTED, WHAT SHOULD I DO?

- Do not blame yourself.
- Seek medical help.
- Seek help from a rape crisis center via a hotline and/or call the police.

CHAPTER **15** HANDOUTS

Women and HIV

WHAT IS HIV?

HIV stands for human immunodeficiency virus. HIV is the virus that causes AIDS, or acquired immunodeficiency syndrome. Many people who acquire HIV develop AIDS. AIDS is considered to be a fatal disease. HIV alters the immune system, the system that fights off diseases, and the infected person dies of an AIDS-related disease such as cancer or serious infection.

Many people live for years after AIDS is diagnosed. The sooner a person gets treated after initial infection, the better the chances of postponing AIDS.

Women of reproductive age are the fastest-growing segment of the AIDS population. In the United States, AIDS is the sixth leading cause of death in women aged 25–44.

HOW DOES A PERSON GET HIV?

In its early stages, infection with HIV causes no outward symptoms so that you cannot tell if a partner is infected. Having unprotected sex puts you at serious risk for the development of HIV infection that can lead to AIDS.

A person becomes infected by coming in contact with body fluids (blood, semen, vaginal fluids, breast milk) of an infected person. A woman can become infected by having unprotected vaginal, anal, or oral sex. Women can get HIV by sharing needles with an infected person. Pregnant women infected with HIV can pass the infection on to their babies.

WHO SHOULD BE TESTED?

- Any woman who has injected drugs into herself with a needle
- Any woman who has had sex with an intravenous (IV) drug user
- Any woman diagnosed with a sexually transmitted disease
- Any woman who had a blood transfusion between 1970 and 1985
- Any woman who has been raped
- Any woman who has had unprotected sex
- Any woman who is pregnant or thinking about becoming pregnant

HOW DO I PROTECT MYSELF FROM HIV?

To protect yourself against HIV infection, never have unprotected sex with anyone. Use a latex condom every time you have sex.

HOW DO I GET TESTED FOR HIV?

A simple blood test will tell you if you have been exposed to HIV. Look for an anonymous testing site. Anonymous testing means that your name is not used. There is no way to trace your name, address, or social security number. Many anonymous testing sites provide the testing service free of charge. The law requires that test results are kept confidential. Confidential means that your test results are told only to you.

WHAT IF THE TEST IS POSITIVE?

- Take steps to make sure that you do not pass on the virus.
- Get medical care so that you can stay healthy longer.
- Get treatment early for any illness that may occur.

WHAT IF THE TEST IS NEGATIVE?

- Your HIV counselor will discuss when to be retested
- Your HIV counselor will discuss ways to decrease the risk of contracting HIV.

CHAPTER **16** HANDOUT

Painful Menses

Painful menses is a crampy feeling in the lower abdomen (belly) that occurs with a period. Cramping with periods is typically diagnosed in adolescents. The pain starts before the period begins but is most severe during the first day of bleeding. The pain is usually confined to the lower abdomen but can extend to the thighs and back. At times, fatigue, nausea, or vomiting accompany the cramping.

The first choice for relief is ibuprofen; 200 to 400 mg every 4 to 6 hours will relieve the hypercontractions of the uterus and relieve the pain. (This medication should be taken with food.)

In women who desire contraception and have severe cramping with their periods, birth control pills are indicated. This form of birth control provides relief from painful menses for 90% of women.

Other pain-relief methods include:

- Exercise
- Increased fiber in the diet
- Increased water intake
- Heating pads or warm baths
- Relaxation techniques

In women who did not have painful menses as a young adult but begin to experience them in the third and fourth decades of life, the cramping may indicate a pelvic problem. An appointment is required with a health-care provider to address this problem.

Women and Headache

There are many kinds of headaches, but the most common ones that plague women are tension headaches and migraines.

TENSION HEADACHES

What causes tension headaches is poorly understood. Ninety percent of women's headaches fall into this category. These headaches usually occur during times of stress and tension. When they occur on a daily basis, they are often associated with depression and require treatment for depression for relief of the headaches. Usually no diagnostic tests are indicated for tension headache. The history of the headache makes the diagnosis.

Tension headaches are not associated with any negative consequences. Ibuprofen is the drug of choice for relief.

MIGRAINE HEADACHES

Migraine headaches are recurrent and may be accompanied by visual or gastrointestinal disturbance. In this type of headache, spasms in vessels of the head cause the pain. Migraine produces unilateral throbbing pain (on one side only), often accompanied by nausea and frequently creates discomfort in bright light. Frequently women with migraine headache have a family history of migraines.

There is a range of medication prescribed for migraine. Some women require medication to prevent migraine "attacks." Stress or certain foods can trigger migraines.

FACTORS RELATED TO HEADACHE IN WOMEN

- **Diet:** Although unrelated to tension headache, diet is related to migraine headache.
- **Family history:** This factor is positive for migraine headache, but negative for tension headache,
- **Menses:** Migraine can be strongly related to menstrual patterns. Of female migraine sufferers, 60% to 70% have migraines around the time of menses, and 50% have a reduction of migraines during pregnancy. Headache prior to menses can be related to falling estrogen levels, allowing migraine inducers to create a headache.

CHAPTER **17** HANDOUT

Genetic Screening during Pregnancy

History is the most valuable tool for identifying couples at risk for a child with a genetic abnormality. When you begin pregnancy care, the obstetrician or midwife will ask many questions about your and your partner's family health histories. These questions help to detect health-related abnormalities that may be genetic in origin. Be sure to bring to the practitioner's office health information about your parents, siblings, children, grandparents, uncles, aunts, nephews, nieces, and first cousins. Your and your partner's ethnic backgrounds are important in assigning risk for genetic disease.

Your age also affects the risk for genetic abnormalities. If you are over age 35, genetic counseling will be recommended.

COMMON GENETIC TESTS

Amniocentesis

Amniocentesis is a safe procedure in which fluid from around the unborn baby is collected and analyzed. The fluid contains cells shed by the baby. These cells can be examined for genetic abnormalities. The fluid is obtained with a needle under ultrasound guidance.

Chorionic Villus Sampling

Chorionic villus sampling (CVS) can be performed earlier than amniocentesis. In this test, cells from the placenta (afterbirth) are collected and analyzed for genetic defects. This procedure is performed under ultrasound guidance.

Triple Screen

Triple screen is a blood test that combines three different measures to evaluate for certain genetic defects.

Ultrasound

Ultrasound performed during pregnancy screens for genetic defects.

Triple Screen

Triple screen is a blood test designed to screen for particular genetic defects. There are three tests involved in a triple screen—thus its name. The first test is called alpha-fetoprotein (AFP), the second is human chorionic gonadotropin (HCG), and the third is an estrogen level. AFP is excreted by the fetus (unborn baby) into the fluid surrounding the baby and into the pregnant woman's bloodstream. The function of AFP is unknown, but the levels that are expected to be present in the mother's blood at each week of pregnancy are known. The function of HCG is to maintain pregnancy; therefore, HCG is the basis for pregnancy tests. HCG is produced by the unborn baby and released into the mother's bloodstream at rates dependent upon the number of weeks of pregnancy. Estriol is the type of estrogen measured as part of the screen. These three levels are determined from a sample of a pregnant woman's blood and calculated with the age of the pregnant women, her ethnicity, and certain health factors to predict her risk for certain genetic diseases. Triple screen is performed at 16 to 18 weeks of pregnancy.

The results of a triple screen are reported as a "risk" for one of the many defects that are associated with an abnormal test. High levels indicate a risk for some genetic defects and low levels indicate a risk for other genetic defects. Of all tested pregnant women, 5% have an abnormal test result.

Many more than 5% of pregnant woman have an unusual test result the first time blood is drawn. The reason for this is that the test is very sensitive to the number of weeks of pregnancy. Many pregnant women are not aware of how many weeks of pregnancy have passed prior to their giving blood for the test. Approximately 12% of women will have abnormal test results related to inaccurate reporting of the number of weeks of pregnancy.

When a triple screen indicates risk, correction for error must be determined by accurate reporting of the number of weeks of pregnancy. This is accomplished by ultrasound. Ultrasound will correctly determine the number of weeks of pregnancy, and the test can be repeated. Ultrasound can also rule out many genetic abnormalities suggested by an abnormal triple screen.

If, after adjustment for weeks of pregnancy, the triple screen is still showing increased risk for genetic defects, the obstetrician or midwife will schedule further testing to rule out or verify genetic abnormalities.

The triple screen is just as its name implies—a screen. Further testing must be done for verification of a genetic abnormality. Testing may include an ultrasound by a perinatologist, a specialist in the health of unborn babies, or an amniocentesis in which cells are retrieved from the fluid around the unborn baby.

The triple screen is a useful test, but not a perfect one. Its sensitivity, meaning its level of accuracy in screening, is approximately 80%. In statistical terms, 80% is far from 100% accurate. Approximately 1 in 30 women with an abnormal triple screen is actually carrying a baby with a problem. The other 29 are carrying a normal baby. In other words, many women will have a triple screen that is abnormal but are carrying a healthy baby. An abnormal triple screen indicates a need for further testing and little else.

Medications during Pregnancy

Prescription and over-the-counter (OTC) drugs, including alcohol and cigarettes, have the potential to affect unborn babies. They can affect the unborn babies' growth and development and/or create injury.

The first rule to be applied to medication and pregnancy is: *Discuss any medication with you obstetrician or midwife before taking it.* This includes prescription and OTC drugs.

Although much has been learned about which drugs can and cannot be taken safely during pregnancy, many new drugs being released have not been tested, and many combinations of drugs have not been tested. It is wise to consult with your midwife or obstetrician before consuming any drug.

It is not just what is taken, but when it is taken and in what quantity. The most dangerous time for the unborn baby to be exposed to drugs is in the first few weeks of pregnancy. It is, therefore, wise to consult your practitioner about drugs while trying to conceive. Remember that you are a few weeks' pregnant when the test becomes positive. During this time, the unborn baby should not be exposed to any drugs, alcohol, or cigarettes.

If there is a prescription medication that you must take to maintain your health, discuss this medication with your obstetrician or midwife prior to becoming pregnant. Risks to the unborn baby may be reduced by a change in the type of medication or the dose of medication.

Revisit an obstetrician or midwife to begin care as soon as you know that you are pregnant.

Take medication while pregnant or attempting to conceive only when absolutely necessary. When you must use an OTC drug, choose one that has a single ingredient. This greatly reduces the chance of it causing a problem for the unborn baby, and it makes the consultation with your obstetrician or midwife more accurate.

Alcohol and cigarettes are hazardous to unborn babies and should not be consumed. Talk to your practitioner about ways to quit smoking and ways to give up alcohol.

A partial list of medications that affect unborn children is:

- Anesthetics
- Androgens
- Anticancer drugs
- Benzodiazepines
- Carbamazepine (Tegretol)
- Warfarin (Coumadin)
- Diethylstilbestrol
- Valproic acid (Depakote)
- Iodine
- Isotretinoin (Accutane)
- Lithium

- Phenytoin (Dilantin)
- Quinolones
- Tetracyclines
- Thyroid agents

Nutritional Requirements during Pregnancy

Food	Number of Servings per Day
Protein	4
Meat, poultry	
Beans and nuts or seeds	
Eggs	
Milk products	4
Milk	
Yogurt	
Cheese	
Tofu	
Grains	6
Bread and rolls	
Macaroni, rice, noodles, cereal	
Wheat germ	
Vitamin C fruits and vegetables	2
Oranges and grapefruits	
Tomatoes	
Green peppers	
Broccoli and cauliflower	
Cabbage	
Green leafy vegetables	1–2
Brussel sprouts	
Asparagus	
Greens and lettuce	
Watercress	
Vitamin A fruits and vegetables	3
Apples	
Carrots	
Green beans	
Bananas	
Sweet potatoes	
Fats and oils	3
Butter and margarine	
Salad dressing	
Cream cheese	

Exercise during Pregnancy

GUIDELINES FOR EXERCISE DURING PREGNANCY

- Exercise on a routine, 3-to-4-time weekly basis.
- Drink water before, during, and after the exercise.
- Do not exercise when ill.
- Do not exercise outdoors in hot and humid weather.
- Take 5 to 10 minutes prior to exercise to warm up and/or stretch and 5 to 10 minutes after exercise to cool down.
- Keep your heart rate under 140 bpm.
- Restrict the most intense portion of the exercise (heart rate at 140 bpm) to 15 to 20 minutes.
- Avoid high-impact exercises.
- Avoid sit-ups and leg raises or other exercises that make use of abdominal muscles.
- Avoid exercises that require uncomfortable positions.
- Do not lie on your back for longer than a few minutes at time.
- Get up slowly.
- Stop exercising if you experience pain related to the specific exercise, bleeding, dizziness, back pain, or pelvic pressure.

SPORTS TO AVOID DURING PREGNANCY

- Skiing—snow or water
- Scuba diving
- Skating—ice or roller
- Any sport performed at high altitudes

Saunas, hot tubs, and whirlpools commonly used after exercise should be avoided during pregnancy. Dizziness can result from the change in circulation due to the high temperatures.

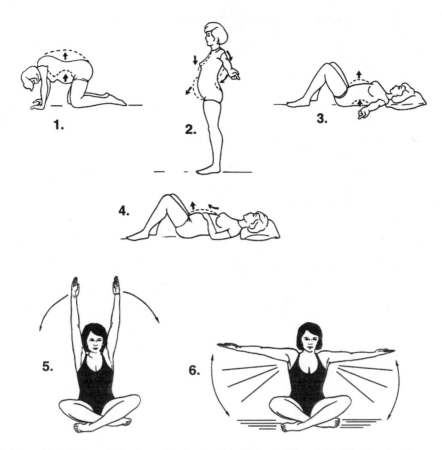

Pelvic rocking (1, 2, and 3) relieves low back ache. Abdominal breathing (4) aids relaxation and lifts abdominal wall from uterus. Flying exercise (5 and 6) promotes relaxation and reduces discomforts such as heartburn and shortness of breath.

Source: Bobak, Jensen, & Zalar: Maternity and Gynecologic Care: The Nurse and the Family. CV Mosby, St. Louis, 1989.

Pregnancy exercises.

Danger Signals during Pregnancy

- Visual disturbance: blurred vision, spots, or double vision
- Swelling of the face
- Severe headache
- Severe muscle irritability or seizures
- Severe stomach ache
- Persistent vomiting
- Fluid discharge from the vagina
- Fever
- Burning upon urination
- Severe diarrhea
- Pain in the abdomen
- Change in fetal movements: any change in usual movement pattern

Pregnancy and Work

In general, women can work until delivery if they have an uncomplicated pregnancy and if the number of hazards in the workplace is low. Every woman should inform her employer about her pregnancy as soon as possible so that modifications in her work can be considered.

WORK MODIFICATIONS NEEDED DURING PREGNANCY

- Hours should not be longer than 8 per day.
- The woman should take two 10-minute breaks per day and one meal break.
- The woman should have a place to rest in a reclining position and she should have a place to elevate her legs.
- A pregnant woman who must sit or stand for most of her workday should be permitted a short time every hour or two to walk
- The pregnant woman should avoid smoking, chemical fumes, extremes in temperature, and any activities that require good balance or could risk trauma to the abdomen.
- Lifting should be limited to 10 lb to 15 lb, and proper lifting techniques should be implemented.

Several physical conditions associated with pregnancy can create the need for further work modifications. Discuss your work environment with your obstetrician or midwife.

REPRODUCTIVE HAZARDS BY OCCUPATION

Lead	Auto workers, ceramic workers, electronics workers, painters
Pesticides	Agricultural workers
Benzene	Chemical manufacturers
Anesthetic gases	Operating room workers, dental workers
Infections	Health-care workers, teachers, day-care workers, parents
Radiation exposure	Health-care workers

Source: Adapted from Younkin and Davis: Women's Health. Appleton & Lange, Norwalk, Conn, 1994.

CHAPTER **18** HANDOUT

Postpartum Exercises

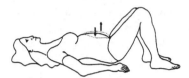

Abdominal Breathing. Lie on back with knees bent. Inhale deeply through nose. Keep ribs stationary and allow abdomen to expand upwards. Exhale slowly but forcefully while contracting the abdominal muscles; hold for 3 to 5 seconds while exhaling. Relax.

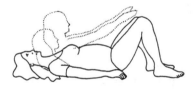

Reach for the Knees. Lie on back with knees bent. While inhaling deeply lower chin onto chest. While exhaling, raise head and shoulders slowly and smoothly and reach for knees with arms outstretched. The body should only rise as far as the back will naturally bend while waist remains on floor or bed (about 6 to 8 inches). Slowly and smoothly lower head and shoulders back to starting position. Relax.

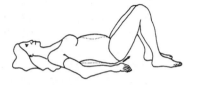

Combined Abdominal Breathing and Supine Pelvic Tilt (Pelvic Rocks). Lie on back with knees bent. While inhaling deeply, roll pelvis back by flattening lower back on floor or bed. Exhale slowly but forcefully while contracting abdominal muscles and tightening buttocks. Hold for 3 to 5 seconds while exhaling. Relax.

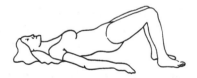

Buttocks Lift. Lie on back with arms at sides, knees bent and feet flat. Slowly raise buttocks and arch back. Return slowly to starting position.

Postpartum exercises.

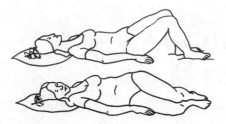

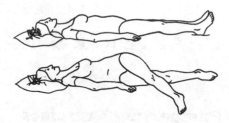

Double Knee Roll. Lie on back with knees bent. Keeping shoulders flat and feet stationary, slowly and smoothly roll knees over to the left to touch the floor or bed. Maintaining a smooth motion, roll knees back over to the right until they touch the floor or bed. Return to starting position and relax.

Single Knee Roll. Lie on back with right leg straight and left leg bent at the knee. Keeping shoulders flat, slowly and smoothly roll left knee over to the right to touch the floor or bed and then back to starting position. Reverse position of legs. Roll right knee over to the left to touch floor or bed and return to starting position. Relax.

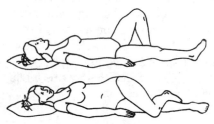

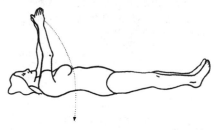

Leg Roll. Lie on back with legs straight. Keeping shoulders flat and legs straight, slowly and smoothly lift left leg and roll it over to touch the right side of floor or bed and return to starting position. Repeat, rolling right leg over to touch left side of floor or bed. Relax.

Arm Raise. Lie on back with arms extended at 90° angle from back. Raise arms so they are perpendicular and hands touch. Lower slowly.

Source: Bobak, Jensen, & Zalar: Maternity and Gynecologic Care: The Nurse and the Family. CV Mosby, St. Louis, 1989.

Postpartum exercises. *Continued*

After-Delivery Guidelines

There is so much to remember once you and the baby are home after delivery.

CHECKLIST BEFORE LEAVING THE HOSPITAL

- Know how to take care of yourself; include care of the vaginal discharge and breast care.
- Know how to care for the infant; include bathing, feeding, and nurturing.
- Know the danger signs that should alert you to call your obstetrician or midwife.
- Discuss birth control methods and when and how to use them.
- If you are breastfeeding, be comfortable with the method, and identify support systems to call if needed.
- Develop a support system for cooking, cleaning, shopping, and so forth.
- Know whom to call, day or night, if you have questions or concerns.
- Schedule a follow-up appointment for yourself and for the baby.

DANGER SIGNS FOR NEW MOTHERS

- Fever
- Foul-smelling or irritating discharge
- Excessive vaginal discharge
- Bright red vaginal bleeding after the discharge has been brown
- A swollen area on the leg that is painful, red, or hot
- Burning upon urination
- Pelvic pain

INDEX

An *f* following a page number indicates a figure; a *t* indicates a table.